Registries for Evaluating Patient Outcomes: A User's Guide

Prepared for:

Agency for Healthcare Research and Quality
U.S. Department of Health and Human Services
540 Gaither Road
Rockville, MD 20850
www.ahrq.gov

Contract Nos. HHSA29020050035I TO1 and 290-02-0025 TO1

Prepared by:

Outcome Sciences, Inc., d/b/a Outcome
Cambridge, MA

Senior Editors

Richard E. Gliklich, M.D.
Nancy A. Dreyer, M.P.H., Ph.D.

Associate Editors

David Matchar, M.D.
Gregory Samsa, Ph.D.
Duke Evidence-based Practice Center

AHRQ Publication No. 07-EHC001-1
April 2007

Acknowledgments

The editors would like to acknowledge the efforts of Brian Edwards, Senior Medical Adviser and Deputy Qualified Person for pharmacovigilance of the Benefit Risk Management Division of Janssen Cilag UK; Mary Lou Skovron, Group Director, Pharmacoepidemiology, at Bristol-Myers Squibb; Kathryn Starzyk, Lili Beit, and Allie McGinty of Outcome Sciences, Inc.; Leslye K. Fitterman and Rosemarie Hakim of the Centers for Medicare & Medicaid Services; and Elise Berliner, Scott R. Smith, and Margaret Rutherford of the Agency for Healthcare Research and Quality.

Preface

This project was performed under a contract from the Agency for Healthcare Research and Quality (AHRQ) in collaboration with the Centers for Medicare & Medicaid Services (CMS) through the Developing Evidence to Inform Decisions about Effectiveness (DEcIDE) Network of AHRQ's Effective Health Care (EHC) Program. The purpose of the project was to produce a handbook that would serve as a reference for establishing, maintaining, and evaluating the success of registries created to collect data about patient outcomes.

Following award of the project on September 29, 2005, we created a draft outline for the document that was posted for public comment on AHRQ's Effective Health Care Web site (www.effectivehealthcare.ahrq.gov) from January through March 2006. During that same period, we worked with AHRQ to create a process for selecting contributors and reviewers. We broadly solicited recommendations from a range of stakeholders, including government agencies, industry groups, medical professional societies, and other experts in the field; conducted a review of the pertinent literature; and contacted the initial list of contributors to confirm their interest and area of expertise and to seek further recommendations. Through that process and in collaboration with AHRQ and CMS, we arrived at a set of contributors and reviewers based on subject/content expertise, practical experience, and interest and availability, with balanced representation from key stakeholder groups for nearly all chapters. In addition, a request for submission of real-world case examples that could be used in the handbook to illustrate issues and challenges in implementing registries was posted on the Effective Health Care Web site. The primary selection criteria for these examples were their utility in illustrating a practical challenge and its resolution.

An initial meeting of contributors was convened in February 2006. A second meeting including contributors and chapter reviewers was held in June 2006, following creation of an initial draft document and focused review by the reviewers. The collaborative efforts of contributors, reviewers, and editors resulted in a draft document that was posted for public comment on the Effective Health Care Web site in October and November 2006. In all, 39 contributors and 35 individual reviewers participated. These contributors and reviewers participated as individuals and not necessarily as representatives of their organizations. We are grateful to all those who contributed to the document and who reviewed it and shared their comments.

To begin the discussion of registries, we would like to clarify some distinctions between registries and clinical trials. While this is further discussed in Chapter 1, from a high-level perspective, we offer the following distinctions: The clinical trial is an experiment in which an active intervention intended to change a human subject's outcome is implemented, generally through a randomization procedure that takes decisionmaking away from the practitioner. The research protocol describes inclusion and exclusion criteria that are used to select the patients who will participate as human subjects, focusing the experiment on a homogeneous group. Human subjects and clinical researchers agree to adhere to a strict schedule of visits and to conduct protocol-specific tests and measurements.

In contrast, registries use an observational study design that does not specify treatments (although a specific treatment may be an inclusion criterion) and observe without requiring any therapies intended to change patient outcomes. There are generally few inclusion and exclusion criteria in an effort to study a broad range of patients to make the results more generalizable. Patients are typically observed as they present for care and the data collected generally reflect whatever tests and measurements a provider customarily uses.

Patient registries represent a useful tool for a number of purposes. Their ideal use and their role in evidence development, design, operations, and evaluation resemble but differ from clinical trials in a number of substantive ways, and therefore they should not be evaluated with the same constructs. This handbook presents what the contributors and reviewers consider to be good registry practices. Many registries today may not meet even the basic practices described. On the whole, registry science is in an active state of development. This document is an important step in developing this field.

This book is divided into three sections: Creating, Operating, and Evaluating Registries. The first two sections provide basic information on key areas of registry development and operations, highlighting the spectrum of practices in each of these areas and their potential strengths and weaknesses. Section I, "Creating Registries," includes six chapters. "Patient Registries" defines and characterizes types of registries, their purposes, and uses, and describes their place within the scope of this document. "Planning a Registry" focuses on the recommended steps in planning a registry, from determining if a registry is the right option to describing goals and objectives. "Registry Design" examines the specifics of designing a registry once the goals and objectives are known. "Data Elements for Registries" provides an approach to selecting data elements that is both scientific and practical. "Data Sources for Registries" addresses how existing data sources (administrative, pharmacy, other registries, etc.) may be used to enhance the value of patient registries. "Principles of Registry Ethics, Data Ownership, and Privacy" reviews several key legal and ethical issues that should be considered in creating or operating a registry.

Section II, "Operating Registries," provides a practical guide to the day-to-day operational issues and decisions for producing and interpreting high-quality registries. "Patient and Provider Recruitment and Management" describes strategies for recruiting and retaining providers and patients. "Data Collection and Quality Assurance" reviews key areas of data collection, cleaning, storing, and quality assurance for registries. "Adverse Event Detection, Processing, and Reporting" examines relevant practical and regulatory issues. "Analysis and Interpretation of Registry Data To Evaluate Outcomes" addresses key considerations in analyzing and interpreting registry data.

Interspersed throughout the first two sections of the handbook are case examples. As discussed above, the choice of examples was limited to those submitted for consideration during the public submission period. The purpose of their inclusion is solely to illustrate specific point(s) in the text from real-world examples, regardless of whether the source of the example is within the scope of the handbook as described in Chapter 1. Inclusion of a case example in this handbook is not intended as an endorsement of the quality of the particular registry, nor do the case examples necessarily present registries that meet all the criteria described in Chapter 11 as basic elements of good practice. Rather, case examples are introduced to provide the reader with a richer description of the issue or question being addressed in the text. In some cases, we have no independent information on the registry other than what has been provided by the contributor.

Section III is "Evaluating Registries." This final chapter summarizes key points from the earlier chapters in a manner that can be used to review the structure, data, or interpretations of patient registries. It describes good registry practice in terms of "basic elements" and "potential enhancements." This information might be used by a person developing a registry, or by a reviewer or user of registry data or interpretations derived from registries.

Richard E. Gliklich
Nancy A. Dreyer
Senior Editors

Contents

v

Contents

Contents

Case Examples

Executive Summary

Patient Registries

The purpose of this document is to serve as a guide to the design, implementation, analysis, interpretation, and evaluation of the quality of a registry for understanding patient outcomes. For the purpose of this handbook, a patient registry is an organized system that uses observational study methods to collect uniform data (clinical and other) to evaluate specified outcomes for a population defined by a particular disease, condition, or exposure, and that serves a predetermined scientific, clinical, or policy purpose(s). The registry database is the file (or files) derived from the registry.

Although registries can serve many purposes, this handbook focuses on registries that are created for one or more of the following purposes: to describe the natural history of disease, to determine clinical effectiveness or cost effectiveness of health care products and services, to measure or monitor safety and harm, and/or to measure quality of care. Registries are classified according to how the populations are defined. For example, product registries include patients who have been exposed to biopharmaceutical products or medical devices. Health services registries consist of patients who have had a common procedure, clinical encounter, or hospitalization. Disease or condition registries are defined by patients having the same diagnosis, such as cystic fibrosis or heart failure.

Planning

There are several key steps in planning a patient registry, including articulating the purpose of the registry, determining whether the registry is an appropriate means for addressing the research question, identifying stakeholders, defining the scope and target population, assessing feasibility, and securing funding. The registry team and advisors should be selected based on expertise and experience. The plan for registry governance and oversight should clearly address such issues as overall direction and operations, scientific content, ethics, safety, data access, publications, and change management. It is also helpful to plan for the entire lifespan of a registry, including how and when the registry will end and any plans for transitioning the registry at that time.

Registry Design

A patient registry should be designed with respect to its major purpose, with the understanding that different levels of rigor may be required for registries that are designed to address focused analytical questions to support decisionmaking, in contrast to those intended primarily for descriptive purposes. The key points to consider in designing a registry include formulating a research question; choosing a study design; translating questions of clinical interest into measurable exposures and outcomes; choosing patients for study, including deciding whether a comparison group is needed; determining where data can be found; and deciding how many patients need to be studied and for how long. Once these key design items have been determined, the registry design should be reviewed to evaluate potential sources of bias (systematic error); these should be addressed to the extent that is practical and achievable.

The specific research questions of interest will guide the registry design, identification of exposures and outcomes, and definitions of the target population (the population to which the findings are meant to apply). The registry population should be designed to approximate the characteristics of the target population as much as possible. The number of study subjects desired and length of observation (followup) should be planned in accordance with the overall purpose of the registry. The desired study size (in terms of subjects or person-years of observation) is determined by specifying the magnitude of an expected clinically meaningful effect or the desired precision of effect estimates.

Study size determinants are also affected by practicality, cost, and whether or not the registry is intended to support regulatory decisionmaking. Depending on the purpose of the registry, internal, external, or historical comparison groups strengthen the understanding of whether the observed effects are indeed real and, in fact, different from what would have occurred under other circumstances.

Registry study designs often restrict eligibility for entry to individuals with certain characteristics to assure that they will assemble enough information for analysis (e.g., age restriction) or use some form of sampling—random selection, systematic sampling, or a haphazard, nonrandom approach. The potential for bias refers to opportunities for systematic errors to influence the results. The information value of a registry is enhanced by its ability to provide an assessment of the potential for bias and to quantify how this bias could affect the study results.

Data Elements

The selection of data elements requires balancing such factors as their importance for the integrity of the registry and for the analysis of primary outcomes, their reliability, their contribution to the overall burden for respondents, and the incremental costs associated with their collection. Selection begins with identifying relevant domains. Specific data elements then are selected with consideration for established clinical data standards, common data definitions, and the use of patient identifiers. It is important to determine which elements are absolutely necessary and which are desirable but not essential. In choosing measurement scales for assessing patient-reported outcomes, it is preferable to use scales that have been appropriately validated, when such tools exist. Once data elements have been selected, a data map should be created, and the data collection tools should be pilot tested. Testing allows assessment of respondent burden, accuracy, and completeness of questions, and potential areas for missing data. Inter-rater agreement for data collection instruments can also be assessed,

especially in registries that rely on chart abstraction. Overall, choice of data elements should be guided by parsimony, validity, and a focus on achieving the registry's purpose.

Data Sources

A single registry may integrate data from various sources. The form, structure, availability, and timeliness of the required data are important considerations. Data sources can be classified as primary or secondary. Primary data are collected for direct purposes of the registry. Secondary data are comprised of information that has been collected for purposes other than the registry, and they may not be uniformly structured or validated with the same rigor as primary data. Sufficient identifiers are necessary to guarantee an accurate match between secondary sources and registry patients. Furthermore, a solid understanding of the original purpose of the secondary data and how they were collected is advised, because the way that those data were collected and verified or validated will help shape their use in a registry. Common secondary sources of data linked to registries include medical records systems, institutional or organizational databases, administrative health insurance claims data, death and birth records, census databases, and related existing registry databases.

Ethics, Data Ownership, and Privacy

Critical ethical and legal considerations should guide the development and use of patient registries. The Common Rule is the uniform set of regulations on the ethical conduct of human subjects research from the Federal agencies that fund such research. Institutions that conduct research agree to comply with the Common Rule for federally funded research and may opt to apply that rule to all human subjects activities conducted within their facilities or by their employees and agents, regardless of the source of funding. The Health Insurance Portability and Accountability Act of 1996 (HIPAA) and its implementing regulations (collectively, the Privacy Rule) are the legal protections for the privacy of individually identifiable health information created and maintained by health care providers, health plans, and health care clearinghouses (called "covered entities"). The research purpose of a registry, the status of its developer, and the extent to which registry data are individually identifiable largely determine applicable regulatory requirements. Other important ethical and legal concerns include transparency of activities, oversight, and data ownership.

Patient and Provider Recruitment and Management

Recruitment and retention of providers (as registry sites) and patients are essential to the success of a registry. Recruitment typically occurs at several levels, including facilities (hospital, practice, pharmacy), providers, and patients. The motivating factors for participation at each level and the factors necessary to achieve retention differ according to the registry. Factors that motivate participation include the perceived relevance, importance, or scientific credibility of the registry, as well as the risks and burdens of participation and any incentives for participation. Because provider and patient recruitment and retention can affect how well a registry accurately represents the target population, well-planned strategies for enrollment and retention are critical. Goals for recruitment, retention, and followup should be explicitly laid out in the registry planning phase, and deviations during the conduct of the registry should be continuously evaluated for their risk of introducing bias.

Data Collection and Quality Assurance

The integrated system for collecting, cleaning, storing, monitoring, reviewing, and reporting on registry data determines the utility of those data for meeting the registry's goals. A broad range of data collection procedures and systems are available. Some are more suitable than others for particular purposes. Critical factors in the ultimate quality of the data include how data elements are structured and defined, how personnel are trained, and how data problems are handled (e.g., missing, out-of-range, or logically inconsistent values). Registries may also be required to conform to guidelines or standards of specific end users of the data (e.g., 21 Code of Federal Regulations, Part 11). Quality assurance aims to affirm that the data were, in fact, collected in accordance with established procedures and that they meet the requisite standards of quality to accomplish the registry's intended purposes and the intended use of the data.

Requirements for quality assurance should be defined during the registry's inception and creation. Because certain requirements may have significant cost implications, a risk-based approach to developing a quality assurance plan is recommended. It should be based on identifying the most important or likely sources of error or potential lapses in procedures that may impact the quality of the registry in the context of its intended purpose.

Adverse Event Detection, Processing, and Reporting

The U.S. Food and Drug Administration defines an adverse event (AE) as any untoward medical occurrence in a patient administered a pharmaceutical product, whether or not related to or considered to have a causal relationship with the treatment. AEs are categorized according to the seriousness and, for drugs, the expectedness of the event. Although AE reporting for all marketed products is dependent on the principle of "becoming aware," collection of adverse event data falls into two categories: those events that are intentionally solicited (meaning data that are part of the uniform collection of information in the registry) and those that are unsolicited (meaning that the AE is volunteered or noted in an unsolicited manner).

Determining whether the registry should use a case report form to collect AEs should be based on the scientific importance of the information for evaluating the specified outcomes of interest.

3

Regardless of whether or not AEs constitute outcomes for the registry, it is important to develop a plan for detecting, processing, and reporting AEs for any registry that has direct patient interaction. If the registry receives sponsorship, in whole or in part, from a regulated industry (for drugs or devices), the sponsor has mandated reporting requirements, and the process for detecting and reporting AEs should be established and registry personnel trained on how to identify AEs and to whom they should be reported. Sponsors of registries designed specifically to meet requirements for surveillance of drug or device safety are encouraged to hold discussions with health authorities about the most appropriate process for reporting serious AEs.

Analysis and Interpretation

Analysis and interpretation of registry data begin with answering a series of core questions. Who was studied? How were the data collected, edited, and verified, and how were missing data handled? How were the analyses performed? Four populations are of interest in describing who was studied: the target population, the accessible population, the intended population, and the population actually studied (the "actual population"). The representativeness of the actual population to the target population is referred to as generalizability.

Analysis of registry outcomes first requires an analysis of the completeness of data collection and data quality. Considerations include an evaluation of completeness for most if not all important covariates and an understanding of how missing data were handled and reported. Analysis of a registry should provide information on the characteristics of the patient population, the exposures of interest, and the endpoints. Descriptive registry studies focus on describing frequency and patterns of various elements in a patient population, whereas analytical studies concentrate on associations between patients or treatment characteristics and health outcomes of interest. A statistical analysis plan describes the analytical plans and statistical techniques that will be used to evaluate the primary and secondary

objectives specified in the study plan. Interpretation of registry data should be provided so that the conclusions can be understood in the appropriate context and so that any lessons from the registry can be applied to the target population and used to improve patient care and outcomes.

Evaluating Registries

Although registries can provide useful information, there are levels of rigor that enhance validity and make the information from some registries more useful for guiding decisions than the information from others. The term "quality" can be applied to registries to describe the confidence that the design, conduct, and analysis of the registry can be shown to protect against bias and errors in inference—that is, erroneous conclusions drawn from a registry. Although there are limitations in any assessment of quality, this handbook uses a quality component analysis to evaluate high-level factors that may affect results and differentiates between research quality (which pertains to the scientific process) and evidence quality (which pertains to the data/findings emanating from the research process). Quality components are classified as either "basic elements of good practice," which can be viewed as a basic checklist that should be considered for all patient registries, or as "potential enhancements to good practice" that may strengthen the information value in particular circumstances. The results of such an evaluation should be considered in the context of the disease area(s), the type of registry, and the purpose of the registry, and should also take into account feasibility and affordability.

Section I.
Creating Registries

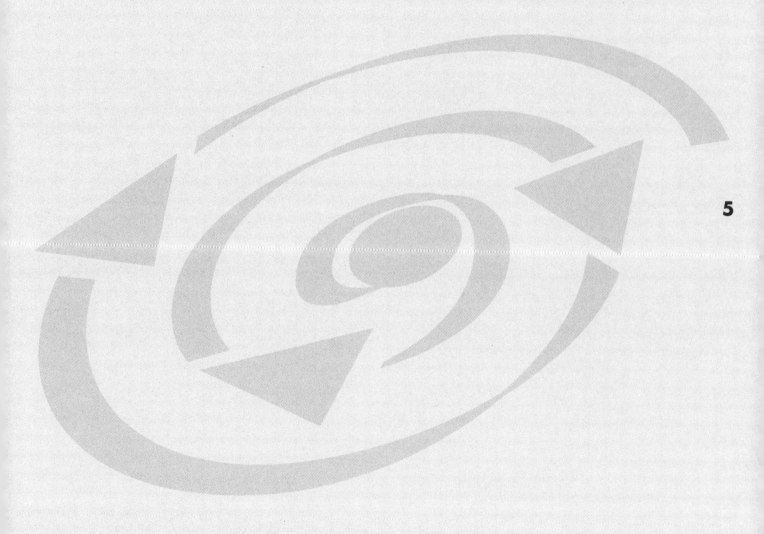

Chapter 1. Patient Registries

The purpose of this document is to serve as a guide for the design and use of patient registries for scientific, clinical, and health policy purposes. Properly designed and executed, patient registries can provide a real-world view of clinical practice, patient outcomes, safety, and comparative effectiveness. This handbook primarily focuses on practical design and operational issues, evaluation principles, and best practices. Where topics are well covered in other materials, references and/or links are provided. The goal of this document is to provide stakeholders in both the public and private sectors with information that they can use to guide the design and implementation of patient registries, the analysis and interpretation of data from patient registries, and the evaluation of the quality of a registry or one of its components. Where useful, case examples have been incorporated to illustrate particular points or challenges.

The term "registry"[1] is defined both as the act of recording or registering and as the record or entry itself. Therefore, "registries" can refer to both programs that collect and store data and the records that are so created.

The term "patient registry" is generally used to distinguish registries focused on health information from other record sets, but there is no consistent definition in current use. E.M. Brooke, in a 1974 publication of the World Health Organization, further delineated registries in health information systems as "a file of documents containing uniform information about individual persons, collected in a systematic and comprehensive way, in order to serve a predetermined purpose."[2]

The National Committee on Vital and Health Statistics[3] describes registries used for a broad range of purposes in public health and medicine as "an organized system for the collection, storage, retrieval, analysis, and dissemination of information on individual persons who have either a particular

disease, a condition (e.g., a risk factor) that predisposes [them] to the occurrence of a health-related event, or prior exposure to substances (or circumstances) known or suspected to cause adverse health effects."

This handbook focuses on patient registries that are used for evaluating patient outcomes. It is not intended to address several other types or uses for registries (although many of the principles may be applicable), such as geographically based population registries (not based on a disease, condition, or exposure); registries created for public health incidence reporting (without tracking outcomes); or listing registries that are used solely to identify patients with particular diseases in clinical practices but are not used for evaluating outcomes. This handbook is also not intended to address the wide range of studies that utilize secondary analyses of data collected for other purposes.

In the narrower context of patient registries used for evaluating patient outcomes, this handbook uses the following definitions:

- A *patient registry* is an organized system that uses observational study methods to collect uniform data (clinical and other) to evaluate specified outcomes for a population defined by a particular disease, condition, or exposure, and that serves one or more predetermined scientific, clinical, or policy purposes.

- The *patient registry database* describes a file (or files) derived from the registry.

Based on these definitions, the handbook focuses on patient registries in which the following are true (although exceptions may apply):

- The data are collected in a naturalistic manner such that the management of patients is determined by the caregiver and patient together and not by the registry protocol.

- The registry is designed to fulfill specific purposes, and these purposes are defined before collecting and analyzing the data. In other words, the data collection is purpose driven rather than the purpose being data driven (meaning limited to or derived from what is already available in an existing data set).

- The registry captures data elements with specific and consistent data definitions.

- The data are collected in a uniform manner for every patient. This consideration refers to both the types of data and the frequency of their collection.

- The data collected include data derived from and reflective of the clinical status of the patient (e.g., history, examination, laboratory test, or patient-reported data). Registries include the types of data that clinicians would use for the diagnosis and management of patients.

- At least one element of registry data collection is active, meaning that some data are collected specifically for the purpose of the registry (usually collected from the patient or clinician) rather than inferred from sources (administrative, billing, pharmacy databases, etc.) that are collected for another purpose. This does not exclude situations where registry data collection is a specific, but not the exclusive, reason data are being collected, such as might be envisioned with future uses of electronic health records, as described in Chapter 8. It also does not exclude the incorporation of other data sources, as discussed in Chapter 5. Registries can be enriched by linkage with extant databases (e.g., to determine deaths and other outcomes or to assess pharmacy use or resource utilization).

Current Uses for Patient Registries

A patient registry can be a powerful tool to observe the course of disease; to understand variations in treatment and outcomes; to examine factors that influence prognosis and quality of life; to describe care patterns, including appropriateness of care and disparities in the delivery of care; to assess effectiveness; to monitor safety; and to change behavior through feedback of data.[4] Different stakeholders perceive and may benefit from the value of registries in different ways. For example, for a clinician, registries can collect data about disease presentation and outcomes on large numbers of patients rapidly, thereby producing a real-world picture of disease. For a physician organization, a registry might assess the degree to which clinicians are managing a disease in accordance with evidence-based guidelines, focus attention on specific aspects of a particular disease that might otherwise be overlooked, or provide data for clinicians to compare themselves with their peers.[5] From a payer's perspective, registries can provide detailed information from large numbers of patients on how procedures, devices, or pharmaceuticals are actually used and on their effectiveness in different populations. This information may be useful for determining coverage policies. For a drug or device manufacturer, a registry might demonstrate the performance of a product in the real world, meet a postmarketing study commitment, develop hypotheses, or identify patient populations that will be useful for product development, clinical trials design, and patient recruitment. The U.S. Food and Drug Administration (FDA) has noted that "through the creation of registries, a sponsor can evaluate safety signals identified from spontaneous case reports, literature reports, or other sources, and evaluate the factors that affect the risk of adverse outcomes such as dose, timing of exposure, or patient characteristics."[6]

Evaluating Patient Outcomes

Patient registries and randomized controlled trials (RCTs) have important and complementary roles in evaluating patient outcomes. Patient registries collect data in a comprehensive manner (with few excluded patients) and therefore produce outcome results that may be generalizable to a wide range of patients. They also evaluate care as it is actually provided, because care is not assigned, determined, or even recommended by a protocol. As a result,

8

the outcomes reported may be more representative of what is achieved in real-world practice. Patient registries also offer the ability to evaluate patient outcomes when clinical trials are not practical (e.g., very rare diseases), and they may be the only option when clinical trials are not ethically acceptable. They are a powerful tool when RCTs are difficult to conduct, such as in surgery or when very long-term outcomes are desired.

RCTs are controlled experiments designed to test hypotheses that can ultimately be applied to real-world care. Because RCTs are conducted under strict constraints, with detailed inclusion and exclusion criteria, they are sometimes limited in their generalizability. If RCTs are not generalizable to the populations to which the information will be applied, they may not be sufficiently informative for decisionmaking. Conversely, patient registries that observe real-world clinical practice may collect all of the information needed to assess patient outcomes in a generalizable way, but interpreting this information correctly requires analytic methodology geared to addressing the potential sources of bias that challenge all observational studies. Interpreting patient registry data also requires checks of internal validity and sometimes the use of external data sources to validate key assumptions (such as comparing the key characteristics of registry participants with external sources to demonstrate the comparability of registry participants to the ultimate reference population). Patient registries, RCTs, other study designs, and other data sources should all be considered tools in the toolbox for evidence development, each with its own advantages and limitations.[7]

Hierarchies of evidence. One question that arises in a discussion of this type is where to place patient registries within the hierarchies of evidence that are frequently used in developing guidelines or decisionmaking. As observational studies, registries would be placed in a subordinate position to RCTs in some commonly used hierarchies.[8]

However, much debate currently exists in the evidence community regarding these traditional methods of grading levels of evidence and some of

their underlying assumptions, their shortcomings in assessing certain types of evidence (e.g., benefit vs. harm), and inter-scale consistency in evaluating the same evidence.[9,10]

The Grading of Recommendations Assessment, Development, and Evaluation (GRADE) Working Group has proposed a more robust approach that addresses some of the decisionmaking issues described in this handbook. As noted by the GRADE collaborators:

> [R]andomised trials are not always feasible and, in some instances, observational studies may provide better evidence, as is generally the case for rare adverse effects. Moreover, the results of randomised trials may not always be applicable–for example, if the participants are highly selected and motivated relative to the population of interest. It is therefore essential to consider study quality, the consistency of results across studies, and the directness of the evidence, as well as the appropriateness of the study design.[11]

As the methods for grading evidence for different purposes continue to evolve, this handbook can serve as a guide to help such evaluators understand study quality and identify well-designed registries. Beyond the evidence hierarchy debate, users of evidence understand the value of registries for providing complementary information that can extend the results of clinical trials to populations not studied in those trials, for demonstrating the real-world effects of treatments outside of the research setting and potentially in large subsets of affected patients, and for providing long-term followup when such data are not available from clinical trials.

Defining patient outcomes. The focus of this handbook is the use of registries to evaluate patient outcomes. An outcome may be thought of as an end result of a particular health care practice or intervention. According to the Agency for Healthcare Research and Quality (AHRQ), end results include effects that people experience and about which they care.[12] The National Cancer Institute further clarifies that "final" endpoints are those that matter to decisionmakers: patients,

9

providers, private payers, government agencies, accrediting organizations, or society.[13,14] Examples of these outcomes include biomedical outcomes, such as survival and disease-free survival, health-related quality of life, satisfaction with care, and economic burden.[15] Although final endpoints are ultimately what matter, it is sometimes more practical when creating registries to collect intermediate outcomes (such as whether processes or guidelines were followed) and clinical outcomes (such as whether a tumor regressed or recurred) that predict success in improving final endpoints.

In *Crossing the Quality Chasm*,[16] the Institute of Medicine (IOM) describes the six guiding aims of health care as safe, effective, efficient, patient-centered, timely, and equitable. While these aims are not outcomes per se, they generally describe the dimensions of results that matter to decisionmakers in the use of health care products and services. Is it safe? Does it produce greater benefit than harm? Is it clinically effective? Does it produce the desired effect in real-world practice? Is it cost effective or efficient? Does it produce the desired effect at a reasonable cost relative to other potential expenditures? Is it patient oriented, timely, and equitable? These last three aims focus on the delivery and quality of care. Does the right patient receive the right therapy or service at the right time? Most of the patient outcomes that registries evaluate reflect one or more of these guiding aims. For example, a patient presenting with an ischemic stroke to an emergency room has a finite window of opportunity to receive a thrombolytic drug, and the patient outcome, whether or not the patient achieves full recovery, is dependent not only on the product dissolving the clot but also the timeliness of its delivery.[17,18]

Purposes of Registries

As discussed throughout this handbook, registries should be designed and evaluated with respect to their intended purpose(s). Registry purposes can be broadly described in terms of patient outcomes. While there are a number of potential purposes for registries, this document primarily discusses four major purposes: describing the natural history of disease, determining clinical and/or cost effectiveness, assessing safety or harm, and measuring or improving quality of care. Other purposes of patient registries mentioned but not discussed in detail in this document are for public health surveillance and disease control. An extensive body of literature from the last half century of experience with cancer and other disease surveillance registries is available.

Natural history of disease. Registries may be established to evaluate the natural history of a disease, meaning its characteristics, management, and outcomes with and/or without treatment. The natural history may be variable across different groups or geographic regions, and it often changes over time. In many cases, the natural histories of diseases are not well described. Furthermore, the natural history of diseases may change after the introduction of certain therapies. As an example, patients with rare diseases, such as the lysosomal storage diseases, who did not previously survive to their twenties, may now be entering their fourth and fifth decades of life, and this uncharted natural history is being first described through a registry.[19]

Determining effectiveness. Registries may be developed to determine clinical effectiveness or cost effectiveness in real-world clinical practice. Multiple studies have demonstrated disparities between the results of clinical trials and results in actual clinical practice.[20,21] Furthermore, efficacy in a clinical trial for a well-defined population may not be generalizable to other populations or subgroups of interest. As an example, many important heart failure trials have focused on a predominantly white male population with a mean age of approximately 60 years, whereas actual heart failure patients are older, more diverse, and have a higher mortality rate than the patients in these trials.[22] Similarly, underrepresentation of older patients has been reported in clinical trials of 15 different types of cancer (e.g., studies with only 25 percent of patients age 65 years and over, while the expected rate is greater than 60 percent).[23] Registries may also be particularly useful for tracking effectiveness outcomes for a longer time period than is typically feasible with clinical trials. For example, some growth hormone registries have tracked children well into adulthood.

In addition to clinical effectiveness, registries can be used to assess cost effectiveness. Cost effectiveness is a means to describe the comparative value of a health care product or service in terms of its ability to achieve a desired outcome for a given unit of resources.[24] Registries can be designed to collect cost data and effectiveness data for the same patients to use in modeling cost effectiveness. A cost-effectiveness analysis examines the incremental benefit of a particular intervention and the costs associated with achieving that benefit. Cost-effectiveness studies compare costs with clinical outcomes measured in units such as life expectancy or disease-free periods. Cost-utility studies compare costs with outcomes adjusted for quality of life (utility), such as quality-adjusted life years (QALYs). Utilities allow comparisons to be made across conditions because the measurement is not disease specific.[25] It should be noted that for both clinical and cost effectiveness, differences between treatments are indirect and must be inferred from data analysis, simulation modeling, or some mixture.

Measuring or monitoring safety and harm.
Registries may be created to assess safety vs. harm. Safety here refers to the concept of being free from danger or hazard. One goal of registries in this context may be to quantify risk or to attribute it properly. Broadly speaking, patient registries can serve as an active surveillance system for the occurrence of unexpected or harmful events for products and services. Such events may range from patient complaints about minor side effects to severe adverse events such as drug reactions or patient falls in the hospital.

Patient registries offer several advantages for active surveillance. First, the current practice of spontaneous reporting of adverse events relies on a nonsystematic recognition of an adverse event by a clinician and the active effort by the clinician to make a report to manufacturers and health authorities. Second, these events are generally reported without a denominator (i.e., the exposed population), and therefore an incidence level is difficult to determine. Because patient registries can provide systematic data on adverse events and the incidence of these events, they are being used with increasing frequency in the areas of health care products and services.

Measuring quality. Registries may be created to measure quality of care. The IOM defines quality as "the degree to which health services for individuals and populations increase the likelihood of desired health outcomes and are consistent with current professional knowledge." Quality-focused registries are being used increasingly to assess differences between providers or patient populations based on performance measures that compare treatments provided or outcomes achieved with "gold standards" (e.g., evidence-based guidelines) or comparative benchmarks for specific health outcomes (e.g., risk-adjusted survival or infection rates). Such programs may be used to identify disparities in access to care, demonstrate opportunities for improvement, establish differentials for payment by third parties, or provide transparency through public reporting. There are multiple examples of such differences in treatment and outcomes of patients in a range of disease areas.[26]

Multiple purposes. While each of these purposes may drive the creation of a registry, many registries will be developed to serve more than one purpose.

Taxonomy for Patient Registries

Even limited to the definitions described above, the breadth of studies that might be included as patient registries is large. Patients in a registry are typically selected based on a particular disease, condition (e.g., a risk factor), or exposure. This handbook utilizes these common selection criteria to develop a taxonomy or classification based on how the populations for registries are defined. Three general categories with multiple subcategories and combinations account for the majority of registries

11

that are developed for evaluating patient outcomes. These categories include observational studies, in which the patient has a particular disease or condition or has had an exposure to a product or service or various combinations thereof.

Product Registries

In the case of a product registry, the patient is exposed to a health care product, such as a drug or a device. The exposure may be brief, as in single dose of a pharmaceutical product, or extended, as in an implanted device or chronic usage of a medication.

Device registries may include all or a subset of patients who receive the device. A registry for all patients who receive an implantable cardioverter defibrillator, a registry of patients with hip prostheses, or a registry of patients who wear contact lenses are all examples of device registries.

Biopharmaceutical product registries similarly have several archetypes, which may include all or subsets of patients who receive the biopharmaceutical product. Again, the duration of exposure may range from a single event to a lifetime of use. Eligibility for the registry includes the requirement that the patient received the product or class of products (e.g., COX-2 inhibitors). In some cases, such registries are mandated by public health authorities to ensure appropriate use of medications. Examples include registries for thalidomide, clozapine, and isotretinoin.

Pregnancy registries represent a separate class of biopharmaceutical product registries that focus on possible exposures during pregnancy and the neonatal consequences. The FDA has a specific guidance focused on pregnancy exposure registries, which is available at http://www.fda.gov/CbER/gdlns/pregexp.htm. This guidance uses the term "pregnancy exposure registry" to refer to "a prospective observational study that actively collects information on medical product exposure during pregnancy and associated pregnancy outcomes."

Health Services Registries

In the context of evaluating patient outcomes, another type of exposure that can be used to define registries is exposure to a health care service. Health care services that may be utilized to define inclusion in a registry include individual clinical encounter(s), such as office visits or hospitalizations, procedures, or full episodes of care. Examples include registries enrolling patients undergoing a procedure (e.g., carotid endarterectomy, appendectomy, or primary coronary intervention) or admitted to a hospital for a particular diagnosis (e.g., community-acquired pneumonia). In these registries, one purpose of the registry is to evaluate the health care service with respect to the outcomes. Health care service registries are sometimes used to evaluate the processes and outcomes of care for quality measurement purposes (e.g., Get With The Guidelines℠ of the American Heart Association, National Surgical Quality Improvement Program of the Department of Veterans Affairs).

Disease or Condition Registries

Disease or condition registries use the state of a particular disease or condition as the inclusion criterion. In disease or condition registries, the patient may always have the disease (e.g., a rare disease, such as cystic fibrosis or Pompe disease, or a chronic illness, such as heart failure, diabetes, or end-stage renal disease) or may have the disease or condition for a more limited period of time (e.g., infectious diseases, some cancers, obesity). These registries typically enroll the patient at the time of a routine health care service, although patients also can be enrolled through voluntary self-identification processes that do not depend on utilization of health care services (such as Internet recruiting of volunteers.) In other disease registries, the patient has an underlying disease or condition, such as atherosclerotic disease, but is enrolled only at the time of an acute event or exacerbation, such as hospitalization for a myocardial infarction or ischemic stroke.

Combinations

Complicating this classification approach is the reality that these categories can be overlapping in many registries. For example, a patient with ischemic heart disease may have an acute myocardial infarction and undergo a primary coronary intervention with placement of a drug-eluting stent and postintervention management with clopidogrel. This patient could be enrolled in an ischemic heart disease registry longitudinally tracking all patients with this disease, a myocardial infarction registry cross-sectionally collecting patients who present to hospitals with acute myocardial infarction, a primary coronary intervention registry that includes management with and without devices, a coronary artery stent registry limited to ischemic heart disease patients, or a clopidogrel product registry that includes patients undergoing primary coronary interventions.

Duration of Observation

The duration of the observational period for a registry is also a useful descriptor. Observational periods may be limited to a single episode of care (e.g., a hospital discharge registry for diverticulitis), or they may extend for as long as the lifetime of a patient with a chronic disease (e.g., cystic fibrosis or Pompe disease) or receiving novel therapy (e.g., gene therapy). The period of observation or followup depends on the outcomes of interest.

From Registry Purpose to Design

As will be discussed extensively in this document, the purpose of the registry defines what the registry will focus on (e.g., product vs. disease) and therefore the registry type. A registry created for the purpose of evaluating outcomes of patients receiving a particular coronary artery stent might be designed as a single product registry if, for example, the purpose is to systematically collect adverse event information on the first 10,000 patients receiving the product. However, the registry might alternatively be designed as a health care service registry for primary coronary intervention if a purpose is to collect comparative effectiveness or safety data on other treatments or products within the same registry.

Patient Registries and Policy Purposes

In addition to the growth of patient registries for scientific and clinical purposes, registries are receiving increasing attention for their potential role in policymaking or decisionmaking.[27,28] As stated earlier, registries may offer a view of real-world health care that is typically inaccessible from clinical trials or other data sources and may provide information on the generalizability of the data from clinical trials to populations not studied in those trials.

The utility of registry data for decisionmaking is related to three factors: the stakeholders, the primary scientific question, and the context. The stakeholders are those associated with the disease or procedure that may be affected from a patient, provider, payer, regulator, or other perspective. The primary scientific question for a registry may relate to effectiveness, safety, or practice patterns. The context includes the scientific context (e.g., previous randomized trials and modeling efforts that help to more precisely define the primary scientific question), as well as the political, regulatory, funding, and other issues that provide the practical parameters around which the registry is developed. In identifying the value of information from registries, it is essential to look at the data with specific reference to the purpose and focus of the registry and in that context.

From a policy perspective, there are several scenarios in which the decision to develop a registry may arise. One possible scenario is as follows. An item or service is considered for use. Stakeholders in the decision collaboratively define "adequate data in support of the decision at hand." Here, "adequate data" refers to information of sufficient relevance and quality to permit an informed decision. An evidence development strategy is selected from one of many potential strategies (RCT, practical clinical trial, registry, etc.) based on the quality of the evidence provided by each design, as well as the burden of data collection and the cost that is imposed. This tradeoff of the quality of evidence vs. cost of data collection for each possible design is

13

termed the "value of information" exercise (Figure 1). Registries should be preferred in those circumstances where they provide sufficiently high-quality information for decisionmaking and a sufficiently low cost (relative to other "acceptable" designs).

One set of policy determinations that may be informed by a patient registry centers on the area of payment for items or services. For example, in the

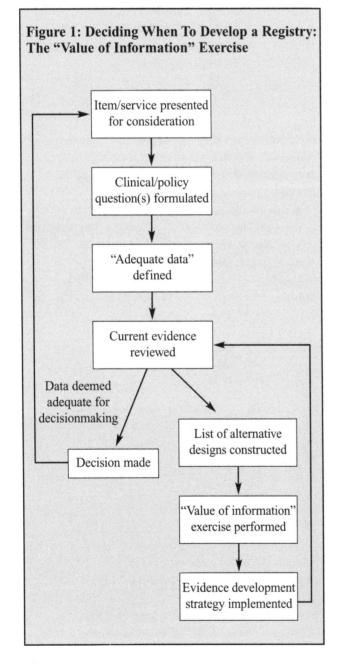

Figure 1: Deciding When To Develop a Registry: The "Value of Information" Exercise

Item/service presented for consideration

↓

Clinical/policy question(s) formulated

↓

"Adequate data" defined

↓

Current evidence reviewed

Data deemed adequate for decisionmaking

Decision made

List of alternative designs constructed

↓

"Value of information" exercise performed

↓

Evidence development strategy implemented

Centers for Medicare & Medicaid Services (CMS) Guidance on National Coverage Determinations With Data Collection as a Condition of Coverage,[28] CMS describes several examples of how data collected in a registry might be used in the context of coverage determinations. As described in the Guidance:

> [T]he purpose of CED [Coverage with Evidence Development] is to generate data on the utilization and impact of the item or service evaluated in the NCD [National Coverage Determination], so that Medicare can a) document the appropriateness of use of that item or service in Medicare beneficiaries under current coverage; b) consider future changes in coverage for the item or service; c) generate clinical information that will improve the evidence base on which providers base their recommendations to Medicare beneficiaries regarding the item or service.

The Guidance provides insight into when registry data may be useful to policymakers. These purposes range from demonstrating that a particular item or service was provided appropriately to patients meeting specific characteristics to collecting new information that is not available from existing clinical trials. CED based on registries may be especially relevant when current data do not address relevant outcomes for Medicare beneficiaries, off-label or unanticipated uses, important patient subgroups, or operator experience or other qualifications.

In many countries, policy determinations on payment rely on cost-effectiveness and cost-utility data and therefore can be informed by registries as well as clinical trials.[29] These data are used and reviewed in a variety of ways. In some countries, there may be a threshold above which a payer is willing to pay for an improvement in patient outcomes.[30] In these scenarios—particularly for rare diseases, when it can be difficult to gather clinical effectiveness data together with quality-of-life data in a utility format—the establishment of disease-specific data registries has been recommended to facilitate the process of technology assessment and improving patient care.[31]

Consider the clinical question of carotid endarterectomy surgery for patients with a high degree of stenosis of the carotid artery. Randomized trials, using highly selected patients and surgeons, indicate a benefit of surgery over medical management in the prevention of stroke. However, that benefit may be exquisitely sensitive to the surgical complication rates (i.e., a relatively small increase in the rate of surgical complications is enough to make medical management the preferred strategy instead), and the studies of surgical performance in a variety of hospitals may suggest substantial variation in surgical mortality and morbidity for this procedure. In such a case, a registry to evaluate treatment outcomes, adjusted by hospital and surgeon, might be considered to support a policy decision as to when the procedure should be reimbursed (e.g., only when performed in medical centers resembling those in the various randomized trials, or only by surgeons or facilities with an acceptably low rate of complications).[32]

Global Registries

As many stakeholders have international interests in diseases, conditions, and health care products and services, it is not surprising that interest in patient registries is global. While some of the specific legal and regulatory discussions in this handbook are intended for and limited to the United States, most of the concepts and specifics are more broadly applicable to similar activities worldwide. Chapters 6 and 9 are perhaps the most limited in their applicability outside the United States. In addition, there may be differences or additions to be considered in data element selection (Chapter 4) stemming from differences ranging from medical training to use of local remedies; the types of data sources that are available outside the United States (Chapter 5); the issues surrounding physician and patient recruitment and retention in different health systems and cultures (Chapter 7); and specific data collection and management options and complexities (Chapter 8) ranging from available technologies to languages.

Summary

A patient registry is an organized system that uses observational study methods to collect uniform data (clinical and other) to evaluate specified outcomes for a population defined by a particular disease, condition, or exposure and that serves predetermined scientific, clinical, or policy purpose(s). Well-designed and well-performed patient registries can provide a real-world view of clinical practice, patient outcomes, safety, and comparative effectiveness and serve a number of evidence development and decisionmaking purposes. In the chapters that follow, this handbook presents practical design and operational issues, evaluation principles, and good registry practices.

15

Chapter 2. Planning a Registry

Registries are considered or created for a number of reasons, and there is tremendous variability in the size, scope, and resource requirements of the various registries that currently exist. Registries may be large or small in their numbers of patients or participating sites. They may target rare or common conditions and exposures, and they may require the collection of narrow or extensive amounts of data. There may be significant or limited resources supporting the registry. In addition, the scope and focus of a registry may be adapted over time to reflect updated information, to reach broader or different populations, to assimilate additional data, to focus on or expand to different geographical regions, or to add new research questions. While this degree of flexibility confers enormous potential, registries require good planning to be successful.

The initial steps in planning a registry should include: articulating the purpose and objective(s) of the registry; determining if the data being sought have already been collected elsewhere; deciding whether a registry is the most appropriate means for addressing the research question; identifying the stakeholders; defining the scope of the registry, including the planned representativeness of the target population and the characteristics of the data to be collected; and assessing if the proposed registry is feasible and likely to be successful. Once a decision is made to proceed, the next considerations in planning concern funding and what types of advisors, teams, and oversight are appropriate for the registry purpose. Plans must also be made to manage change through an orderly and predefined process. Finally, registry planners should determine what will happen when the registry ends. The *Guidelines for Good Pharmacoepidemiology Practice* from the International Society of Pharmacoepidemiology is a useful resource for registry planners.[33] The *Updated Guidelines for Evaluating Public Health*

Surveillance Systems may also be useful to planners, especially the appendixes, which provide various checklists.[34]

Purpose

One of the first steps in planning a registry is defining and establishing a registry purpose. Having a clearly defined purpose and supporting rationale makes it easier to evaluate whether a registry is the right vehicle for capturing the information of interest.[35] In addition, a clearly defined purpose helps clarify the need for certain data, including their scope and level of detail. Conversely, having a clear sense of how the data may be used will help refine the stated purpose.

A registry may have a singular focus, or it may serve many purposes.[36] In either case, the overall purpose should be translated into specific objectives or questions to be addressed through the registry. This process needs to take into account the interests of those collaborating in the registry and the key audiences to be reached.[37] Clear objectives are essential to define the structure and process of data collection and to ensure that the registry effectively addresses the important questions through the appropriate outcomes analyses. Specific objectives also help the registry to avoid collecting large amounts of data of limited value. The time and resources needed to collect and process data in a registry setting can be substantial,[38] and the identification of a core data set is essential. The benefits of any data element included in the registry must outweigh the costs of including it.

Registry planners can begin to establish specific objectives by considering what key questions the registry needs to answer. Critical consideration needs to be given to defining the key questions in order to evaluate how best to proceed, as these questions will help to establish the type of registry, the data points to be captured, and the type of analysis that will be planned. Examples of key, or driving, questions are:

- What is the natural course of a disease in different geographic locations?

- Does a treatment lead to long-term benefits or harm, including delayed complications?

- How successful is a "comprehensive" childhood immunization program?

- How is disease progression affected by available therapies?

- What is the safety profile of a specific therapy?

- Is a specific product or therapy teratogenic?

- How do clinical practices vary when treating a specific disease?

- What characteristics or practices enhance compliance and adherence?

- Do quality improvement programs affect patient outcomes, and, if so, how?

- What are significant predictors of poor outcomes?

- What clinical outcomes should be measured to improve quality of patient care?

- Are there disparities in the delivery of care?

- Should a particular procedure or product be a covered benefit in a particular population?

Two of the case examples in this chapter provide examples of how key questions have shaped registries. (See Case Examples 1 and 2.)

Once the key questions have been identified, the focus turns to practical issues, such as determining if relevant data already exist to answer these questions in a rigorous way or if an entirely new data collection effort needs to be initiated. In some situations, adding new data to an existing registry rather than setting up an entirely new registry may be possible.

18

Case Example 1: Developing a Registry To Determine Policy	
Description	The ICD Registry™ collects detailed information on implantable cardioverter defibrillator (ICD) implantations and tracks the relationship between physician training and in-hospital patient outcomes. The registry meets the Centers for Medicare & Medicaid Services (CMS) Coverage with Evidence Development policy for data collection on ICD implantations.
Sponsor	The Heart Rhythm Society and the American College of Cardiology Foundation
Year Started	2005
Year Ended	Ongoing
No. of Sites	1,448 hospital participants
No. of Patients	Over 100,000 patients annually

Challenge

In March 2004, a manufacturer requested that CMS reconsider its prior coverage decision on ICDs, using the new evidence from the Sudden Cardiac Death in Heart Failure Trial (SCD-HeFT). CMS agreed to this request and reviewed evidence from SCD-HeFT, as well as outcomes from other trials. CMS concluded that "the available evidence does not provide a high degree of guidance to providers to target these devices to patients who will clearly derive benefit." In other words, the evidence did not clearly support the appropriateness of the procedure for Medicare patients, who, with a median age of 70-75 years,

(continued)

Case Example 1: Developing a Registry To Determine Policy (continued)

are significantly older than the patients in the SCD-HeFT trial, where the median age was 60 years. In addition, CMS raised questions about the relationship between the expanding physician specialties implanting ICDs and patient outcomes, stating, "As with any invasive procedure, physicians who insert ICDs must be appropriately trained and fully competent to perform the implantation." While CMS had clear concerns, the evidence from the randomized controlled trials presented strong evidence that ICDs are effective for primary prevention of sudden cardiac death. CMS needed to make a coverage determination that would be in the best interest of its beneficiaries, but the gaps in the evidence made this difficult.

Proposed Solution

In September 2004, CMS proposed that a national registry be developed as a condition for coverage for Medicare beneficiaries receiving ICDs for primary prevention. The Heart Rhythm Society convened a new National ICD Registry Working Group, which consisted of physician associations, health insurance providers, government officials, medical device manufacturers, and members-at-large with expertise in registry development, to determine how best to develop and implement the registry.

In October 2005, CMS announced that the ICD Registry™ satisfies the data reporting requirements for the national coverage determination. All hospitals that implant ICDs for primary prevention in Medicare beneficiaries are required as a condition for coverage to routinely submit data to the registry. While hospitals can limit their data entry to Medicare beneficiaries for primary prevention, the preferred approach is to enter all

patients receiving ICDs. Through the National ICD Registry, CMS hopes to gain information to "determine whether primary prevention ICD implantation procedures are appropriate for Medicare beneficiaries who meet the clinical conditions as identified in the Agency's national coverage determination" (Hammill, 2006).

Results

With 1,448 hospitals participating, the registry collected over 100,000 patients in its first year. Many hospitals entered all patients receiving ICDs. CMS will have data to conduct analysis and shape its ICD coverage decision, and the first outcome reports that compare the hospital participants with their peers are planned to be released in April 2007.

Key Point

Observational registries can quickly accumulate large amounts of data on real-world practice and effectiveness of new treatments and procedures. Physicians and hospitals can use these data to further quality improvement efforts at a local level, and physician associations can evaluate data to determine the effectiveness of existing clinical guidelines. Payers can use these data to inform coverage decisions and shape public policy, particularly in cases where the clinical trial population differs from the potential beneficiaries.

For More Information

Hammill S, Phurrough S, Brindis R. The National ICD Registry: now and into the future. Heart Rhythm 2006 Apr;3(4):470-3.

CMS National Coverage Determination: http://www.cms.hss.gov/mcd/viewdecisionsmemo. asp?id=148

19

Case Example 2: Using Registries To Understand Rare Diseases	
Description	The International Collaborative Gaucher Group (ICGG) Gaucher Registry aims to enhance understanding of the variability, progression, and natural history of Gaucher disease, with the ultimate goals of better guiding and assessing therapeutic intervention and providing recommendations on patient care to the medical community.
Sponsor	Genzyme Corporation
Year Started	1991
Year Ended	Ongoing
No. of Sites	732 (as of January 2007)
No. of Patients	4,620 (as of January 2007), with open-ended followup

Challenge

Rare diseases pose special research challenges. The small number of affected patients often results in limited clinical experience within individual centers. Therefore, the clinical description of rare diseases may be incomplete or skewed. The medical literature often consists of individual case reports or small case series, limiting understanding of the natural history of the disease. Furthermore, randomized controlled trials with adequate sample size and length of followup to assess treatment outcomes may be extremely difficult or not feasible. The challenge is even greater for rare diseases that are chronic in nature, where long-term followup is especially important. As a result, rare diseases are often incompletely characterized and lack published data on long-term treatment outcomes.

Gaucher disease, a rare enzyme deficiency affecting fewer than 10,000 known patients worldwide, illustrates many of the challenges facing researchers of rare diseases. Physicians who encounter patients with Gaucher disease typically have one or two patients in their practice; only a few physicians around the world have more than 10 to 20 patients in their care. Understanding Gaucher disease is further complicated by the fact that it is a highly heterogeneous and rare disorder, and a patient cohort from a single center may represent a subset of the entire spectrum of disease phenotypes.

The rarity and chronic nature of Gaucher disease also pose challenges in conducting clinical research. The clinical trial that led to U. S. Food and Drug Administration approval of enzyme replacement therapy (ERT) for Gaucher disease (Ceredase®, alglucerase injection) in 1991 was a single-arm, open-label study involving only 12 patients followed for 9-12 months. In 1994, a recombinant form of enzyme replacement therapy was approved (Cerezyme®, imiglucerase for injection), based on a randomized two-arm clinical trial comparing Ceredase and Cerezyme in 30 patients (15 in each arm) followed for 9 months.

Proposed Solution

With planning initiated in 1991, the registry is an international, longitudinal disease registry, open voluntarily to all physicians caring for patients with all subtypes of Gaucher disease, regardless of treatment status or treatment type. Data on patient demographics; clinical characteristics; treatment regimen; and laboratory, radiologic, and quality-of-

(continued)

Case Example 2: Using Registries To Understand Rare Diseases (continued)

life outcomes are entered and analyzed to address the research challenges of this rare disease. Responsibility for the use, integrity, and objectivity of the data and analyses is invested in the ICGG board, which is comprised of physician-investigators who are not employees of the sponsor.

Results

With an aggregated, international database, analysis of data from the registry has provided a much more complete clinical description of Gaucher disease and its natural history, with longitudinal data on more than 4,600 patients from over 700 centers in more than 55 countries. The registry has an open-ended followup period, with the length of followup currently ranging from zero to 15 years. The registry has collected approximately 23,000 patient-years of followup over the past 15 years.

With these extensive followup data, analysis of the registry has increased knowledge of longer term treatment outcomes for enzyme replacement therapy. In 2002, the ICGG published the clinical outcomes of 1,028 patients treated with ERT with up to 5 years of followup. A clinical trial of this size and duration would not be feasible for such a rare disease. As the registry database continues to grow in size and duration, further analyses of clinically significant long-term treatment outcomes are being conducted.

A rare disease registry can also help foster the formation of an international community of expert physicians who can collaboratively develop recommendations on the clinical management of

patients. The collective clinical experience of the ICGG led to the development of recommendations for evaluation and monitoring of patients with Gaucher disease. The analysis of registry data on treatment outcomes has facilitated the establishment of therapeutic goals for patients with type 1 Gaucher disease. Together, these publications have formed the foundation for a consensus- and evidence-based disease management approach, something usually only possible for much more common diseases.

Key Point

For rare or ultra-rare diseases such as Gaucher disease, an international, longitudinal disease registry may be the best or only feasible way to comprehensively increase knowledge about the clinical characteristics and natural history of the disease and assess the long-term outcomes of treatment.

For More Information

Charrow J, Esplin JA, Gribble TJ et al. Gaucher disease – recommendations on diagnosis, evaluation, and monitoring. Arch Intern Med 1998;158:1754-60.

Charrow J, Andersson HC, Kaplan P et al. The Gaucher Registry: demographics and disease characteristics of 1698 patients with Gaucher disease. Arch Intern Med 2000;160:2835-43.

Appropriateness for Answering the Key Questions

Advances in epidemiological and biostatistical methods have broadened the scope of questions that can be addressed through observational designs. Stratification, propensity score matching, and risk adjustment are increasingly useful approaches for addressing confounding issues and for creating comparably homogeneous subgroups for analysis within registry data sets (Chapters 3 and 10).[39,40] These techniques may allow registries to conduct informative and reliable analyses to support investigations of comparative safety and effectiveness. Including data quality measures such as source data verification as part of registry operations can strengthen scientific rigor. A careful evaluation of the possibilities for data collection and registry design, the degree of certainty required, and the timeframe in which this certainty is expected can help in selecting an appropriate study design. It is important to note that, historically, there has been a lack of consensus standards for conducting and reporting methods and results for registries. Therefore, registries have tended to be more variable in implementation and are generally harder to assess for quality than randomized controlled trials.

Other Sources of Accessible Data

Because there may be alternative ways to access data and/or analyses, an important question needs to be asked very early in planning a registry: Do these data already exist and, if so, are they accessible? In some cases, the required data have already been collected through another source, or research may be underway. For example, relevant data could be extracted from electronic medical records or administrative health insurance claims data. In such cases, registries might avoid re-collecting data that have already been collected elsewhere and are accessible. Thought should be given to adapting the registry (based on extant data) and/or linking to other relevant data sources (including "piggy-backing" onto other registries).

When the required data have not been sufficiently collected or are not accessible for the desired purpose, it is appropriate to consider creating a new registry.

Stakeholders

Once registry planners have decided that a new registry is the most appropriate method of data collection, they should consider to whom the data matter. It is important to recognize the potential stakeholders at an early stage, as these stakeholders may have important input into the type and scope of data to be collected, they may ultimately be users of the data, or they may have a key role in disseminating the results of the registry.

One or more parties could be considered stakeholders of the registry. These parties could be as specific as a regulatory agency that will be monitoring postmarketing studies or as broad as the general population. Often, a stakeholder's input directly influences whether a registry design can proceed. A regulatory agency looking for management of a therapeutic with a known toxicity profile may require a different level of rigor than a manufacturer with general questions about how a product is being used.

Typically, there are primary and secondary stakeholders for any registry. A primary stakeholder is usually responsible for creating and funding the registry. The party that requires the data, such as a regulatory authority, may also be considered a primary stakeholder. A secondary stakeholder may be a party that would benefit from knowledge of the data (or would be impacted by the results) but that is not instrumental in establishing the registry. Treating physicians and their patients could be considered secondary stakeholders. A partial list of possible stakeholders follows:

- Regulatory authorities.
- Product manufacturers.

- Health care service providers.
- Payer or commissioning authorities.
- Patients and/or advocacy groups.
- Treating physician groups.
- Universities or professional societies.

Once the stakeholders have been established, consideration should be given to how the registry will be funded. Depending on the sources of funding for the registry, this process may identify a new stakeholder. This process of stakeholder definition will become relevant in a later section of this chapter, which discusses issues of oversight and governance for registries.

Although interactions with the potential stakeholders will vary, the registry will be best supported by defined interactions and communications with these parties. Defining these interactions during the planning stage will ensure that adequate dialog occurs and appropriate input is received to support the overall value of the registry. Interactions throughout the entire duration of the registry can also assure stakeholders that the registry is aligned with the purposes and goals that were set out during the planning stages and that the registry complies with all required guidances, rules, and/or regulations.

Characteristics of Data and Target Population

Scope of Data Required

After the registry purpose has been established and the registry stakeholders identified, the registry planners can proceed with determining the scope of the data required to address the key questions. The scope of a registry may be viewed in terms of size, setting, duration, geography, and financing. The purpose and objectives of the registry should frame the scope, but other factors (aside from feasibility and cost) may ultimately shape it. For example, the scope may be affected by:

- Regulatory requirements, such as those imposed by the U.S. Food and Drug Administration (FDA) as a condition of product marketing.
- Reimbursement decisions, such as national coverage decisions by the Centers for Medicare & Medicaid Services.
- National research interests, such as those driven by the National Institutes of Health (NIH).
- Public health policy, such as policy of the Centers for Disease Control and Prevention (CDC) and immunization policy.
- Manufacturers' interests.

The scope is also affected by the degree of uncertainty that is acceptable to the primary stakeholders, with that uncertainty being principally driven by the quantity, quality, and detail of the data collection balanced against its considered importance and value. Therefore, it is critical to understand the potential questions that may or may not be answerable because of the quantity and quality of the data.

Specific variables. Some of the specific variables that can characterize the scope of a registry include:

- *Size:* This may refer to the number and complexity of data points or to the enrollment of investigators and patients. A registry with a large number of complex data points may allow for detailed and thoughtful analyses but may be so burdensome as to discourage investigator and patient enrollments. In turn, a small registry with few patients and data points may be easier to execute, but the data could lack depth and be less meaningful.[41] Size also determines the precision with which measures of risk or risk difference can be calculated.

- *Setting:* This refers to the specific setting through which the registry will recruit investigators and patients as well as collect data (e.g., hospital, doctor's office, pharmacy, home).

- *Duration:* The planning of a registry must reflect the length of time that the registry is expected to collect the data to achieve its

23

purpose and provide analysis of the data collected. An example of a relevant factor is whether a product is nearing the end of the life of its patent.

- *Geography:* The setup, management, and analysis of a locally run registry represent a very different scope than a global registry. The geographic scope impact includes many challenges (e.g., language, cultural, time zone, regulatory) that must be taken into consideration in the planning process.

- *Financial investment:* The scope of a registry will determine the cost of creating, managing, and analyzing the registry. Budgetary constraints must be carefully considered before moving from conception to reality. Additionally, the value of the information weighs in on the financial decisions. The cost of the registry should be less than (or at a minimum, equal to) the projected value gained through the information generated. Some choices in planning, such as building on existing infrastructure and/or linking to data sources relevant to the purposes of the registry, may increase the net return.

- *Richness of clinical data needed:* In some situations, the outcome may be relatively simple to characterize (e.g., death). In other cases, the focus of interest may be a complex set of symptoms and measurements (e.g., for Churg-Strauss Syndrome) or may require specialized diagnostic testing or tissue sampling to confirm (e.g., sentinel node in melanoma). Some outcomes may require assessment by an independent third party. (See "Scientific Rigor," below.)

When data need to be available for analysis. Meaningful data on disease progression or other long-term patient outcomes may not be available through a registry for many years, whereas safety data could be analyzed on a rolling basis. Therefore, the type of data on patient outcomes and when they will be available for analysis should be addressed from the perspective of the intended uses of the data in both the short term and long term.

Scientific rigor. The content of the data to be collected should be driven by the scientific analyses that are planned for the registry, which in turn are determined by the objectives of the registry. A registry that is designed primarily for monitoring drug safety will inevitably contain different data elements from one that is designed primarily for monitoring drug effectiveness. Similarly, the extent to which data need to be validated will depend on the purpose of the registry and the complexity of the clinical information being sought. Some outcomes may require formal adjudication by a committee, while others may require obtaining supporting documents from referrals or biopsies. Generally, registries that are undertaken for regulatory decisionmaking will merit increased attention toward diagnostic confirmation (i.e., enhanced scientific rigor).

Defining the Core Data Set

Elements of data to be included must have potential value in the context of the current scientific and clinical climate and be chosen by a team of experts, preferably with input from experts in biostatistics and epidemiology. Each data element should be chosen for a reason related to the purpose of the registry. Ideally, each data element should address the central questions for which the registry was designed. While a certain number of speculative fields may be desired to generate and explore hypotheses, these must be balanced against the risk of overburdening sites with capturing superfluous data.

The core data set variables ("need to know") define the information set needed to address the critical questions for which the registry was created. At a minimum, when calculating the resource needs and overall design of the registry, registry planners must account for these fields. If additional noncore variables ("nice to know") are included, such as exploratory variables, it is important that such data elements align with the goals of the registry and take into account the burden of data collection and entry at the site level. A parsimonious use of "nice to know" variables is important for several reasons.

24

First, when data elements change, there is a cascade effect to all dependent components of the registry process and outputs. For example, the addition of new data elements may require changes to the data collection system, retraining of site personnel on data definitions and collection practices, adjustments to the registry protocol, and amendment submissions to institutional review boards. Such changes often require additional financial resources. Ideally, the registry would both limit the total number of data elements and include at the outset data elements that might change from "nice to know" to "need to know" during the course of the registry. In practice, this is a difficult balance to achieve, so most registries should plan for some resources to be used for change management.

Second, a registry should not try to accomplish too many goals, or its burden will outweigh its usefulness to the clinical sites and researchers. Examples exist, however, of registries that serve multiple purposes successfully without overburdening clinicians. (See Case Example 3.)

Third, even "need-to-know" variables can sometimes be difficult to collect reliably (e.g., use of illegal substances) or without substantial burden (e.g., unusual laboratory tests). Even with a limited core data set, feasibility must still be considered. (See Chapter 4.)

Defining Patient Outcomes

The outcomes of greatest importance should be identified early in the concept phase of the registry. Having to delineate these outcomes (e.g., primary or secondary endpoints) forces registry designers to establish priorities. Prioritization of interests in the planning phase will help focus the work of the registry and will guide study size requirements. (See Chapter 3.) Identifying the patient outcomes of the greatest importance will also help to guide the selection of the data set. Avoiding the temptation to collect "nice to know" data that are likely of marginal value is of paramount importance, but some registries that accomplish their purposes do in fact need to collect large amounts of data. Having adequate data to properly address potential

confounders during analyses is one reason that extensive data collection is sometimes required.[42]

Methods to ascertain the principal outcomes should be clearly established. The diagnostic requirements, level of data detail, and level of data validation and/or adjudication should also be addressed. As noted below in the context of identifying a target population, relying on established guidelines and standards to aid in defining outcomes of interest has many benefits and should be considered.

The issues of ascertainment noted here are important to consider because they will have a bearing on some attributes by which registries may be evaluated.[43] These attributes include sensitivity (the extent to which the methods identify all outcomes of interest) and external validity (generalizability to similar populations), among others.

Defining the Target Population

The target population is the population to which the findings of the registry are meant to apply. It must be defined for two basic reasons. First, the target population serves as the foundation for how to plan the registry. Second, it also represents a major constituency that will be impacted by the results of the registry.

Criteria for defining the target population should be established. Since one of the goals for registry data may be to enable generalization of conclusions from clinical research on narrowly defined populations to broader ones, the inclusion criteria for most (although not all) registries are relatively broad. As an example, screening criteria for a registry may allow inclusion of elderly patients, patients with multiple comorbidities, patients on multiple therapies, patients who switch treatments during the period of observation, or patients who are using products "off label." The definition of the target population will depend on many factors (e.g., scope and cost) but ultimately will be driven by the purpose of the registry.

As with defining patient outcomes, target population criteria and/or definitions should be consistent with

25

established guidelines and standards within the therapeutic area. Achieving this goal enhances the potential utility of the registry by leveraging other data sources (historical or concurrent) with different information on the same target population and enhancing statistical power if similar information is collected on the target population.

In establishing target population criteria, consideration should be given to the feasibility of access to that population. One should try to distinguish the ideal from the real. Some questions to consider in this regard are:

- How common is the exposure or disease of interest?
- Can eligible persons be readily identified?
- Are other sources competing for the same patients?
- Is care centralized or dispersed (e.g., in a referral or tertiary care facility)?
- How mobile is the target population?

Ultimately, methods to ascertain members of the target population should be carefully considered (e.g., use of screening logs that identify all potential patients and indicate whether they participate and, if not, why not), as well as use of sources outside the registry (e.g., patient groups). Greater accessibility of the target population will reap benefits in terms of enhanced representativeness and statistical power.

Lastly, thought should be given to comparison (control) groups either internal or external to the registry. Again, much of this consideration will be driven by the purpose of the registry, as detailed in its objectives and questions. For example, no need for controls exists in natural history registries, but controls are especially desirable for registries created to evaluate comparative effectiveness or safety.

Registry Funding

Registries that meet the attributes described in this handbook will most likely require funding. The degree of expense incurred will be determined by the scope of the purpose of the registry and the rigor of data collection and audit that is required. The larger the scope of data collected and the greater the need for representation from a wide variety of patient characteristics, the larger is the expense. In addition, the method of data collection will contribute to expense, with electronic collection being more expensive to implement but generally less expensive to maintain compared with fax and scan or mailed forms.[44] Funding will be affected by whether other relevant data sources and/or infrastructures exist that capture some of the information of interest, whether the registry adapts to new issues over time, and whether multiple funding sources participate. Funding needs also should be examined in terms of the projected life of the registry and/or its long-term sustainability. If de-identified data will be accessible to either internal or external groups after the registry closes, it is important to clarify how that activity will be managed and supported.

There are many potential funding sources for registries. Funding sources are likely to want to share in planning and provide input for the many choices that will need to be made in the implementation plans. Funding sources may negotiate to receive access to de-identified data as a requirement for their participation. For a variety of reasons, some funding sources (as is also the case in clinical trials) may require that such access be restricted or exclusive outside of addressing the scientific questions in the registry protocol. Funding models for registries may vary significantly, and a preferred approach does not exist. Rather, the funding model for a registry should be dictated by the needs of the registry.

Potential sources of funding include:

- *Government*: The branches of the government, such as NIH, CDC, and State agencies, may be interested in a registry to determine long-term outcomes of agents, devices, or groups of drugs. While the pharmaceutical industry or device manufacturers collect most long-term data on drug and device safety, many research questions arise that could potentially be suitable for government funding in the context of sponsored Phase IV safety studies mandated by FDA. To

26

determine if there is interest in funding a registry, look for Requests for Proposals (RFPs) on the Web site of the funding agency. Direct contact with the study section secretary is also advisable to determine if there is potential interest in a registry to fill a niche need that may not be posted on the agency Web site. An RFP posting or direct posting with NIH study section personnel would provide a great deal of specific information as to how a submission will be judged and what specific criteria would be needed in order for a proposal to be favorably ranked.

- *Product manufacturers*: Product manufacturers may be interested in studying the natural history of the disease for which they have (or are developing) a product, demonstrating the effectiveness and/or safety of existing products in real-world use, or assisting providers in evaluating or improving quality of care.

- *Foundation funding*: National disease foundations may be in a position to award applications for registry design and implementation from competitive grant applications. The need for a disease-specific registry is dependent on what already exists and whether the perceived need is being met by other organizations. Inquiries from investigators to foundation study section personnel are appropriate in order to determine the climate for a registry proposal to a foundation source.

- *Private funding*: Private philanthropic individuals may be identified within the community who might have an interest in furthering research to better understand the effects of a particular intervention or sets of interventions on a disease process.

- *Professional societies*: Health care professional associations often have scientific committees that could determine whether it is in the interest of the society to develop a registry. Such efforts have been rare because of competing needs for other activities (e.g., meetings, conferences).

- *Professional society/pharmaceutical industry "hybrid"*: Situations may exist in which a product manufacturer funds a registry that would be designed and implemented by a professional society to gain insight into a set of research questions.

- *Health plan providers*: Under certain circumstances, health plan providers may be interested in funding a registry, as practical clinical research is increasingly viewed as a useful tool for providing evidence for health coverage and health care decisions.[45]

- *Multiple sponsors*: Several registries may meet the goals of multiple stakeholders, and such stakeholders may each have an interest in funding. Registries for isotretinoin and antiretrovirals in pregnancy are examples, but many others exist. Such registries can decrease the costs for each funding source.

Recently, there have been several proposals for increasing postmarketing programs such as registries as a path to improved safety monitoring and for streamlining the cost of the drug development process.[46,47,48] At this stage, it is not clear how such efforts would be funded.

Registry Team

Several different kinds of technical expertise and skills are needed to plan and implement a registry. In a small registry run by a single individual, consultants may be able to provide the critical levels of expertise needed to plan all components of the registry. In a large registry, a variety of individuals may work together as a team to contribute the necessary components of expertise. Depending on the size, scope, and purpose of the registry, few, some, or all of the individuals representing the components of expertise described below may be included at the time of the planning process. Whatever number of individuals is eventually assembled, it is important to build a group that can work together as a collegial team to accomplish the goals of the registry. Additionally, the team participants must understand the data sources. By understanding the goals and data sources, the

27

registry team will enable the data to be utilized in the most appropriate context for the most appropriate interpretation.

The different kinds of expertise and experience that are useful include the following:

- *Subject matter*: A registry must be designed so that it contains the appropriate data to meet its goals as well as the needs of its constituents. For example, experts in the treatment of the clinical disease to be studied who are also familiar with the potential toxicities of the treatment(s) to be studied are critical to the success of the registry. Clinical experts must be able to apply all of the latest published clinical, toxicity, and outcome data to components of the registry and determine which elements are necessary, desirable, or superfluous. The importance of this activity to the overall success of the venture cannot be overemphasized.

- *Registry science*: Epidemiology and biostatistics expertise specific to the subtleties of patient registries is useful in the design, implementation, and analysis of registry data. Epidemiologists can provide the study design and can work in collaboration with biostatisticians to develop a mutual understanding of the research objectives. These scientists should work with the subject matter experts to ensure that appropriate analytic methods are being used to address the clinical issues relevant to achieving the goals of the registry.

- *Data collection and database management*: The decision to include various data elements can be made in consultation with experts in this field to place "critical fields" in a prominent and logical position on the data form for both paper-based and electronic data collection tools. A final determination of what is usable and workable for data collection tools should be approved by all members of the team. These experts may also need to write specific programs so that the data received from the registry are grouped, stored, and identified. They may generate reports for individuals who track registry

participation, and they may provide data downloads periodically to registry analysts. This team will also be responsible for implementing and maintaining firewalls to protect the data according to accepted levels of security for similar collections of sensitive data.

- *Legal/patient privacy*: In the present legal climate, it is critical that either information that identifies individual patients be excluded or specific consent be sought to include information on the identity of a patient. This topic is quite complex and is dealt with in detail in Chapter 6. Legal and privacy expertise is needed to protect the patients and the owners of the database by ensuring that the registry complies with all national and local laws applicable to patient information.

- *Quality assurance*: As discussed in Chapter 8, quality assurance of procedures and data is another important component of registry success. Expertise in quality assurance will help in planning a good registry. The goals for quality assurance should be established for each registry, and the efforts made and results achieved should be described.

- *Project management*: Project management will be needed to coordinate the components of the registry; to manage timelines, milestones, deliverables, and budgets; and to ensure communication with sites, stakeholders, oversight committees, and funding sources. Ongoing oversight of the entire process will require a team approach. (See the next section.)

Registry Governance and Oversight

Governance refers to guidance and high-level decisionmaking, including concept, funding, execution, and dissemination of information. The composition and relative mix of internal and external stakeholders and experts relate largely to the purpose of the registry. For example, if the purpose of the registry is to determine a comparative effectiveness or reimbursement policy, those impacted by the policy should not solely govern the registry. Broad stakeholder involvement is most desirable in governance boards when there are many stakeholders.

Depending on the size of the registry, governance may be assumed by various oversight committees made up of interested individuals who are part of the design team (internal governance) or who remain external to the day-to-day operations of the registry (external governance). Differences in the nature of the study questions, the overall resources being consumed by the registry, the soundness of the underlying data sources, and many other factors will influence the degree of involvement and role of oversight groups. In other words, the purpose of the committee functions described below is to lay out the roles that need to be assumed by the governance structure of many registries, but these should be individualized for a particular registry. It is also possible, if methods are clear and transparency self-evident, that oversight requirements may be minimal.

Registries fulfill governance roles in a variety of ways. Many of the roles, for example, could be assumed by a single committee (e.g., a steering committee) in some registries. Whatever model is adopted, it must accommodate all of the working constituencies and provide a mechanism for these individuals to work together to achieve the goals of the registry.

All aspects of governance should be codified in a written format that can be reviewed, shared, and refined over time. In addition, governance is a dynamic process, subject to change in policy as evidence emerges that is likely to lead to improvements in the process.

Governance and oversight functions that may be considered include:

- *Executive or steering*: This function assumes responsibility for the major financial, administrative, legal/ethical, and scientific decisions that determine the direction of the registry. These decisions are made with appropriate input from legal, scientific, and administrative experts. Depending on their

capabilities and the size and resources of the registry, the group serving the steering function may also assume some of the functions described below.

- *Scientific*: This function may include experts ranging from database content, to general clinical research, to epidemiology and biostatistics. This function may determine the overall direction of database inquiries and recommend specific analyses to the executive or steering group. It is strongly desirable that the reports that emerge from a registry be scientifically based analyses that are independent and transparent.[49] To enhance credibility and in the interest of full disclosure, the role of all stakeholders in the publication process should be specified and any potential conflicts of interest identified.

- *Liaison*: In large registries, a function may be specified to focus on maintaining relationships with the funding source, health care providers, and patients who utilize the database. The group serving this function may develop monitoring and satisfaction tools to assure that the day-to-day operations of the registry remain healthy.

- *Adjudication*: Adjudication is used to review and confirm cases (outcomes) that may be difficult to classify. Individuals performing this function are generally blinded to the exposure (product or process) under study so that the confirmation of outcomes is made without knowledge of exposure.

- *Data Safety Monitoring Board (DSMB)*: The majority of registries will not have a need for a DSMB, since a DSMB is commonly used to monitor the safety of drugs and devices in development and is rarely used in studies of marketed products and services. There may be situations in which the registry is responsible for the primary accumulation of safety data on a particular intervention; in such situations, it is possible that a DSMB would be appropriate.

- *Data access, use, and publications*: A process by which registry investigators access and perform analyses of registry data for the purpose of submitting abstracts to scientific meetings and developing manuscripts for peer-reviewed journal submission should be addressed by this function. Authorship (including registry sponsors) in scientific publications should satisfy the conditions of the Uniform Requirements for Manuscripts Submitted to Biomedical Journals.[50] The rules governing authorship may be affected by the funding source, as in the case of NIH or foundation funding, or by the biomedical journal. (See Case Example 3.) Other investigators may request permission to access the data. For example, a Ph.D. candidate at an institution might seek registry-wide aggregate data for the purposes of evaluating a new scientific question. A process for reviewing and responding to such requests from other investigators should be considered in some registries that may generate broad external interest if the registry stakeholders and participants are agreeable to such use.

An example of a way to respond to these requests is the following: Proposals for data analysis are submitted using a uniform submission format that describes the hypothesis to be tested, methods to be utilized in the analysis, likely significance of the results of the analysis, and publication plans. These uniform submissions can be evaluated in a blinded manner by members of a designated group and assigned a numerical ranking, with input from epidemiologists or biostatisticians as to the feasibility of the proposal.

What Happens When the Registry Ends?

Most registries have a finite lifespan. A registry that tests the safety of a product used during pregnancy will have a different lifespan from one that examines the effectiveness of new interventions in a chronic disease. Sponsors and registry participants should have an understanding of the proposed lifespan of the registry at the time of its inception.

The determination of who owns the data at the end of the natural lifespan of the registry and where the data are to be stored should also be defined at the time of registry inception. Possibilities include the principal investigator, the sponsor or funding source, or a related professional society. Chapter 6 discusses issues in ownership.

Registries that generate continuing societal value, such as quality improvement programs and safety programs, might consider transitions that continue the registry functions after the original funding sources have expired.

Case Example 3: Creating a Registry To Fulfill Multiple Purposes and Using a Publications Committee To Review Data Requests	
Description	The National Registry of Myocardial Infarction (NRMI) collects, analyzes, and disseminates data on patients experiencing acute myocardial infarction. Its goal is improvement of patient care at individual hospitals through the hospital team's evaluation of data and assessment of care delivery systems.
Sponsor	Genentech, Inc.
Year Started	1990
Year Ended	Ongoing
No. of Sites	451 hospitals (NRMI 5). Over 1,700 hospitals have participated in NRMI over the past 16 years.
No. of Patients	2,472,218

Challenge

Over the past 20 years, there have been significant changes in the treatment of acute myocardial infarction (AMI) patients. Evidence from large clinical trials has led to the introduction of new guidelines and therapies for treating AMI patients, including fibrinolytic therapy and percutaneous coronary intervention. While these treatments can improve both morbidity and mortality for AMI patients, they are time sensitive and must be administered very soon after hospital arrival in order to be most effective.

After the release of its first fibrinolytic therapy product in 1987, the sponsor's field representatives learned from their discussions with emergency department physicians, cardiologists, and hospital staff that most clinicians believed they were treating patients quickly, although there was no documentation or benchmarking to confirm this

assumption or to identify and correct delays. At that time, many emergency departments did not have readily available diagnostic tools (such as angiography labs) and hospitals with AMI-specific decision pathways and treatment protocols were the exception rather than the rule.

In addition, since fibrinolytic therapy was being widely used for the first time, the sponsor wanted to gather safety information related to its use in real-world situations and in a broader range of patients than those treated in the controlled environment of a clinical trial.

Proposed Solutions and Results

The sponsor decided to create the National Registry of Myocardial Infarction to fulfill the multiple purposes of identifying treatment patterns, promoting time-to-treatment and other quality improvements, and gathering real-world safety data. The scope of the data collection necessary to meet these needs could have made such a registry impracticable, so the NRMI team faced the sizable challenge of balancing the data needs with the feasibility of the registry.

The sponsor formed a Scientific Advisory Board with members representing the various clinical stakeholders (emergency department, cardiology, nursing, research, etc.). The Scientific Advisory Board developed the data set for the registry, keeping a few guiding principles in mind. These principles emphasized maintaining balance between the clinical research and the feasibility of the registry. The first principle was to determine whether the proposed data element was necessary by asking several key questions: How will the data element be used in generating hospital feedback reports or research analyses? Is the data element already collected? If not, should it be collected? If it should be collected, is it feasible to collect those data? The second principle focused on using existing data standards whenever possible. If a data standard did not exist, the team tried to collect the data in the simplest possible way. The third principle emphasized data consistency and making the registry user friendly by continually refining

31

(continued)

Case Example 3: Creating a Registry To Fulfill Multiple Purposes and Using a Publications Committee To Review Data Requests (continued)

data element definitions until they were as clear as possible.

In 1990, the sponsor launched the registry. Over the past 16 years, the registry has proven that the advisory board's efforts to create a feasible multipurpose registry were successful. To date, the registry has collected data on the clinical presentation, treatment, and outcomes of over 2.4 million patients with AMI from more than 1,700 participating sites.

The success of the registry presented a new challenge for the registry team. The sponsor receives a large volume of requests to analyze the registry data, often for research topics that fall outside of the standardized reports developed for the registry. As a guiding principle, the registry team is committed to making the data available for research projects, but it has limited resources to support these requests. The team needed to develop a process that would allow outside researchers to access the registry data without overburdening the registry team.

The registry team created a publication process to determine when another group could use the data for research. The team set high-level criteria that all data requests must meet. The request must be feasible given the data in the registry, and the request must not represent a duplication of another research effort.

To review the requests the registry team involved its Scientific Advisory Board, made up of cardiologists, emergency department physicians, nurses, research scientists, pharmacists, and reviewers with specialties in biostatistics and statistical programming, in creating a publication Review Committee. The role of the Review Committee is to evaluate all research proposals to determine originality, interest to peers, feasibility, appropriateness, and priority. The Review Committee limits its review of research proposals to a set number of reviews per year, and it schedules the reviews and deadlines around the

abstract deadlines for the major conferences. Research analyses must be intended to result in peer-reviewed presentations and publications. Researchers are asked to submit proposals that include well-defined questions and an analysis plan. If the proposal is accepted, the researchers discuss any further details with the biostatisticians and statistical programmers who will perform the analyses (and who are employed at an independent clinical research organization). The results are sent directly to the researchers.

The Scientific Advisory Board and Review Committee remain involved in the process once a data request has been granted. All authors must submit their abstracts to the Review Committee before sending them to conferences. The Review Committee reviews the abstracts and offers constructive criticism to help the authors improve them. The Review Committee also reviews manuscripts before journal submission to help identify any issues or concerns that the authors should address.

The publication process has enabled the wealth of data collected in this registry to be used in over 150 scientific abstracts and 100 peer-reviewed articles, addressing each of the purposes of the registry as well as other research topics. By involving the Scientific Advisory Board and providing independent biostatistical support, the registry team has developed an infrastructure that enhances the credibility of the research uses of this observational database.

Key Points

Registries can be developed to fulfill more than one purpose, but this added complexity requires careful planning to ensure that the final registry data collection burden and procedures are feasible. Making sure that the advisory board includes representatives with clinical and operational perspectives can help the board to maintain its focus on feasibility.

(continued)

32

Case Example 3: Creating a Registry To Fulfill Multiple Purposes and Using a Publications Committee To Review Data Requests (continued)

As a registry database gains large amounts of data, the registry team will likely receive research proposals from groups interested in using the data. The registry team may want to set up a publication process during the registry design phase.

For More Information

Roe MT, Parsons LS, Pollack CV et al. Quality of care by classification of myocardial infarction: treatment patterns for ST-segment elevation vs non-ST-segment elevation myocardial infarction. Arch Intern Med 2005 Jul 25;65 (14):1630-6.

McNamara RL, Herrin J, Bradley EH et al. Hospital improvement in time to reperfusion in patients with acute myocardial infarction, 1999 to 2002. J Am Coll Cardiol 2006;47:45-51.

33

Chapter 3. Registry Design

Once the purpose of the registry has been established and the registry team, funding, and stakeholders have been determined, the task of specific registry design may begin. Seven key aspects of registry design should be considered and evaluated in the context of the registry purpose, be it clinical effectiveness, cost effectiveness, safety, or natural history, as shown in Table 1.

Table 1: Considerations for Study Design	
Construct	**Relevant questions**
Research question	What are the clinical and/or public health questions of interest?
Study design	What types of study designs can be used in registries?
Exposures and outcomes	How do the clinical questions of interest translate into measurable exposures and outcomes?
Study population	What types of patients are needed for study? Is a comparison group needed? How should patients be selected for study?
Data sources	Where can the necessary data be found?
Study size and duration	For how long should data be collected, and for how many patients?
Potential for bias	What is the potential for bias, and how does this affect generalizability (external validity)?

This chapter is intended as a high-level practical guide to the application of epidemiological methods that are particularly useful in the design of registries that evaluate patient outcomes. It is not intended to replace a basic textbook on epidemiologic design. Throughout the design process, registry planners may want to discuss options and decisions with the registry stakeholders and relevant experts to ensure that sound decisions are made. The choice of groups to be consulted during the design phase generally depends on the nature of the registry, the registry funding source, and the funding mechanism.

Research Questions That Are Appropriate for Registries

The questions typically addressed in registries range from purely descriptive questions aimed at understanding the characteristics of people who develop a disease and how the disease generally progresses, to highly focused questions that are intended to support decisionmaking. Registries focused on determining clinical or cost effectiveness or assessing safety or harm are generally hypothesis driven and concentrate on evaluating the effects of specific treatments on patient outcomes.

Registries are often considered as alternatives to conducting randomized controlled trials (RCTs). While these can be complementary research methodologies, some research questions are better answered by one method than the other. RCTs are generally considered to provide the highest grade evidence for evaluating whether a drug has the ability to bring about an intended effect in optimal or "ideal world" situations, a concept also known as "efficacy."[51] Registries may be preferable designs for studies of effectiveness—that is, whether a drug, device, procedure, or program in fact achieves its desired effect in the real world. This is particularly true when the factors surrounding the decision to treat are part of what is intended to be studied.

In many situations, nonrandomized comparisons either are sufficient to address the research question or, in some cases, may be necessary because of the following issues with randomized treatment:

- *Equipoise*: Can providers ethically introduce randomization between treatments when the treatments are not necessarily considered clinically equivalent?

- *Ethics*: If reasonable suspicion about the safety of a product has become known, would it be ethical to conduct a trial that deliberately exposes patients to potential harm? Is it reasonable to subject patients to "sham" surgery in an effort to blind investigators to treatment? How can pregnant women be ethically exposed to drugs that may be teratogenic? (See Case Example 4.)

- *Practicality*: Will patients enroll in a study where they might not receive the treatment? How can compliance and adherence to a treatment be studied, if not by observing what people do in real-world situations?

Registries are particularly suitable for situations where experimental research is not feasible or practical, such as:

- Natural history studies where the goal is to observe clinical practice and patient experience but not to introduce any intervention.

- Measures of clinical effectiveness, especially as related to compliance, where the purpose is to learn about what patients actually do and how that affects outcomes, if at all, rather than to observe the effects of products used according to a study protocol.

- Studies of heterogeneous patient populations, since unlike randomized trials, registries generally have much broader inclusion criteria and fewer exclusion criteria. These characteristics lead to studies with greater generalizability (external validity).

- Followup for delayed or long-term benefits or harm, since registries can extend over much longer periods than most clinical trials (because of their generally lower costs to run and lesser burden on participants).

Case Example 4: Assessing the Safety of Products Used During Pregnancy

Description	The Antiretroviral Pregnancy Registry is the oldest ongoing pregnancy exposure registry. This multisponsor, international collaborative registry monitors prenatal exposures to all marketed antiretroviral drugs, which include several drug classes and multiple drugs in each class.
Sponsor	Abbott Laboratories; Agouron Pharmaceuticals, Inc., a Pfizer Company; Aurobindo Pharma Ltd.; Barr Laboratories, Inc.; Boehringer Ingelheim Pharmaceuticals, Inc.; Bristol-Myers Squibb Company; Gilead Sciences, Inc.; GlaxoSmithKline; F. Hoffmann-La Roche Ltd.; Merck & Co., Inc.; Ranbaxy, Inc.
Year Started	1989
Year Ended	Ongoing
No. of Sites	Not site based; open to all health care providers. Over 1,200 health care providers have enrolled patients.
No. of Patients	10,000

Challenge

Data on the teratogenic effects of pharmaceutical products is often difficult to obtain. Most clinical trials exclude pregnant women because of the ethical concerns of potentially exposing the fetus to harm. While data on the teratogenic risk is available from preclinical animal testing, this information is not always predictive of the effects of a drug taken during human pregnancy. As a result, data to help patients and physicians understand the potential risk and benefits of continuing a treatment during pregnancy are often lacking.

(continued)

36

Case Example 4: Assessing the Safety of Products Used During Pregnancy (continued)

There is a great need for this information, as pregnant women may receive drugs for various reasons. For example, a pregnant woman may need drugs to treat an illness that arises during pregnancy or to treat a chronic mental or physical illness. Women may also become pregnant while taking a drug, resulting in an unintended exposure. This last scenario is particularly likely, given that 50 to 60 percent of all pregnancies in the United States are unintended, and most are not recognized until late in the first trimester.

Antiretroviral treatments represent an area of particular concern, as women may need to take the drugs during pregnancy to manage their HIV infection. In addition, these drugs can reduce the risk of transmitting HIV to the infant, but that benefit must be weighed against the possible risk of teratogenic effects. Because of these factors, it is extremely important for clinicians and patients to understand the potential risks of using antiretroviral drugs during pregnancy in order to make an informed decision. However, ethical and practical concerns make a randomized trial to gather these data difficult, if not impossible.

Proposed Solution

In 1989, the first manufacturer of an antiretroviral drug voluntarily initiated a pregnancy exposure registry to track outcomes of women who had used its product during pregnancy. The purpose of the registry is to collect information on any teratogenic effects of the product by prospectively enrolling women during the course of their pregnancy and following up with them to determine the outcome of the pregnancy. Physicians enroll a patient by providing information on the pregnancy dates, characteristics of the HIV infection, drug dosage, length of therapy, and trimester of exposure to the antiretroviral drug. Information on the pregnancy outcome is gathered through a followup form sent to the physician after the expected delivery date.

In 1993, the registry expanded to include all antiretroviral drugs, as other manufacturers voluntarily joined the registry once their drugs were on the market. The registry is international in scope and allows any health care provider to enroll a patient who has intentional or unintentional use of an antiretroviral drug during pregnancy. The U.S. Food and Drug Administration (FDA), which has used this registry as a model for new pregnancy registries, now requires participation in the registry for all new and generic antiretroviral drugs.

Results

Since its inception 13 years ago, the registry has provided many lessons in how to monitor the safety of these drugs during pregnancy. The registry has developed processes to monitor and assess the safety of these drugs in pregnancy. To ensure both rigor and consistency, it has predefined analytic methods and criteria for recognizing a potential teratogenic signal.

The monitoring system developed by the registry includes several groups, which provide different levels of the monitoring. The groups include:

- Steering Committee (comprised of all groups below).

- Scientific Advisory Committee (comprised of FDA, Centers for Disease Control and Prevention, National Institutes of Health, and academic experts).

- Birth Defect Review Committee (comprised of representatives from the other groups).

- Sponsor Committee (comprised of epidemiologists and safety experts).

- Consultants (geneticist and pharmacoepidemiologist).

- Coordinating Center staff (epidemiologist, project manager, and clinical research associates).

Tools for coding and classifying birth defects have been developed specifically for the registry to maximize identification of a teratogenic signal.

37

(continued)

38

Case Example 4: Assessing the Safety of Products Used During Pregnancy (continued)

This unique system groups birth defects by etiology or embryology rather than by general location or category, as in the Medical Dictionary for Regulatory Activities (MedDRA). Grouping like defects together increases the likelihood of detecting a potential signal. Another unique aspect of this registry that aids in signal detection is coding the temporal association between timing of exposure and formation of the birth defect.

Specific monitoring criteria have been developed for evaluating signals at various levels, including:

- Individual and composite data.

- Primary analysis (statistical considerations, including power/relative risk calculation and statistical probabilities associated with detecting various birth defects).

- Complementary data, including clinical studies in pregnancy, retrospectively reported data, other registries or epidemiological studies, published studies, and case studies.

These efforts to monitor and study the teratogenic effects of antiretroviral use during pregnancy have produced many publications. Registry data have been used in seven publications, four abstracts, and nine presentations, and the registry design and operation have been the subject of many publications and presentations. The registry data and publications can help to provide clinicians and patients with information to make informed decisions regarding use of antiretroviral drugs during pregnancy.

Key Point

An observational registry can collect data to answer research questions in cases where a randomized trial is not feasible for ethical or practical reasons. For pregnancy exposure registries, the observational model allows the researchers to gather data on women and infants exposed to products during pregnancy without deliberately introducing the exposure.

For More Information

Watts D, Covington D, Beckerman K et al. Assessing the risk of birth defects associated with antiretroviral exposure during pregnancy. Am J Obstet Gynecol 2004;191:985-92.

Covington D, Tilson H, Elder J et al. Assessing teratogenicity of antiretroviral drugs: monitoring and analysis plan of the Antiretroviral Pregnancy Registry. Pharmacoepidemiol Drug Saf 2004;13:537-45.

Scheuerle A, Covington D. Clinical review procedures for the Antiretroviral Pregnancy Registry. Pharmacoepidemiol Drug Saf 2004; 13:529-36.

- Surveillance for rare events or of rare diseases.

- Studies for treatments in which randomization is unethical, such as intentional exposure to potential harm (as in safety studies of marketed products that are suspected of being harmful).

- Studies for which blinding is challenging or unethical (e.g., studies of surgical interventions, acupuncture).

- Studies of rapidly changing technology.

- Studies of conditions with complex treatment patterns and treatment combinations.

- Studies of health care access and barriers to care.

- Evaluation of actual standard medical practice. (See Case Example 5.)

A benefit of registries is the ability to conduct embedded substudies. These substudies can have various designs (e.g., highly detailed prospective data collection on a subset of registry participants, case-control study focused on either incident or prevalent cases identified within the registry). (See Case Example 6.) The registry can also be used as a sampling frame for randomized controlled trials. (See Case Example 7.)

Case Example 5: Designing a Registry To Study Outcomes	
Description	The Carotid Artery Stenting with Emboli Protection Surveillance Post-Marketing Study (CASES-PMS) was designed to assess the outcomes of carotid artery stent procedures for the treatment of obstructive artery disease during real-world use. The primary purpose of the registry was to evaluate outcomes in the peri-approval setting, including the use of a detailed training program for physicians not experienced in carotid artery stenting.
Sponsor	Cordis Corporation
Year Started	2004
Year Ended	2006
No. of Sites	74
No. of Patients	1,493

Challenge

In 2004, the sponsor received approval for a carotid stent procedure from the U.S. Food and Drug Administration (FDA), largely because of the results of the Stenting and Angioplasty With Protection in Patients at HIgh Risk for Endarterectomy (SAPPHIRE) clinical trial. The SAPPHIRE trial studied the results of stent procedures performed by experts in the field. While the trial provided strong data to support the approval of the carotid stent, FDA and the Centers for Medicare & Medicaid Services (CMS) both questioned whether the outcomes of the trial were generalizable to procedures performed by physicians without prior experience in carotid artery stenting.

To respond to FDA and CMS requests, the sponsor needed to design a study to confirm the safety and effectiveness of carotid artery stenting in a variety of settings. The study needed to gather data from

academic and nonacademic settings, from physicians with various levels of carotid stenting experience, from settings with varying levels of carotid stenting volume, and from a geographically diverse mix of sites. The study would also need to examine the effectiveness of a training program that the sponsor had designed to teach physicians about the stenting procedure.

Proposed Solution

The sponsor designed a comprehensive training program for physicians and other health care professionals. The training program, which began in 2004, included didactic review, case observations and simulation training, and hands-on experience. To study the effectiveness of the training program and to provide data on the clinical safety and effectiveness of carotid stenting in a variety of settings, the sponsor designed and launched the registry in 2004.

The registry was a multicenter, prospective, observational study designed to assess stenting outcomes in relation to the outcomes of the SAPPHIRE trial (historic comparison group). The study enrolled 1,493 patients from 74 sites, using inclusion and exclusion criteria that matched those of the SAPPHIRE trial. The patients in the study were high-surgical-risk patients with de novo atherosclerotic or postendarterectomy restenotic obstructive lesions in native carotid arteries. Study participants completed clinical followups at 30 days and again at 1 year after the procedure. The 30-day assessments included a neurological examination by an independent neurologist and an evaluation of adverse events. The study defined the 30-day major adverse event rate as the 30-day composite of all deaths, myocardial infarctions, and strokes.

Results

The 30-day major adverse event rate of 5.0 percent met the criteria for noninferiority to the outcomes of stented patients from the pivotal SAPPHIRE trial. Outcomes were similar across levels of physician experience, carotid stent volume, geographic location, and presence/absence of the

39

(continued)

40

Case Example 5: Designing a Registry To Study Outcomes (continued)
training program. The initial findings show that a comprehensive, formal training program in carotid stenting enables physicians from multiple specialties with varying levels of experience in carotid stenting to achieve outcomes similar to those achieved by the experts in the clinical trial.
Key Point
An observational registry can provide the necessary data for a postmarket evaluation of devices that are dependent on newly acquired skills. The registry can provide data to assess both the clinical safety of the device and the effectiveness and success of a training program.
For More Information
Yadav JS, Wholey MH, Kuntz RE et al. Protected carotid-artery stenting versus endarterectomy in high-risk patients. N Engl J Med 2004;351:1493-501.

Case Example 6: Analyzing Clinical Effectiveness and Comparative Effectiveness in an Observational Study	
Description	The National Cooperative Growth Study (NCGS) collects data on children with growth disorders who are treated with a specific growth hormone (GH). The purpose of the multicenter, observational, postmarketing surveillance registry is to collect long-term safety and efficacy information on the GH preparations, with the goal of better understanding the growth response to GH therapy.
Sponsor	Genentech, Inc.
Year Started	1985
Year Ended	Ongoing
No. of Sites	More than 500 centers have participated over the life of the registry
No. of Patients	47,226

Challenge

Clinical trials of GH therapy for short children without GH deficiency and without known etiology for their growth failure (idiopathic short stature, or ISS) have generally only included a small number of patients. The registration trial for the sponsor's GH therapy for the ISS condition was comprised of 118 children at baseline. While the trial demonstrated the efficacy of the treatment and an indication was obtained, physicians and families had lingering concerns about the applicability (safety and effectiveness) of the results to clinical practice.

Proposed Solution

To provide further safety and effectiveness data, the sponsor compared the data in the registration trial with data in the existing NCGS registry. In the 18-year period used in the analysis, the

(continued)

Case Example 6: Analyzing Clinical Effectiveness and Comparative Effectiveness in an Observational Study (continued)

registry contained 8,018 children without GH deficiency and with no identified etiology for their growth failure. The analysis team extracted the data from these 8,018 children as a comparator to the 118 children in the sponsor's clinical registration trial.

For the purposes of the safety analysis, the analysis team summarized all reportable adverse events, serious adverse events, and certain targeted adverse events specified by the protocol for the registry cohort and compared these data with data from the clinical trial cohort. For the purposes of effectiveness, the analysis team selected children from the registry who matched the clinical characteristics of the trial cohort (age 5 years or older, prepubertal, maximum stimulated GH 10 ng/ml or more, no text report of contraindicating diagnosis, naïve to previous therapy, and receiving a dose of GH similar to that in the clinical trial). The team found 1,721 patients who had at least 1 year of treatment data reported. The team compared these data with the growth rates of the children in the registration trial by year of treatment.

In addition, the team performed an analysis to look at children in the registry younger than those in the registration trial to provide clinical data that would be useful to clinicians but could not be obtained easily in a clinical trial. Lastly, the team completed an analysis on children in puberty, another group that could not be studied in the registration trial because of the confounding variable of the puberty group and insufficient numbers in the trial to account for this variable vs. the effect of GH alone.

Results

The results of these analyses using the registry data and the sponsor's registration trial data demonstrated that ISS patients in a clinical setting had a significant increase in height similar to that of patients in the registration trial, with no new safety signals. Children in groups not studied in the registration trial had characteristic growth patterns that could be used by clinicians as comparators not available from the registration trial. Finally, the lack of new safety signals from any of the groups in the registry provided data in numbers and in years of exposure to GH that could never be obtained from a small registration trial.

Key Point

A large registry can provide a resource of study subjects for focused investigations. Inclusion and exclusion criteria can be designed to match those of a registration trial to provide more robust data on outcomes and safety.

For More Information

Kemp SF, Kuntze J, Attie KM et al. Efficacy and safety results of long-term growth hormone treatment of idiopathic short stature. J Clin Endocrinol Metab 2005;90:5247-53.

41

42

Case Example 7: Using a Registry To Recruit Patients for Clinical Trials

Description	The Alpha-1 Antitrypsin Deficiency Research Registry is an observational registry of individuals diagnosed with Alpha-1 Antitrypsin Deficiency and individuals identified as Alpha-1 carriers. The objective of the registry is to serve as a resource for investigators seeking individuals with Alpha-1 to participate in clinical trials and to promote the development of improved treatments and a cure for Alpha-1.
Sponsor	Alpha-1 Foundation
Year Started	1997
Year Ended	Ongoing
No. of Sites	One central recruitment site
No. of Patients	3,000

Challenge

Alpha-1 Antitrypsin Deficiency (Alpha-1) is a hereditary, genetic condition that can cause serious lung and/or liver disease over the life of an individual. Alpha-1 results from a lack of the protein alpha-1 antitrypsin (AAT) in the blood. The AAT protein, which protects the lungs from inflammation caused by infection and inhaled irritants, is produced in the liver. In individuals with Alpha-1, the protein is not released from the liver at the normal rate, resulting in both low blood levels of AAT and a buildup of AAT in the liver, which can lead to liver disease.

Although the exact number of affected individuals is unknown, current evidence suggests that up to 100,000 people in the Unites States have Alpha-1, which is commonly misdiagnosed as asthma or smoking-related chronic obstructive pulmonary disease. Because Alpha-1 is a hereditary, genetic condition, the patient population is highly sensitive to confidentiality and genetic discrimination issues. To prevent these concerns from limiting Alpha-1 research, the Alpha-1 Foundation, a patient-founded and patient-run nonprofit research foundation, needed to develop a method of facilitating research while protecting patient privacy.

Proposed Solution

The Foundation established the registry in 1997 to promote Alpha-1 research and the development of new treatments. The registry collects data from individuals with Alpha-1 and those identified as carriers through a central recruitment site. Data on the unaffected spouses of individuals with Alpha-1 is also collected for use as controls. The patient-reported data include a three-page enrollment questionnaire and a yearly followup questionnaire, and patients are asked to submit their latest lung function testing (FEV1) result from their physician. Individuals who agree to participate in the registry also consent to be contacted regarding clinical studies for which they may qualify.

Scientific and medical investigators are encouraged to utilize the registry as a source of patients for clinical research and as a source of demographic information on the patient population. However, the registry uses a strict process to ensure patient confidentiality. Investigators who wish to recruit through the registry must apply to a committee made up of patients, scientists, and bioethicists. If the request is approved, the registry team matches the proposed inclusion and exclusion criteria against the registry database to identify potentially qualifying subjects. The registry team then contacts the potential subjects with information about the proposed study, usually by mail. Subjects can decide if they wish to participate and, if so, contact the study sites directly. The registry never provides subject contact information to the investigators.

(continued)

Case Example 7: Using a Registry To Recruit Patients for Clinical Trials (continued)

Results

By using a model that emphasizes patient privacy and promotes research on new treatments, the registry has collected data on over 3,000 patients and several hundred controls. The registry has helped many investigators with recruitment for clinical trials, and the registry has used its database to conduct research for publications on the cost of care to patients with Alpha-1, liver disease in Alpha-1 patients, and perceptions regarding genetic discrimination.

Key Point

A registry can serve as a source of potential subjects for clinical trials, particularly in cases where the population of interest is difficult to recruit directly or through health care providers.

For More Information

Mayer A, Stoller J, Bucher Bartelson B et al. Occupational exposure risks in individuals with PI*Z alpha(1)-antitrypsin deficiency. Am J Respir Crit Care Med 2000;162(2 Pt 1):553-8.

Bowlus C, Willner I, Zern M et al. Factors associated with advanced liver disease in adults with alpha1-antitrypsin deficiency. Clin Gastroenterol Hepatol 2005;3(4):390-6.

Eden E, Strange C, Holladay B et al. Asthma and allergy in alpha-1 antitrypsin deficiency. Respir Med 2006;100(8):1384-91.

Study Designs for Registries

While registries are, by definition, observational studies, the framework for how the data will be analyzed drives the data collection. The conventional study models of cohort, case-control, and case-cohort are commonly applied to registry data and are described briefly here. Other models that are also useful in some situations, but are not covered here, include case-crossover studies, which are efficient designs for studying the effects of intermittent exposures (e.g., use of erectile dysfunction drugs) on conditions with sudden onset, and quasi-experimental studies in which providers are randomized as to which intervention or quality improvement tools they use, but patients are observed without further intervention. Also, there has been recent interest in applying the concept of adaptive clinical trial design to registries. An adaptive design has been defined as a design that allows adaptations or modifications to some aspects of a clinical trial after its initiation without undermining the validity and integrity of the trial.[52] While many long-term registries are modified after initiation, applying the more formal aspects of adaptive trial design to registries is an interesting area for future exploration but is not covered in this chapter.

Determining what framework will be used to analyze the data is important in designing the registry and registry data collection procedures. Readers are encouraged to consult textbooks of epidemiology and pharmacoepidemiology for more information. (Many of the references in Chapter 10 relate to study design and analysis.)

Cohort

Cohort studies follow over time a group of people who possess a characteristic to see if they develop a particular endpoint or outcome. Cohort studies are used for descriptive studies as well as for studies seeking to evaluate comparative effectiveness and/or safety and quality of care. Cohort studies may include only people with exposures (such as to a particular drug or class of drugs) or disease of interest. Cohort studies may also include one or

43

more comparison groups, in which data are collected using the same methods during the same period. A single cohort study may, in fact, include multiple cohorts, each defined by a common disease or exposure. Cohorts may be small, such as those focused on rare diseases, but often they target large groups of people (e.g., safety studies), such as all users of a particular drug or device. Some limitations of registry-based cohort studies may include limited availability of treatment data and underreporting of outcomes if a patient leaves the registry or is not adequately followed up.[53] These pitfalls should be considered and addressed when planning a study.

Case-Control

A case-control study design may be applied in registries when one anticipates the need to determine what proportion of persons with or without a certain outcome has or had an exposure or characteristic of interest. In a case-control design, one gathers "cases" of patients who have a particular outcome or who have suffered an adverse event and "controls" who have not but are considered otherwise comparable.[54] This design is optimal for understanding the etiology of rare diseases.[55]

Depending on the outcome or event of interest, cases and controls may be identifiable within a single registry. For example, in the evaluation of restenosis after coronary angioplasty in patients with end-stage renal disease, investigators identified both cases and controls from an institutional percutaneous transluminal coronary angioplasty registry; in this example, controls were randomly selected from the registry and were matched by age and gender.[56] Alternatively, cases can be identified in the registry and controls from outside the registry. Care must be taken, however, that the controls chosen from outside the registry are derived from the same base population. Matching, which ensures that certain patient characteristics such as age and gender are similar in the cases and their controls, must also be planned carefully to avoid potential confounding (if the matching factors are associated with the exposure) and overmatching, which is an inefficient use of the data.

Properly executed, a case-control design can prove highly efficient if more extensive data are collected by the registry *only* for the smaller number of subjects selected for the case-control study. This design is sometimes referred to as a "nested" case-control study, since subjects are taken from a larger cohort. Nested case-control studies have been conducted in a wide range of patient registries, from studying the association between oral contraceptives and various types of cancer using the Surveillance Epidemiology and End Results (SEER) program[57,58,59] to evaluating the possible association of depression with Alzheimer's disease. As an example, in the latter case-control study design, probable cases were enrolled from an Alzheimer's disease registry and compared to randomly selected nondemented controls from the same base population.[60]

Case-Cohort

Case-cohort design is a variant of a case-control study. In traditional case-control studies, each person in the source population has a probability of being selected as a control that is, ideally, in proportion to his or her person-time contribution to the cohort; in a case-cohort study, however, each control has an equal probability of being sampled from the source population.[61] This allows for collection of pertinent exposure data for the subcohort and the cases only, instead of the whole cohort. For example, in a case-cohort study of histopathologic and microbiological indicators of chorioamnionitis, including the identification of specific microorganisms in the placenta, cases consisted of extreme preterm infants with cerebral palsy. Controls, which can be thought of as a randomly selected subcohort of subjects at risk of the event of interest, were selected from all infants enrolled in a long-term study of preterm infants.[62] The type of sampling used for controls in case-cohort studies is sometimes referred to as "density sampling."[61] By way of contrast, in a traditional case-control study, control selection is not random and is affected by the length of followup (person-time at risk).

44

Translating Clinical Questions Into Measurable Exposures and Outcomes

The specific clinical questions of interest in a registry will guide the definitions of study subjects, exposure, and outcome measures, as well as the study design, data collection, and analysis. The clinical questions of interest can be defined by reviewing published clinical information, soliciting experts' opinions, and evaluating the expressed needs of the marketplace. Examples of research questions, key outcome and exposure variables, and sources of data are shown in Table 2.

As these examples show, the outcomes (generally beneficial or deleterious outcomes) are the main endpoints of interest posed in the research question. Relevant exposures also derive from the main research question and relate to why a patient might experience benefit or harm. Evaluation of an exposure often includes the exposure of interest as well as information that affects or augments the main exposure, such as dose, duration of exposure, route of exposure, or adherence. In the context of registries, the term "exposure" is used broadly to include treatments and procedures, health care services, diseases, and conditions. Other exposures of interest include independent risk factors for the outcomes of interest (e.g., comorbidities, age), as well as variables, known as potential confounding

variables, that are related to both the exposure and the outcome and are necessary for clarifying analyses. Confounding can result in the statistical detection of a significant association between the study variables where no real association between them exists. For example, in a study of asthma medications, prior history of treatment resistance should be collected or else results may be biased. The bias could occur because treatment resistance may relate both to the likelihood of receiving the new drug (meaning that doctors will be more likely to try a new drug in patients who have failed other therapies) and the likelihood of having a poorer outcome (e.g., hospitalization). Refer to Chapter 4 for a discussion of selecting data elements.

Choosing Patients for Study

The purpose of a registry is to provide information about a specific patient population to whom all study results are meant to apply. Studies can be conducted of people who share common characteristics, with or without including comparison groups. For example, for the purposes of evaluating patient outcomes, studies can be conducted of:

- Those with a particular disease/outcome or condition. (These are person focused.)
  - Examples include studies of the occurrence of cancer or rare diseases, quality of life, utilization of health services, pregnancy

45

Table 2: Examples of Research Questions and Key Outcomes and Exposures		
Research question	**Key outcome (source of data)**	**Key exposure (source of data)**
What is the expected time to rejection for first kidney transplants among adults, and how does that differ according to immunosuppressive regimen?	Organ rejection (clinician)	All immunosuppressants, including dosage and duration (clinician)
Are patients using a particular treatment better able to perform activities of daily living than others?	Ability to independently perform key activities related to daily living (patient)	Treatments for the disease of interest (clinician)
Are patients using a particular drug more likely to have serious adverse pregnancy outcomes?	Pregnancy outcome (clinician or patient)	Drug use by mother during pregnancy (clinician or patient)

outcomes, and recruitment pools for clinical trials.

- Those with a particular exposure. (These exposures may be to a product, procedure, or other health service.)
    - Examples include general surveillance, pregnancy registries for particular drug exposures, and studies of exposure to medications and devices, such as stents.[63] They also include studies of people who were treated under a quality improvement program, as well as studies of a particular exposure that requires controlled distribution, such as drugs with serious safety concerns (e.g., isotretinoin, clozapine, natalizumab [Tysabri®]), where the participants in the registry are identified because of their participation in a controlled distribution/risk management program.
- Those who were part of a program evaluation, disease management effort, or quality improvement project.
    - An example is the evaluation of the effectiveness of evidence-based program guidelines on improving treatment.

Target Population

Selecting patients for registries can be thought of as a multistage process that begins with understanding the target population (the population to which the findings are meant to apply, such as all patients with a disease or a common exposure) and then selecting subpopulation(s) for study. The decision about studying subpopulations relates to the accessibility of people for study, the subset of those who can actually be identified and invited for study, and the actual population who participate in the study.[64] While it is desirable for the patients who participate in the study to be representative of the target population, it is rarely possible to study groups that are fully representative from a statistical sampling perspective, either for budgetary reasons or reasons of practicality. For example, it is important to consider the ethical and legal challenges of studying select, important populations, such as children and

fetal exposures. While the information about such sensitive subgroups is often important and relevant, it is not always reasonable to expect that it will be ethical or that study budgets will be sufficient to meet the additional requirements of institutional review boards and other oversight groups.

As with any research study, very clear definitions of the inclusion and exclusion criteria are necessary and should be clearly documented, including the rationale for these criteria. A common feature of registries is that they typically have few inclusion and exclusion criteria, thus enhancing their applicability to broader populations. These criteria will largely be driven by the study objectives and any sampling strategy. For a more detailed description of target populations and their subpopulations, and how these choices affect generalizability and interpretation, see Chapter 10.

Once the patient population has been identified, attention shifts to selecting the groups from which patients will be selected (e.g., choosing the institutions and providers). For more information on recruiting patients and providers, see Chapter 7.

Comparison Groups

Once the target population has been selected and the mechanism for their identification (e.g., providers) is decided, the next decision involves determining whether to collect data on comparators (sometimes called parallel cohorts). Depending on the purpose of the registry, internal, external, or historical groups can be used to strengthen the understanding of whether the observed effects are real, and in fact, different from what would have occurred under other circumstances. Comparison groups are most useful in registries where it is important to distinguish between alternative decisions or to assess differences, the magnitude of differences, or the strength of associations between groups. Registries without comparison groups can be used for descriptive purposes, such as characterizing the natural history of a disease or condition.

Although it may be appealing to use more than one comparison group in an effort to overcome the limitations that may result from using a single group, multiple comparison groups pose their own challenges to the interpretation of registry results. For example, the results of comparative safety and effectiveness evaluations may differ depending on the comparison group used. Generally, it is preferable to make judgments about the "best" comparison group for study during the design phase and then concentrate resources on these selected subjects. Alternatively, sensitivity analyses can be used to test inferences against alternative reference groups to determine the robustness of the findings. (See Chapter 10.)

The choice of comparison groups is more complex in registries than in clinical trials. Whereas clinical trials use randomization to try to achieve an equal (or nearly equal) distribution of known and unknown risk factors that can confound the drug-outcome association, registry studies need to use various design and analytic strategies to control for the confounders that they have measured. The concern for observational studies is that people who receive a new drug or device have different risk factors for adverse events than those who choose other treatments or receive no treatment at all. In other words, the treatment choices are often related to demographic and lifestyle characteristics and the presence of coexisting conditions.[65]

Design strategies that are used frequently to assure comparability of groups relate to individual matching of exposed patients and comparators with regard to key demographic factors, such as age and gender. Matching is also achieved by inclusion criteria that could, for example, restrict the registry focus to patients who have had the disease for a similar duration or are receiving their first drug treatment for a new condition. These inclusion criteria make the patient groups more similar but add constraints to the external validity by defining the target population more narrowly. Other design techniques include matching study subjects on the basis of a large number of risk factors, such as by using statistical techniques (e.g., propensity scoring) to create strata of patients with similar risks.

As an example, consider a recent study of a rare side effect in coronary artery surgery for patients with acute coronary syndrome. In this instance, the main exposure of interest was the use of antifibrinolytic agents during revascularization surgery, a practice that had become standard for such surgeries. This practice also complicated the planned design because only the sickest patients, who were most likely to have adverse events, received alternative treatments. To address this, the investigators measured more than 200 covariates (by drug and by outcome) per patient and used this information in a propensity analysis. The results of this large-scale observational study revealed that the traditionally accepted practice (aprotinin) was associated with serious end-organ damage and that the less expensive generic medications were safe alternatives.[66]

Case-control studies present special challenges with regard to control selection. For more information on considerations and strategies, readers are encouraged to consult an excellent set of papers by Wacholder.[67,68,69]

An internal comparison group refers to simultaneous data collection for patients who are similar to the focus of interest (i.e., those with a particular disease or exposure in common) but who do not have the condition or exposure of interest. For example, a registry might collect information on patients with arthritis who are using acetaminophen for pain control. An internal comparison group could be arthritis patients who are using other medications for pain control. Data about similar patients, collected during the same calendar period and using the same data collection methods, are useful for subgroup comparisons, such as for studying the effects in certain age categories or among people with similar comorbidities. However, the information value and utility of these comparisons depend largely on having adequate sample sizes within subgroups, and such analyses may need to be specified a priori to ensure that recruitment supports them. Internal comparisons are particularly useful because data are collected during the same observation period as for all study subjects, which will account for time-related influences that may be external to the study. For example, if an important scientific article is published that affects general clinical practice and the publication occurs during the period in which the study is being conducted, clinical practice may change. The effects may be comparable for groups observed during the same period through the same system, whereas information from historical controls, for example, would be expected to reflect different practices.

An external comparison group refers to patients who are similar to the focus of interest but who do not have the condition or exposure of interest and for whom relevant data that have been collected outside of the registry are available. For example, the SEER program maintains national data about cancer and has provided useful comparison information for many registries.[70] External comparison groups can provide informative benchmarks for understanding effects observed as well as for assessing generalizability. Also, large clinical and administrative claims databases can contribute useful information on comparable subjects for a relatively low cost. The drawback of external comparison groups is that the data are generally not collected the same way and the same information may not be available. In addition, plans to merge data from other databases require the proper privacy safeguards to comply with legal requirements for patient data; Chapter 6 covers patient privacy rules in detail.

A historical comparison group refers to patients who are similar to the focus of interest but who do not have the condition or exposure of interest and for whom information was collected in the past (such as before the introduction of an exposure or treatment or development of a condition). Historical controls may actually be the same patients who later become exposed, or they may consist of a completely different group of patients. This design provides weak evidence because symmetry is not assured (i.e., the patients in different time periods may not be as similar as desirable). Historical controls are susceptible to bias by changes over time in uncontrollable, confounding risk factors, such as differences in climate, management practices, and nutrition. Bias stemming from differences in measuring procedures over time may also account for observed differences.

There are several situations in which conventional prospective design is impossible and historical controls may be considered:

- When one cannot ethically continue the older practices or when physicians and/or patients refuse to continue old practices, thus preventing the researcher from identifying relevant sites using the "older" practices.

- When conventional treatment has been consistently unsuccessful and the effect of new intervention is obvious and dramatic (e.g., first use of a new product for a previously untreatable condition).

- When collecting the control data is too expensive.

- When the Hawthorne effect (a phenomenon that refers to changes in the behavior of subjects because they know they are being studied or observed) makes it impossible to replicate actual practice in a comparison group during the same period.

- When the desired comparison is to usual care or "expected" outcomes at a population level, and data collection is too expensive because of the distribution or size of that population.

Sampling

Various sampling strategies can be considered. Each of these has tradeoffs in terms of validity and information yield. The less representative the study population is of the broader target population, the more questions will be raised about the external validity of the study. In contrast, more broadly representative studies often suffer from insufficient information in subcategories of interest. Reviewing and refining the research question can help to define an appropriate target population and a realistic strategy for subject selection.

Registry studies often restrict eligibility for entry to individuals within a certain range of characteristics to assure that enough meaningful information will be available for analysis. Alternatively, they may use some form of sampling: random selection, systematic sampling, or a nonrandom approach. Often-used sampling strategies include the following:

- *Restriction (specification)*: Eligibility for entry is restricted to individuals within a certain range of values for a confounding factor, such as age, to reduce the effect of the confounding factor when it cannot otherwise be controlled. Restriction limits the external validity (generalizability) to those with the same confounder values but maximizes the information yield for the patients under study.

- *Probability sampling*: Some form of random selection is used, and each person in the population must have a known (often equal) probability of being selected. Despite their best intentions, humans cannot choose a sample in a random fashion without a formal randomizing mechanism. Examples are:

  - *Census*: A census sample includes every individual in a population or group (e.g., all known cases). A census is not feasible when the group is large relative to the costs of obtaining information from individuals.

  - *Simple random sampling*: The sample is selected in such a way that each person has the same probability of being sampled.

  - *Stratified sampling*: The group from which the sample is to be taken is first stratified into subgroups on the basis of an important, related characteristic (e.g., age, parity, weight) such that each individual in a subgroup has the same probability of being included in the sample, but the probabilities for different subgroups or strata are different. Stratified random sampling assures that the different categories of the characteristic that is the basis of the strata are sufficiently represented in the sample, but the resulting data must be analyzed using more complicated statistical procedures (such as Mantel-Haenszel) in which the stratification is taken into account.

  - *Systematic sampling*: Every n^{th} person in a population is sampled.

  - *Cluster (area) sampling*: The population is divided into clusters, these clusters are randomly sampled, and then some or all patients within selected clusters are sampled. This technique is particularly useful in large geographic areas.

  - *Multistage sampling*: Multistage sampling can include any combination of the sampling techniques described above.

- *Nonprobability sampling*: Selection is systematic or haphazard but not random. The following sampling strategies generally pose more limitations in interpreting results than those described previously but can be useful in situations where probability sampling is not feasible.

  - *Haphazard, convenience, volunteer, or judgmental sampling*: This includes any sampling not involving a truly random mechanism. A hallmark of this form of sampling is that the probability that a given individual will be in the sample is unknown before sampling. The theoretical basis for statistical inference is lost, and the result is inevitably biased in unknown ways.

  - *Modal instance*: The most typical subject is sampled.

  - *Purposive*: Several predefined groups are deliberately sampled.

  - *Expert*: A panel of experts judges the representativeness of the sample or is the source that contributes subjects to a registry.

  - *Consecutive (quota) sampling*: Individuals with a given characteristic are sampled as they are presented until enough people with that characteristic are acquired.

Individual matching of cases and controls is sometimes used as a sampling strategy for controls. Cases are matched with individual controls who have similar confounding factors, such as age, to reduce the effect of the confounding factors on the association being investigated in analytic studies.

49

Patients are recruited in a fashion that accomplishes individual matching. For example, if a 69-year-old "case" participates in the registry, a comparator near in age will be sought. Individual matching for prospective recruitment is challenging and not customarily used. More often, matching is used to create subgroups for supplemental data collection for case-control studies and cohort studies when subjects are limited and/or stratification is unlikely to provide enough subjects in each stratum for meaningful evaluation.

There are a number of other sampling strategies that have arisen from survey research (e.g., snowball, heterogeneity), but they are of less relevance to registries.

Finding the Necessary Data

The identification of key outcome and exposure variables and patients will drive the strategy for data collection, including the choice of data sources. A key challenge to registries is that it is generally not possible to collect all desired data. As discussed in Chapter 4, data collection should be both parsimonious and broadly applicable. For example, while experimental imaging studies may provide interesting data, if the imaging technology is not widely available, the data will not be available for enough patients to be useful in analysis. Moreover, the registry findings will not be generalizable if only sophisticated centers that have that technology participate. Instead, registries focus on collecting relevant data with relatively modest burden on patients and physicians. Registry data can be obtained from patients, clinicians, medical records, and linkage with other sources (in particular, extant databases), depending on the available budget. (See Chapter 8.)

Examples of patient data include quality of life; utilities (i.e., patient preferences); use of over-the-counter (OTC), complementary, and alternative medication; behavioral data (e.g., smoking and alcohol use); family history; and biological specimens. These data have the characteristics of relying on the subjective interpretation and reporting of the patient (e.g., quality of life, utilities); being

difficult to otherwise track (e.g., use of complementary and alternative medication, smoking and alcohol use); or being unique to the patient (e.g., biological specimens). The primary advantage of this form of data collection is that it provides direct information from the entity that is ultimately of the most interest–the patient. The primary disadvantages are that the patient is not necessarily a trained observer and that various forms of bias, such as recall bias, may influence subjective information. For example, people may selectively recall certain exposures because they believe they have a disease that was caused by that exposure, or their recall may be influenced by recent news stories claiming cause-and-effect relations.

Examples of clinician data include clinical impressions, clinical diagnoses, clinical signs, differential diagnoses, laboratory results, and staging. The primary advantage of clinical data is that clinicians are trained observers. Even so, the primary disadvantages are that clinicians are not necessarily accurate reporters of patient perceptions, and their responses may also be subject to recall bias. Moreover, the time that busy clinicians can devote to registry data collection is often limited.

Medical records also are a repository of clinician-derived data. Electronic medical records, when available, improve access to the data within medical records. As discussed further in Chapter 8, the availability of medical records data in electronic format does not by itself guarantee consistency of terminology and coding. For example, certain data, such as data on OTC medications, smoking and alcohol use, complementary and alternative medicines, and counseling activities by the clinician on lifestyle modifications, are often not consistently captured in medical records of any type.

Examples of other data sources include health insurance claims, pharmacy data, laboratory data, other registries, and national data sets, such as Medicare claims data and the National Death Index. These sources can be used to supplement registries with data that may otherwise be difficult to obtain, subject to recall bias, not collected because of loss to followup, or likely inaccurate by self-report (e.g., in those patients with diseases affecting recall, cognition, or mental status). See Table 7 in Chapter 5 for more information on data sources.

Registry Size and Duration

During the registry design stage, it is critical to explicitly state how large the registry should be, how long patients should be followed, and the justifications for these decisions. These decisions are based on the overall purpose of the registry. For example, it is usually desirable to have precise information such that one can confirm or rule out the existence of an important effect and can make policy or practice decisions based on evidence. Precision in measurement and estimation corresponds to the reduction of random error; it can be improved by increasing the size of the study and by modifying the design of the study to increase the efficiency with which information is obtained from a given number of subjects.[71]

Study size determinations are guided by the intended purpose of the registry and are most often tempered by budgetary constraints. Some registries are intended to answer a specific question at a single point in time. For example, if the goal of the registry is to compare the effectiveness of a technologically stable health intervention in typical practice with the efficacy of this intervention obtained in randomized trials (which often include a high degree of selection), then such a registry could (and, indeed, should) include a defined end at which time data collection stops. Safety studies, in contrast, usually are created with specific study size requirements in terms of person-years of observation, and data collection stops when the study size is achieved or the budget runs out. Studies intended to demonstrate equivalence between treatments (or, say, side effect profiles that are no worse than another therapy) are designed to collect enough information so that the upper bound of a confidence interval around the relative risk or risk difference is no greater than an arbitrary, acceptable, and affordable level. At the other end of the spectrum from registries for safety and effectiveness are quality assurance and quality improvement registries, where the goal is to assess

the performance of the participants (e.g., physicians, hospitals). Study size requirements are often more arbitrary for such programs than for safety and effectiveness registries. For example, obtaining a reasonable degree of precision to detect differences between groups of practitioners or within the same groups over time for particular quality measures may drive the study size at the practice level. Registries in which the goal is to assess a health care practice that is changing over time (e.g., a device with multiple versions, each presumably an improvement over the last) generally seek to study as many patients as possible in order to rule out large risks, but they face limitations because the exposure pool is relatively small.

A detailed discussion of the topic of sample size calculations for registries is provided in Appendix A. For the present purposes, it is sufficient to briefly describe some of the critical inputs to these calculations that must be provided by the registry developers:

- The expected timeframe of the registry and the time intervals at which analyses of registry data will be performed

- Either the size of clinically important effects (e.g., minimum clinically important differences) or the required precision associated with registry-based estimates.

- Whether or not the registry is intended to support regulatory decisionmaking. If the results from statistical tests of significance from registry analyses will affect regulatory action—for example, the likelihood that a product may be pulled from the market—then the general approach to the consideration of multiple comparisons is important.

In a classical calculation of sample size, the crucial inputs that must be provided by the investigators include either the size of clinically important effects or their required precision. For example, suppose that the primary goal of the registry is to compare surgical complication rates in general practice with those in randomized trials. The inputs to the power calculations would include the complication rates from the randomized trials (e.g., 4 percent) and the complication rate in general practice that would reflect a meaningful departure from this rate (e.g., 6 percent). If, on the other hand, the goal of the registry is simply to track complication rates (and not to compare the registry with an external standard), then the investigators should specify the required width of the confidence interval associated with those rates. For example, in a large registry, the 95-percent confidence interval for a 5-percent complication rate might extend from 4.5 percent to 5.5 percent. If all of the points in this confidence interval lead to the same decision, then an interval of ±0.5 percent is considered sufficiently precise, and this is the input required for the estimation of sample size.

Specifying the above inputs to sample size calculations is a substantial matter and usually involves a combination of quantitative and qualitative reasoning. However, the issues involved in making this specification are essentially similar for registries and other study designs.

52

One approach to addressing multiple comparisons in the surgical complication rate example above is to use control chart methodology, a statistical approach used in process measurement to examine the observed variability and determine whether out-of-control conditions are occurring. Control chart methodology is used in sample size estimation, largely for studies with repeated measurements, to adjust the sample size as needed to maintain reasonably precise estimates of confidence limits around the point estimate. Accordingly, for registries that involve ongoing evaluation, sample size per time interval could be determined by the precision associated with the associated confidence interval, and decision rules for identifying problems could be based on control chart methodology.

Potential for Bias and External Validity

The potential for bias refers to opportunities for systematic errors to influence the results. Generalizability, also known as external validity, is a concept that refers to the utility of the inferences for the broader population that the study subjects are intended to represent. To understand how the potential for bias affects generalizability, it is useful to consider the differences between RCTs and observational registries, since these are the two principal approaches to conducting clinically relevant research.

The strong internal validity that earns RCTs high grades for evidence comes largely from the randomization of exposures that helps ensure that the groups receiving the different treatments are similar in all measured or unmeasured characteristics. Thus any differences in outcome (beyond those attributable to chance) can be reasonably attributed to differences in the efficacy or safety of the treatments. However, it is worth noting that RCTs are not without their own biases, as illustrated by the "intent-to-treat" analytic approach, in which people are considered to have used the assigned treatment, regardless of actual compliance. The intent-to-treat analyses can minimize a real difference, known as bias toward the null, by including the experience of people who adhered to the recommended study product along with those who did not.

Another principal difference between registries and RCTs is that RCTs are often focused on a relatively homogeneous pool of patients from which significant numbers of patients are consciously excluded at the cost of external validity—that is, generalizability to the target population of disease sufferers. Registries, in contrast, focus on generalizability so that their population will be representative and relevant to decisionmakers.

The strong external validity of registries is achieved by studying more heterogeneous populations. Registries are often evaluated in terms of the extent to which study subjects are representative of the target population. Therefore, registry data represent the course of disease and impact of interventions in actual practice and are likely more relevant than the data derived from the artificial constructs of the clinical trial. In fact, even though registries have more opportunities to introduce bias (systematic error) because of their nonexperimental methodology, well-designed observational studies can approximate the effects of interventions as well as RCTs on the same topic[72,73] and, in particular, in the evaluation of health care effectiveness.[74]

The choice of groups from which patients will be selected directly affects generalizability. No particular method will assure that an approach to patient recruitment is adequate, but it is worthwhile to note that the way that patients are recruited, classified, and followed can either enhance or diminish the external validity of a registry. Some examples of how these methods of patient recruitment and followup can lead to systematic error follow.

If the registry's principal goal is the estimation of risk, it is possible that adverse events or patients experiencing them will be underreported if the reporter will be viewed negatively for reporting them. It is also possible for those collecting data to introduce bias by misreporting the outcome of an intervention if they have a vested interest in doing so. This type of bias is referred to as information bias (also called detection, observer, ascertainment, or assessment bias), and it addresses the extent to which the data that are collected are valid (represent what they are intended to represent) and whether they are accurate. This bias arises if the outcome assessment can be interfered with, intentionally or unintentionally. On the other hand, if the outcome is objective, such as whether or not a patient died or the results of a lab test, then the data are unlikely to be biased.

A registry may create the incentive to enroll only patients who either are at low risk of complications or are known not to have suffered such complications, biasing the results of the registry toward lower event rates. Those registries for which participants derive some sort of benefit from

reporting low complication rates, such as surgical registries, are at particularly high risk for this type of bias. Another example of how patient selection methods can lead to bias is the use of volunteers, which may lead to selective participation from subjects most likely to perceive a benefit, distorting results for studies of patient-reported outcomes. Enrolling patients who share a common exposure history, such as having used a drug that has been publicly linked to a serious adverse effect, could distort effect estimates for cohort and case-control analyses. Registries also have the potential to selectively enroll people who are at higher risk of developing serious side effects, since having a high-risk profile can motivate a patient to participate in a registry.

The term "selection bias" refers to situations where the procedures used to select study subjects lead to an effect estimate among those participating in the study that is different from the estimate that is obtainable from the target population.[75] Selection bias may be introduced if certain subgroups of patients are routinely included or excluded from the registry. Channeling bias, also called confounding by indication, is a form of selection bias, where drugs with similar therapeutic indications are prescribed to groups of patients with prognostic differences.[76] For example, physicians may prescribe new treatments more often to those patients who have failed on traditional, first-line treatments.

One approach to designing studies to address confounding by indication is to conduct a prospective review of cases in which external reviewers are blinded as to the treatments that were employed and are asked to determine whether a particular type of therapy is indicated and to rate the overall prognosis for the patient.[77] This method of blinded prospective review was developed to support research on ruptured cerebral aneurysms, a rare and serious situation. The results of the blinded review were used to create risk strata for analysis so that comparisons could be conducted only for candidates for whom both therapies under study were indicated, a procedure much like applying additional inclusion and exclusion criteria in a clinical trial.

53

If there is any potential for tolerance to affect the use of a product, such that only those who perceive benefit or are free from harm continue, the recruitment of existing users rather than new users may lead to the inclusion of only those who have tolerated or benefited from the intervention and would not necessarily capture the full spectrum of experience and outcomes. Selecting only existing users may introduce any number of biases, including incidence/prevalence bias, survivorship bias, and followup bias. By enrolling new users (an inception or incidence cohort), the study is ensuring that the population will reflect all users of the product, that the longitudinal experience of all users will be captured, and that the ascertainment of their experience will be comparable.[78]

Loss to followup or attrition threatens generalizability if there is differential loss to followup for people with a particular exposure or disease, which could substantially affect the conclusions and interpretation of results. As with loss to followup, attrition is generally a serious concern only when it is nonrandom (that is, when there are systematic differences between those who leave or are lost and those who remain).

Remaining alert for any source of bias is important, and the value of a registry is enhanced by its ability to provide a formal assessment of the likely magnitude of all potential sources of bias. Any information that can be generated regarding nonrespondents, missing respondents, and the like, even if it is just an estimation of their raw numbers, is helpful. As with many types of survey research, an assessment of response rate and differential patient selection can sometimes be undertaken when key data elements are available for both registry enrollees and nonparticipants. Such analyses can easily be undertaken when the initial data source or population pool is that of a health care organization, employer, or practice that would have access to data other than key selection criteria (e.g., demographics, comorbidities). Another tool is the use of sequential screening logs, in which all subjects fitting the inclusion criteria are enumerated and a few key data elements are recorded for all those who are screened. This technique allows quantitative analysis of nonparticipants and assessments of the

effects, if any, on representativeness. Another technique, although not as rigorous as quantitative approaches, is to obtain an informed opinion of how the sample obtained is likely to differ from a true probability sample and why it is likely to differ. So long as this assessment is made explicitly, users have a framework for drawing their own conclusions.

Accordingly, two items that can be reported to help the user assess generalizability are a description of the criteria used to select registry sites and the characteristics of these sites, particularly those characteristics that might have an impact on the purpose of the registry. For example, if a registry for the purpose of assessing adherence to lipid screening guidelines requires that its sites have a sophisticated electronic medical record in order to collect data, it will probably report better adherence than usual practice because this same electronic medical record facilitates the generation of real-time reminders to engage in screening. In this case, a report of rates of adherence to other screening guidelines (for which there were no reminders), even if these are outside the direct scope of inquiry, would provide some insight as to the degree of overestimation.

Finally, and most importantly, whether or not study subjects need to be evaluated on their representativeness depends on the purpose and kind of inference needed. For example, for understanding biological effects, it is not necessary to sample in proportion to the underlying distribution in the population. It is more important to demonstrate to the stakeholders the degree to which patients who are included in a registry are representative of the population from which they were derived.

Summary

In summary, the key points to consider in designing a registry include study design, data sources, patient selection criteria, comparison groups, sampling strategies, considerations of possible sources of bias, and ways to address them to the extent that is practical and achievable.

Chapter 4. Data Elements for Registries

Selection of data elements for a registry requires a balancing of potentially competing considerations. These considerations include the importance of the data elements to the integrity of the registry, their reliability, their necessity for the analysis of the primary outcomes, their contribution to the overall response burden, and the incremental costs associated with their collection. Registries are generally designed for a specific purpose, and data elements that are not critical to the successful execution of the registry or to the core planned analyses should not be collected unless there are explicit plans for their analysis.

The selection of data elements for a registry begins with the identification of the domains that must be quantified to accomplish the registry purpose. The specific data elements can then be selected, with consideration given to clinical data standards, common data definitions, and the use of patient identifiers. Next, the data element list can be refined to include only those elements that are necessary for the registry purpose. Once the selected elements have been incorporated into a data collection tool, the tool can be pilot tested to identify potential issues, such as the time required to complete the form, data that may be more difficult to access than realized during the design phase, and practical issues in data quality (such as appropriate range checks). This information can be used to modify the data elements and reach a final set of elements.

Identifying Domains

Registry design requires an explicit articulation of the goals of the registry and a close collaboration among disciplines, such as epidemiology, statistics, and clinical specialists. Once the goals of the study are determined, the domains most likely to influence the desired outcomes must be defined. Registries generally include personal, exposure, and outcomes information. The personal domain consists of data that describe the patient, such as information on patient demographics, medical history, health status, and any necessary patient identifiers. The exposure domain describes the patient's experience with the product, disease, device, or service of interest to the registry. Exposure can also include other treatments that are known to influence outcome but are not necessarily the focus of the study, so that their confounding influence can be adjusted for in the planned analyses. The outcomes domain collects information on the patient outcomes that are of interest to the registry; this domain should include both the primary endpoints and any secondary endpoints that are part of the overall registry goals.

In addition to the goals and desired outcomes, it is necessary to consider the need to create important subsets when defining the domains. Measuring potential confounding factors (variables that are linked with both the exposure and outcome) should be taken into account in this stage of registry development. Collecting data on potential confounders will allow for analytic or design control. (See Chapters 3 and 10.)

Understanding the time reference for all variables that can change over time is critical in order to distinguish cause-and-effect relationships. For example, a drug taken after an outcome is observed cannot possibly have contributed to the development of that outcome. Time reference periods can be addressed by including start and stop dates for variables that can change; they can also be addressed categorically, as is done in some quality improvement registries. For example, the Paul Coverdell National Acute Stroke Registry organized its patient-level information into categories to reflect the timeframe of the stroke event from onset through treatment to followup. In this case, the domains were categorized as prehospital, emergency evaluation and treatment, in-hospital evaluation and treatment, discharge information, and postdischarge followup.[79]

Selecting Data Elements

Once the domains have been identified, the process of selecting data elements begins with the identification of the data elements that best quantify that domain and the source(s) from which those data elements can be collected. When selecting data elements, gaining consensus among the registry stakeholders is important, but this must be achieved without undermining the purpose of the registry by including elements solely to please a stakeholder. Each data element should support the purpose of the registry and answer a specific scientific question or address a specific issue or need. The most effective way to select data elements is to start with the study purpose and objective and then decide what types of measurements or calculations will be needed to analyze that objective. Once the plan of analysis is clear, it is possible to work backward into the data elements necessary to implement that analysis plan. This process keeps the group focused on the registry purpose and limits the number of extraneous ("nice to know") data elements that may be included.[80] (See Case Example 8.)

The data element selection process can be simplified if clinical data standards for a disease area exist. Currently there are few, if any, consensus or broadly accepted sets of standard data elements and data definitions for most disease areas. Thus, different studies of the same disease state may use different definitions for fundamental concepts, such as the diagnosis of myocardial infarction or the definition of worsening renal function. To address this problem and to support more consistent data elements so that comparisons across studies can be more easily accomplished, some specialty societies are beginning to compile clinical data standards. For example, the American College of Cardiology has created clinical data standards for acute coronary syndromes, heart failure, and atrial fibrillation.[81,82,83] The use of established data standards, when available, is essential so that registries can maximally contribute to evolving medical knowledge.

Case Example 8: Selecting Data Elements for a Registry

Description	The Dosing and Outcomes Study of Erythropoiesis-stimulating Therapies (DOSE) Registry is designed to understand current anemia management patterns and clinical, economic, and patient-reported outcomes in oncology patients treated in various outpatient oncology practice settings across the United States. The prospective design of the DOSE Registry enables the capture of data from oncology patients treated with erythropoiesis-stimulating therapies.
Sponsor	Ortho Biotech Clinical Affairs, LLC
Year Started	2003
Year Ended	Ongoing
No. of Sites	62
No. of Patients	Over 1,500

Challenge

Epoetin alfa was approved for patients with chemotherapy-induced anemia in 1994. In 2002, the U.S. Food and Drug Administration approved a second erythropoiesis-stimulating therapy (EST), darbepoetin alfa, for a similar indication. While multiple clinical trials described outcomes following intervention with ESTs, little information was available on real-world practice patterns and outcomes in oncology patients. To gain this information, the registry team determined that a prospective observational effectiveness study in this therapeutic area was needed. The three key challenges were to make the study representative of real-world practices and settings (e.g., hospital-based clinics, community oncology clinics); to collect data elements that were straightforward to minimize

(continued)

Case Example 8: Selecting Data Elements for a Registry (continued)

potential data collection errors; and to collect sufficient data to study effectiveness while ensuring that the data collection remained feasible and time efficient for outpatient oncology clinics.

Proposed Solution

The registry team began selecting data elements by completing a thorough literature review. Because this would be one of the first prospective observational studies in this therapeutic area, the team wanted to ensure that study results could be presented to health care professionals and decisionmakers in a manner consistent with clinical trials. The team also intended to make the data reports from the study comparable with other study reports. To meet these objectives, data elements (e.g., baseline demographics, dosing patterns, hemoglobin levels) similar to those in clinical trials were selected whenever possible.

For the patient-reported outcomes component of the registry, the team incorporated standard, validated instruments. This decision allowed the team to avoid developing and validating new instruments and supported consistency with clinical trial literature, as many trials had incorporated these instruments. The team selected two instruments, the Functional Assessment of Cancer Therapy–Anemia (FACT-An) tool and the Linear Analog Scale Assessment (LASA) tool, to gather patient-reported data. The FACT-An tool, developed from the FACT-General scale, was previously designed and validated to measure the impact of anemia in cancer patients. The LASA tool measures quality of life by having patients rate their energy level, activity level, and overall quality of life on a scale of zero to 100. Both tools are commonly used to gather patient-reported outcomes data for cancer patients.

Following the literature review, an advisory board was convened to discuss the registry objectives, data elements, and study execution. The advisory board included representatives from the nursing and medical professions. The multidisciplinary board provided insights on both the practical and clinical aspects of the registry procedures and data elements. Throughout the entire process, the registry team remained focused on both the overall registry objectives and user-friendly data collection. In particular, the team worked to make each question clear and unambiguous in order to minimize confusion and to enable a variety of site personnel to complete the registry data collection.

Results

The registry launched in 2003 as one of the first prospective observational effectiveness studies in this therapeutic area. To date, 62 sites and over 1,500 patients have enrolled in the study, with a target accrual of 2,000 patients. The sites participating in the registry represent a wide geographic distribution and a mixture of practice settings.

Key Point

Use of common data elements, guided by a literature review, and validated instruments helps to make the registry data more generalizable, as well as more comparable with trial data. A multidisciplinary advisory board can also help ensure collection of key data elements in an appropriate manner from both a clinical and practical standpoint.

For More Information

Peake C, Wang Q, Chen E et al. Hematologic outcomes and costs in epoetin alfa (EPO)- and darbepoetin alfa (DARB)-treated cancer patients: results of the Dosing and Outcomes Study of Erythropoiesis-Stimulating Therapies (D.O.S.E. Registry) [abstract 205]. Pharmacotherapy 2006;26:1453.

Chen E, Peake C, Buscaino E et al. Hematologic outcomes and erythropoiesis-stimulating therapy costs in epoetin alfa (EPO)- and darbepoetin alfa (DARB)-treated cancer patients: results of the Dosing and Outcomes Study of Erythropoiesis-Stimulating Therapies (D.O.S.E. Registry) [abstract 3340]. Blood 2006;108:953a.

57

Although clinical data standards are important to allow comparisons between studies, there is a concern that overlapping standards may be developed. To consolidate and align standards that have been developed for clinical research, the Clinical Data Interchange Standards Consortium (CDISC) initiated work on the Biomedical Research Integrated Domain Group (BRIDG) model, a domain-analysis model representing biomedical and clinical research. Other groups, including the National Cancer Institute (NCI), Health Level Seven (HL7), and the U.S. Food and Drug Administration, have joined this effort. In 2005, the HL7 Regulated Clinical Research Information Management Technical Committee adopted BRIDG as their domain-analysis model. The purpose of the project is to provide an overarching model that can be used to harmonize standards between the clinical research domain and the health care domain. As development continues on this model, CDISC and NCI have made the BRIDG model freely available to the public as part of an open-source project at www.bridgproject.org. It is hoped that the BRIDG model, when completed, will guide registry creators in selecting approaches that will enable their registry data to be compared with other clinical data.[84,85]

In cases where clinical data standards for the disease area do not exist, established data sets may be widely used in the field. For example, United Network of Organ Sharing (UNOS) collects a large amount of data on organ transplant patients. Creators of a registry in the transplant field should consider aligning their data definitions and data element formats with those of UNOS to simplify the training and data abstraction process for sites. Other examples of widely used data sets are the Joint Commission (formerly JCAHO) and the Centers for Medicare & Medicaid Services (CMS) data elements for hospital data submission programs. These data sets cover a range of procedures and diseases, from heart failure and acute myocardial infarction to pregnancy and surgical infection prevention. Hospital-based registries that collect data on these conditions may want to align their data sets with the Joint

Commission and CMS. However, one limitation of tying elements and definitions to another data collection program rather than a fixed standard is that these programs may change their elements or definitions. With Joint Commission core measure elements, for example, this has occurred with some frequency.

If clinical data standards for the disease area and established data sets do not exist, it is still possible to incorporate standard terminology into a registry. This will make it easier to compare the data with the data of other registries and reduce the training and data abstraction burden on sites. Some examples of standard systems used to classify important data elements are listed in Table 3.[86]

After investigating clinical data standards, registry planners may find that there are no useful standards or established data sets for the registry, or that these standards comprise only a small portion of the data set. In these cases, the registry will need to define and select data elements with the guidance of its project team, which may include an advisory board. When selecting data elements, it is often helpful to gather input from statisticians, epidemiologists, psychometricians, and experts in health outcomes assessment who will be analyzing the data, as they may notice potential analysis issues that need to be considered at the time of data element selection. Data elements may also be selected based on performance or quality measures in a clinical area. (See Case Example 9.)

When beginning the process of defining and selecting data elements, it can be useful to start by considering the registry design. Since many registries are longitudinal, sites often collect data at multiple visits. In these cases, it is necessary to determine which data elements can be collected once and which data elements should be collected at every visit. Data elements that can be collected once are often collected at the baseline visit. In other cases, the registry may be collecting data at an event level, so all of the data elements will be collected during the course of the event rather than in separate visits. In considering when to collect a data element, it is also important to determine the most appropriate order of data collection. Data

58

Table 3: Standard Terminologies

Standard	Acronym	Description	Developer	Web site
Current Procedural Terminology	CPT®	Medical service and procedure codes commonly used in public and private health insurance plans and claims processing.	American Medical Association	http://www.ama-assn.org/ama/pub/category/3113.html
International Classification of Diseases	ICD	International standard for classifying diseases and other health problems recorded on health and vital records. ICD-9-CM, a modified version of the ICD-9 standard, is used for billing and claims data in the United States. ICD-10 is in use in many parts of the world, but has not yet been implemented in the United States.	World Health Organization	http://www.who.int/classifications/icd/en/
Logical Observation Identifiers Names and Codes	LOINC®	Concept-based terminology for lab orders and results.	Regenstrief Institute for Health Care	http://www.regenstrief.org/loinc/
Medical Dictionary for Regulatory Activities	MedDRA	Terminology covering all phases of drug development, excluding animal toxicology. Also covers health effects and malfunctions of devices.	International Conference on Harmonisation	http://www.meddramsso.com
National Drug Code	NDC	Unique 3-segment number used as the universal identifier for human drugs.	U.S. Food and Drug Administration	http://www.fda.gov/cder/ndc/
Systemized Nomenclature of Medicine	SNOMED®	Mapping of clinical concepts with standard descriptive terms.	College of American Pathologists	http://www.snomed.org
Unified Medical Language System	UMLS	Database of 100 medical terminologies with concept mapping tools.	National Library of Medicine	http://www.nlm.nih.gov/research/umls/
World Health Organization Drug Dictionary	WHODRUG	International drug dictionary	World Health Organization	http://www.who.int/druginformation/index.shtml

Case Example 9: Using Performance Measures To Develop a Data Set	
Description	Get With The Guidelines^{SM} (GWTG) is the flagship program for in-hospital quality improvement of the American Heart Association (AHA) and American Stroke Association (ASA). The program uses the experience of the AHA/ASA to ensure the care that hospitals provide for coronary artery disease, heart failure, and stroke is aligned with the latest evidence-based guidelines.
Sponsor	American Stroke Association
Year Started	2003
Year Ended	Ongoing
No. of Sites	890
No. of Patients	348,917

60

Challenge

The primary purpose of the program is to improve the quality of in-hospital care for stroke patients. The program uses the PDSA (Plan, Do, Study, Act) quality improvement cycle, in which hospitals plan quality improvement initiatives, implement them, study the results, and then make adjustments to the initiatives. To help hospitals implement this cycle, the program uses a registry to collect data on stroke patients and generate real-time reports showing compliance with a set of standardized stroke performance and quality measures. The reports also include benchmarking capabilities, enabling hospitals to compare themselves with other hospitals at a national and regional level, as well as with similar hospitals.

In developing the registry, the team faced the challenge of creating a data set that would be comprehensive enough to satisfy evidence-based medicine but manageable by hospitals participating in the program. The program does not provide reimbursements to hospitals entering data, so it needed to keep the data set as small as possible while still maintaining the ability to measure quality improvement.

Proposed Solution

The team began developing the data set by working backward from the performance measures. Performance measures, based on the sponsor's guidelines for stroke care, contain detailed inclusion and exclusion criteria to determine the measure population, and they group patients into the denominator and numerator groups. Using these criteria, the team developed a data set that asked only the questions necessary to determine compliance with each of the guidelines. The team then added a few additional questions to gather information on the patient population characteristics.

Results

By using this approach, the registry team was able to create the minimum necessary data set for measuring compliance with stroke guidelines. The program launched in 2003 and now has 890 hospitals and over 345,000 patient records. The data from the program have been used in several abstracts and publications and have confirmed quality improvement in participating hospitals.

Key Point

Registry teams should focus on the outcomes or endpoints of interest when selecting data elements. In cases where compliance with guidelines or quality measures is the outcome of interest, teams can work backward from the guidelines or measures to develop the minimum necessary data set for their registry.

(continued)

elements that are related to each other in time (e.g., dietary information and a fasting blood sample for glucose or lipids) should be collected in the same visit rather than in different visit case report forms.

International physician and patient participation may be required to meet certain registry data objectives. In such situations, it is desirable to consider the international participation in the context of data element selection, especially if it will be necessary to collect and compare data from individual countries. Examination and laboratory test results or units may differ among countries, and standardization of data elements may become necessary at the data-entry level. Data elements relating to cost-effectiveness studies may be particularly challenging, since there is substantial variation among countries in practice and the costs of medical "inputs," relating largely to differences in national or regional coverage practices and national health policies. Alternatively, if capture of internationally standardized data elements is not desirable or cannot be achieved, registry stakeholders should consider provisions to capture data elements according to local standards. Later,

separate data conversions and merging outside the database for uniform reporting or comparison of data elements captured in multiple countries can be evaluated and performed as needed if the study design ensures that all data necessary for such conversions have been collected.

Table 4 provides a listing of sample baseline data elements. These elements will vary depending on the design, nature, and goals of the registry. Examples listed include patient identifiers (e.g., for linkage to other databases), contact information (e.g., for telephone followup), and residence location of enrollee (e.g., for geographic comparisons). Other administrative data elements that may be collected include the source of enrollment, enrollee sociodemographic characteristics, and information on provider locations.

Depending on the purpose of a registry, other sets of data elements may be required (Table 5). In addition, data elements needed for specific types of registries are outlined below.

- For registries examining questions of safety for drugs, vaccines, procedures, or devices, key information includes history of the exposure and data elements that will permit analysis of potential confounding factors that may affect observed outcomes, such as enrollee characteristics (e.g., comorbidities, concomitant therapies, socioeconomic status, ethnicity, environmental and social factors) and provider characteristics. For drug exposures, data on use (start and stop dates), as well as providing continuing evidence that the drug was actually used (data on medication persistence and/or adherence), may be important. In some instances, it is also useful to record reasons for discontinuation.

- For registries examining questions of effectiveness and cost effectiveness, key information includes the history of exposure and data elements that will permit analysis of

Table 4: Sample Baseline Data Elements	
Enrollee contact information	• Enrollee contact information for registries with direct-to-enrollee contact • Another individual who can be reached for followup (address, telephone, e-mail)
Enrollment data elements	• Patient identifiers (e.g., name [last, first, middle initial], date of birth, place of birth, Social Security Number) • Permission/consent • Source of enrollment (e.g., provider, institution, phone number, address, contact information) • Enrollment criteria • Sociodemographic characteristics, including race, sex, age or date of birth • Education and/or economic status, insurance, etc. • Preferred language • Place of birth • Location of residence at enrollment • Source of information • Country, State, city, county, ZIP Code of residence

potential confounding factors that may affect observed outcomes. In addition to those mentioned above for safety, these may include individual behaviors and provider and/or system characteristics. For assessment of cost effectiveness, information may be recorded on the financial and economic burden of illness, such as office visits, visits to urgent care or the emergency room, and hospitalizations, including length of stay. For some studies, a quality-of-life instrument that can be analyzed to provide quality-adjusted life years (QALYs) or similar comparative data across conditions may be used.

• For registries assessing quality of care and quality improvement, data that categorize and possibly differentiate among the services provided (e.g., equipment, training or experience level of providers, type of health care system) may be sought, as well as information that identifies individual patients as potential candidates for the treatment. In addition, self-reported data are valuable to assess the patients' perception of quality of care.

• For registries examining the natural history of a condition, the selection of data elements would be similar to that for effectiveness registries.

If one goal of a registry is to identify patient subsets that are at higher risk for particular outcomes, more detailed information on patient and provider characteristics should be collected. This information may be important in registries that look at the usage of a procedure or treatment. Quality improvement registries also use this information to understand how improvement differs across many types of institutions.

When selecting patient identifiers, there are a variety of options, including using the patient's name, date of birth, and Social Security Number (or some combination thereof), that are subject to legal and security considerations. When the planned analyses require linkage to other data (such as medical records), more specific patient information may be needed. In selecting patient identifiers, some thought should be given to the possibility that patient identifiers may change during the course of the registry. For example, female patients may change their name during the course of the registry, and patients may move or change their telephone number. Patient identifiers can also be inaccurate because of intentional falsification by the patient (e.g., for privacy reasons in a sexually transmitted disease registry), unintentional misreporting by the patient or a parent (e.g., wrong date of birth), or

Table 5: Sample Additional Enrollee, Provider, and Environmental Data Elements	
Pre-enrollment history	
Medical history	• Morbidities/conditions
	• Onset/duration
	• Severity
	• Treatment history
	• Medications
	• Adherence
	• Health care resource utilization
	• Diagnostic tests and results
	• Procedures and outcomes
	• Emergency room visits, hospitalizations (including length of stay), long-term care, or stays in skilled nursing facilities
	• Genetic information
	• Comorbidities
	• Development (pediatric/adolescent)
Environmental exposures	• Places of residence, employment
Patient characteristics	• Functional status (including ability to perform tasks related to daily living), quality of life, symptoms
	• Health behaviors (alcohol, tobacco use, physical activity, diet)
	• Social history
	• Marital status
	• Family history
	• Work history
	• Employment, industry, job category
	• Social support network
	• Economic status, income, living situation
	• Sexual history
	• Foreign travel, citizenship
	• Legal (e.g., incarceration, legal status)
	• Reproductive history
	• Health literacy
	• Individual understanding of medical conditions and the risks and benefits of interventions
	• Social environment (e.g., community services)
	• Enrollment in clinical trials (if patients enrolled in clinical trials are eligible for the registry)
Provider/system characteristics	• Geographical coverage
	• Access barriers
	• Quality improvement programs
	• Disease management, case management
	• Compliance programs
	• Information technology use (e.g., computerized physician order entry, e-prescribing, electronic medical records)

63

(continued)

Table 5: Sample Additional Enrollee, Provider, and Environmental Data Elements (continued)	
Provider/system characteristics (continued)	• Quality improvement metrics (e.g., health plan level [HEDIS], hospital level [Joint Commission], group level [pay for performance], or individual practitioner [Bridges to Excellence]) • Cultural competency
Financial/economic information	• Disability, work attendance, or absenteeism • Out-of-pocket costs • Health care utilization behavior, including outpatient visits, hospitalizations (and length of stay), and visits to the emergency room or urgent care • Patient assessments of the degree to which they avoid health care because of its cost • Patients' reports of the availability of insurance coverage to assist/cover the costs of outpatient medications • Destination when discharged from a hospitalization (home, skilled nursing facility, long-term care, etc.) • Medical costs, often derived from data on physician office visits, hospitalizations, and/or procedures
Followup	
Key primary outcomes	• Safety: adverse events (see Chapter 9) • Effectiveness and value: intermediate and endpoint outcomes; health care resource use and hospitalizations; diagnostic tests and results. Particularly important are outcomes meaningful to patients, including survival, symptoms, function, and quality of life • Quality measurement/improvement: key selected measures at appropriate intervals • Natural history: progression of disease severity; use of health care services; diagnostic tests, procedures, and results; quality of life; mortality; cause/date of death
Key secondary outcomes	• Economic status • Social functioning
Other potentially important information	• Changes in medical status • Changes in patient characteristics • Changes in provider characteristics • Changes in financial status • Residence • Changes, additions, or discontinuation of exposures (drugs, environment, behaviors, procedures) • Sources of care (e.g., where hospitalized) • Changes in individual attitudes, behaviors
Note: HEDIS = Health plan Employer Data and Information Set.	

typographical errors by clerical staff. In these cases, having more than one patient identifier for linking patient records can be invaluable. In addition, identifier needs will differ based on the registry goals. For example, a registry that tracks children will need identifiers related to the parents, and registries that are likely to include twins (e.g., immunization registries) should plan for the duplication of birth dates and other identifiers. In selecting patient identifiers for use in a registry, registry planners will need to determine what data are necessary for their purpose and plan for potential inaccurate and changing data.

Generally, patient identifiers can simplify the process of identifying patients and tracking patients for followup. Patient identifiers also allow for the possibility of identifying patients who are lost to followup due to death (i.e., through the National Death Index) and linking to birth certificates for studies in children. In addition, unique patient identifiers allow for analysis to remove duplicate patients.

When considering the advantages of patient identifiers, it is important to take into account the potential barriers that patient identifiers can present. Obtaining consent for the use of patient-identifiable information can be an obstacle to enrollment, as it can lead to the refusal of patients to participate. Chapter 6 contains more information on the ethical and legal considerations of using patient identifiers.

In addition to the data points related to primary and secondary outcomes, it is important to plan for patients who will leave the registry. While the intention of a registry is generally for all patients to remain in the study until planned followup is completed, planning for patients to leave the study before completion of full followup may reduce analysis problems. By designing a final study visit form, registry planners can more clearly document when losses to followup occurred and possibly collect important information about why patients left the study. Not all registries will need a study discontinuation form, as some studies collect data on the patient only once and do not include followup information (e.g., in-hospital procedure registries).

Creating explicit data definitions for each variable to be collected is essential to the process of selecting data elements. This is important to ensure internal validity of the proposed study so that all participants in data collection are acquiring the requisite information in the same reproducible way. (See Chapter 8.) The data definitions should also include the ranges and acceptable values for each individual data element, as well as the potential interplay of different data elements. For example, logic checks for the validity of data capture may be created for data elements that should be mutually exclusive.

When deciding on data definitions, it is important to determine which data elements are required and which elements may be optional. This is particularly true in cases where the registry may collect a few additional "nice to know" data elements. Consideration should also be given to how to account for missing or unknown data. In some cases, a data element may be unknown or not documented for a particular patient, and followup with the patient to answer the question may not be possible. Including an option on the form for "not documented" or "unknown" will allow the person completing the case report form to provide a response to each question rather than leaving it blank. Depending on the analysis plans for the registry, the distinction between undocumented data and missing data may be important.

When collecting data for patient outcomes analysis, it is important to use patient-centered outcomes that are valid, reliable, responsive, interpretable, and translatable. Patient-centered outcomes reflect the patients' perceptions of their status and their perspective on health and disease. Patient-centered outcomes have become an increasingly important avenue of investigation, particularly in light of the recent Institute of Medicine report calling for a more patient-centered health care system.[87]

Among the most important patient-centered outcome to quantify is health status. Health status includes the manifestations of a disease—its symptoms; the degree to which a disease limits patients physically, emotionally, and socially; and the impact on patients' quality of life—as seen by

65

the patient. There are several methods for quantifying patients' health status, including the use of generic, disease-specific, and utility measures. Generic health status and utility measures seek to quantify the overall status of a patient's health. Whereas generic health status measures often have several domains,[88] utility measures distill patients' health to a single value between 0 (indicating death) and 1.0 (indicating perfect health) that can be used in economic analyses.[89,90,91,92] In contrast to these approaches that seek to quantify the overall effects of patients' health on their health status, disease-specific measures focus on the specific symptoms, limitations, and quality-of-life impairment associated with a particular disease.[93] Because of the more narrow focus of disease-specific instruments, they are often more sensitive to clinical change[94,95,96] and "actionable" by physicians who are familiar with the clinically oriented domains assessed by these instruments.[97]

Prior to their use, however, patient-centered health status measures need to have appropriate psychometric characteristics. There are at least five key attributes that a health status measure should demonstrate prior to its incorporation into a clinical study or registry. Relevant attributes of a potential instrument (Table 6) include its validity, reliability, responsiveness to change, interpretability, and the availability of translations in other languages.[98] Often, explicit demonstration of these properties prior to the initial use of the instrument is needed to be sure that the results are meaningful.

When no instrument exists and a new one needs to be developed, a series of methodological studies should be performed to ensure that the instrument meets these requisite qualities prior to investing in it for a larger study. While several resources exist for creating new measures, clearinghouses for previously created measures and the literature should be carefully searched before embarking on the lengthy and challenging process of new measure creation. (See Case Examples 10 and 11.)

Registry Data Map

Once data elements have been selected, a data map should be created. The data map identifies all sources of data (Chapter 5) and explains how the sources of data will be integrated. Data maps are useful to defend the validity and/or reliability of the data, and they are typically an integral part of the data management plan (Chapter 8).

Pilot Testing

After the data elements have been selected and the data map created, it is important to pilot test the data collection tools to determine the time needed to complete the form and the resulting subject/abstractor burden. For example, through pilot testing, registry planners might determine that it is wise to collect certain highly burdensome (or "nice to know") data elements in only a subset of participating sites (nested registry) that agree to the more intensive data collection, so as not to endanger participation in the registry as a whole. Pilot testing should also help to identify the missing data rate and any validity issues with the data collection system.

The burden of form collection is a major factor determining a registry's success or failure, with major implications for the cost of participation and for the overall acceptance of the registry by hospitals and health care personnel. Moreover, knowing the anticipated time needed for patient recruitment/enrollment will allow better communication to potential sites of the scope and magnitude of commitment required to participate in the study. Registries that obtain information directly from patients have an additional issue of participant burden, with the potential for participant fatigue, leading to failure to answer all items in the registry. Highly burdensome questions can be collected in a prespecified subset of subjects. The purpose of these added questions should be carefully considered when determining the subset so that useful and accurate conclusions can be achieved.

Pilot testing the registry also allows the opportunity to identify issues and make refinements in the registry data collection tool, including alterations in

66

Table 6: Key Attributes of a Health Status Instrument

Measurement property	Description
Validity	The measure quantifies what it is intended to
Reliability	Reproducible results are obtained when repeatedly given to stable patients
Responsiveness	The measure is sensitive to clinical change
Interpretability	A clinical framework is available to interpret cross-sectional data and changes in scores
Translations exist	Linguistically and culturally appropriate translations are available

Case Example 10: Developing and Validating a Patient-Administered Questionnaire

Description	The Benign Prostatic Hypertrophy (BPH) Registry & Patient Survey is a multicenter, prospective, observational registry examining the patient management practices of primary care providers and urologists and assessing patient outcomes, including symptom amelioration and disease progress. The registry collects patient-reported and clinician-reported data at multiple clinical visits.
Sponsor	Sanofi-Aventis
Year Started	2004
Year Ended	Ongoing
No. of Sites	403
No. of Patients	6,928

Challenge

Lower urinary tract symptoms associated with benign prostatic hyperplasia (LUTS/BPH) have a strong relationship to sexual dysfunction in aging males. Sexual dysfunction includes both erectile dysfunction (ED) and ejaculatory dysfunction (EjD), and health care providers treating patients with symptoms of BPH should evaluate men for both types of dysfunction. Providers can use the Male Sexual Health Questionnaire (MSHQ), a validated, self-administered, sexual function scale to assess dysfunction, but the 25-item scale can be perceived as too long. To assess EjD more efficiently, it was necessary to develop a brief, patient-administered, validated questionnaire.

Proposed Solution

The team used representative, population-based samples to develop a short-form scale for assessing EjD. The team administered the 25-item MSHQ to three populations: a sample of men from the Men's Sexual Health Population Survey, a subsample of men from the Urban Men's Health Study, and a sample of men enrolled in the observational registry.

Using the data from the sample populations, the team conducted a series of analyses to develop the scale. The team used factor analysis to help select the items from the scale that had the highest correlations with the principal factors. Using conventional validation, the team examined reliability (both internal consistency and test-retest repeatability). To assess validity, tests of repeatability and discriminant/convergent validity were used to determine that the short form successfully discriminated between men with no to mild LUTS/BPH and those with moderate to severe LUTS/BPH. Lastly, the team examined the correlation between the 7-item ejaculation domain of the 25-item MSHQ and the new short-form scale using data from the observational registry.

(continued)

67

Case Example 10: Developing and Validating a Patient-Administered Questionnaire (continued)

Results

Based on the results of these analyses, the team selected three ejaculatory function items and one ejaculation bother item for inclusion in the new MSHQ-EjD Short Form. The new scale demonstrates a high degree of internal consistency and reliability, and it provides information to identify men with no to mild LUTS/BPH and those with moderate to severe LUTS/BPH.

Key Point

Developing new instruments for collecting patient-reported outcomes requires careful testing of the new tool in representative populations to ensure validity and reliability. Registries can provide a large sample population for validating new instruments.

For More Information

Althof SE, Rosen RC, Catania J et al. Short-Form Scale to Assess Ejaculatory Dysfunction (EjD): development and validation of a 4-item version of the Male Sexual Health Questionnaire (MSHQ-EjD Short Form). Poster presentation at Society for Sex Therapy and Research (SSTAR) 2006 Meeting. Available at: http://www.sstarnet.org/download/ 2006FinalProgram.pdf. Accessed April 2, 2007.

Rosen R, Altwein J, Boyle P et al. Lower urinary tract symptoms and male sexual dysfunction: the Multinational Survey of the Aging Male. Eur Urol 2003;44:637-49.

Case Example 11: Understanding the Needs and Goals of the Registry Participants

Description	The Prospective Registry Evaluating Myocardial Infarction: Events and Recovery (PREMIER) studied the health status of patients for 1 year after discharge for a myocardial infarction. The registry focused on developing a rich understanding of the patients' symptoms, functional status, and quality of life by collecting extensive baseline data in the hospital and completing followup interviews at 1, 6, and 12 months.
Sponsor	CV Therapeutics and CV Outcomes
Year Started	2003
Year Ended	2004
No. of Sites	19
No. of Patients	2,498

Challenge

With the significant advances in myocardial infarction (MI) care over the past 20 years, many studies have documented the improved mortality and morbidity associated with these new treatments. These studies typically have focused on in-hospital care, with little to no followup component. As a result, information on the transition from inpatient to outpatient care was lacking, as were data on health status outcomes.

PREMIER was designed to address these gaps by collecting detailed information on MI patients during the hospital stay and through followup telephone interviews conducted at 1, 6, and 12 months. The goal of the registry was to provide a rich understanding of patients' health status (their symptoms, function, and quality of life) 1 year after an acute MI. The registry also proposed to

(continued)

Case Example 11: Understanding the Needs and Goals of the Registry Participants (continued)

quantify the prevalence, determinants, and consequences of patient and clinical factors in order to understand how the structures and processes of MI care affect patients' health status.

To develop the registry data set, the team began by clearly defining the phases of care and recovery and identifying the clinical characteristics that were important in each of these phases. These included patient characteristics upon hospital arrival, details on inpatient care, and details on outpatient care. The team felt that information on each of these phases was necessary, since the variability of any outcome over 1 year may be explained by patient, inpatient treatment, or outpatient factors. Health status also includes many determinants beyond the clinical status of disease, such as access to care, socioeconomic status, and social support; the registry needed to collect these additional data in order to understand fully the health status outcomes.

Proposed Solution

While registries often try to include as many eligible patients and sites as possible by reducing the burden of data entry, this registry took an alternative approach. The team designed a data set that included over 650 baseline data elements and over 200 followup interview-assessed data elements. Instead of allowing retrospective chart abstraction, the registry required hospitals to complete a five-page patient interview while the patient was in the hospital. The registry demanded significant resources from the participating sites. For each patient, the registry required about 4 hours of time, with 15 minutes for screening, 2 hours for chart abstraction, 45 minutes for interviews, 45 minutes for data entry, and 15 minutes of a cardiologist's time to interpret the electrocardiograms and angiograms. A detailed, prespecified sampling plan was developed by each

site and approved by the data coordinating center to ensure that the patients enrolled at each center were representative of all of the patients seen by that site.

The registry team developed this extremely detailed data set and data collection process through extensive consultations with the registry participants. The coordinators and steering committees reviewed the data set multiple times, with some sites giving extensive feedback. Throughout the development process, there was an ongoing dialog among the registry designers, the steering committee, and the registry sites.

The registry team also used standard definitions and established instruments whenever possible to enable the registry data to be cross-referenced to other studies and to minimize the training burden. The team used the American College of Cardiology Data Standards for Acute Coronary Syndromes for data definitions of any overlapping fields. To measure other areas of the patient experience, the team used the Patient Health Questionnaire to examine depression, the ENRICHD Social Support Inventory to measure social support, the Short Form-12 to quantify overall mental and physical health, and the Seattle Angina Questionnaire (SAQ) to understand the patients' perspective on how coronary disease affects their life.

Results

The data collection burden posed some challenges. Two of the 19 sites dropped out of the registry early on. Two other sites fell behind on their chart abstractions. Turnover of personnel and multiple commitments at participating sites also delayed the study.

Despite these challenges, the registry experienced very little loss of enthusiasm or loss of sites once it was up and running. The remaining 17 sites

69

(continued)

> **Case Example 11: Understanding the Needs and Goals of the Registry Participants (continued)**
>
> completed the registry and collected data on nearly 2,500 patients. In return for this data collection, sites enjoyed the academic productivity and collaborative nature of the study. The data coordinating center created a Web site that offered private groups for the principal investigators, so each investigator had access to all of the abstract ideas and all of the research that was being done. This structure provided nurturing and support for the investigators, and they viewed the registry as a way to engage themselves and their institution in research with a prominent, highly respected team.
>
> On the patient side, the registry met followup goals. Over 85 percent of patients completed a 1-month followup interview, and 87 percent of surviving patients completed at least part of their 6-month followup interview. The registry team attributed this followup rate to the strong rapport that the interviewers developed with the patients during the course of the followup period.
>
> **Key Point**
>
> This example illustrates that there is no maximum or minimum number of data elements for a successful registry. Instead, a registry can best achieve its goals by ensuring that sufficient information is collected to achieve the purpose of the registry while remaining feasible for the participants. An open, ongoing dialog with the participants or a subgroup of participants can help to determine what is feasible for a particular registry and to ensure that the registry will retain the participants for the life of the study.
>
> **For More Information**
>
> Spertus JA, Peterson E, Rumsfeld JS et al. The Prospective Registry Evaluating Myocardial Infarction: Events and Recovery (PREMIER)–evaluating the impact of myocardial infarction on patient outcomes. Am Heart J 2006 Mar;151(3):589-97.

the format or order of data elements and clarification of item definitions. Piloting may also uncover problems in registry logistics, such as the ability to accurately or comprehensively identify subjects for inclusion.

A fundamental aspect of pilot testing is evaluation of the accuracy and completeness of registry questions and the comprehensiveness of both instructional materials and training in addressing these potential issues. Missing data may cause bias and result in inaccurate or misleading conclusions. For example, time points, such as time to radiologic interpretation of imaging test, may be difficult to obtain retrospectively, and their presence in hospital charting may occur more frequently when the time span is short, making it difficult to evaluate association between time and various clinical or demographic factors.

Pilot testing ranges in practice from ad hoc assessments of the face validity of instruments and materials in clinical sites, to trial runs of the registry in small numbers of sites, to highly structured evaluations of inter-rater agreement. The level of pilot testing is determined by multiple factors. Accuracy of data entry is a key criterion to evaluate during the pilot phase of the registry. When a "gold standard" exists, the level of agreement with a reference standard (construct validity) may be measured.[99] Data collected by seasoned abstractors or auditors following strict operational criteria can serve as the gold standard on which to judge accuracy of abstraction for chart-based registries.[100] In instances where no reference standard is available, reproducibility of responses to registry elements by abstractors (inter-rater reliability) or test-retest agreement of subject responses may be assessed.[101] Reliability and/or validity of data elements should be tested in the pilot phase whenever the element is collected in new populations or for new applications. Similar mechanisms to those used during the pilot phase can be used during data quality assurance (Chapter 8).

Kappa statistic is a measure of how much the level of agreement between two observers exceeds the amount of agreement expected by chance alone. It is the most common method for measuring reliability of categorical and ordinal data. Intra-class correlation coefficient, or inter-rater reliability coefficient, provides information on the degree of agreement for continuous data. It is a proportion that ranges from zero to one. Item-specific agreement represents the highest standard for registries; it has been employed in cancer registries and to assess the quality of data in statewide stroke registries. Other methods, such as the Bland and Altman method,[102] may also be chosen, depending upon the type of data and registry purpose.

Overall, the choice of data elements should be guided by parsimony, validity, and consistent focus on achieving the purpose for which the registry was created.

71

Chapter 5. Data Sources for Registries

Identification and evaluation of suitable data sources should be done within the context of the registry purpose and availability of the data of interest. A single registry may have multiple purposes and integrate data from various sources. When people think of clinical registries, they typically think of data collected directly for registry purposes (primary data collection). However, this is not the only option, as important information can be transferred into the registry from existing databases. Examples include demographic information from a hospital admission, discharge, and transfer system; medication use from a pharmacy database; and disease and treatment information, such as details of the coronary anatomy and percutaneous coronary intervention from a (catheterization) laboratory information system, electronic medical record, or medical claims databases. In addition, observational studies can generate as many hypotheses as they test, and secondary sources of data can be merged with the primary data collection to allow for analyses of questions that were unanticipated when the registry was conceived.

This chapter will review the various sources of both primary and secondary data, comment on their strengths and weaknesses, and provide some examples of how data collected from different sources can be integrated to help answer important questions.

Types of Data

The types of data to be collected are closely linked with the registry design and data collection methods. The form, organization, and timing of required data are important components in determining appropriate data sources. Data elements can be grouped into categories identifying the specific variable or construct they are intended to describe. One framework for grouping data elements into categories follows:

- *Patient identifiers*: Patient identifiers are critical to linkage of all data elements in some registries. Registry data elements are linked to the specific patient through a unique patient identifier or registry identification number.

- *Patient selection criteria*: The eligibility criteria in a registry protocol (or study plan) determine the group that will be included in the registry. These criteria may be very broad or restrictive, depending on the purpose. Criteria often include demographics (e.g., target age group), a disease diagnosis, a treatment, or diagnostic procedures and laboratory tests. Health care provider, health care facility or system, and insurance criteria may also be included in certain types of registries (e.g., following care patterns of specific conditions at large medical centers compared with small private clinics).

- *Treatments and tests*: Treatments and tests are necessary to describe the natural history of patients. Treatments can include pharmaceutical, biotechnology, or device therapies or procedures, such as surgery or radiation. Evaluation of the treatment itself is often a primary focus of registries (e.g., treatment safety and effectiveness over 5 years). Results of laboratory testing or diagnostic procedures may be included as registry outcomes and used in defining a diagnosis or condition of interest.

- *Confounders*: Confounders are elements or factors that have an independent association with the outcomes of interest. These are particularly important because patients are typically not randomized to therapies in registries. Confounders such as comorbidities (disease diagnoses and conditions) can confuse analysis results and interpretation of causality. Information on the health care provider, treatment facility, concomitant therapies, or insurance may also be considered.

- *Outcomes*: The focus of this document is on patient outcomes. Outcomes are end results and are defined for each condition. In some registries, surrogate markers, such as biomarkers or other interim outcomes (e.g., hemoglobin A1C levels in diabetes) that are highly reflective of the longer term end results, are used.

The types of data elements included in this framework are further described below with respect to their source or the utility of the data for linking to other sources. Many of these may be available through data sources outside of the registry system.

Patient identifiers—Depending on the data sources required, registries may utilize certain personal identifiers for patients to locate specific patients and link the data. For example, Social Security Numbers (SSNs), as well as a combination of other personal identifiers, can be utilized to identify individuals in the National Death Index (NDI). Patient contact information, such as address and phone numbers, may be collected to support tracking of participants over time. Information for additional contacts (e.g., family members) may be collected to support followup in cases where the patient cannot be reached. In many cases, patient informed consent and appropriate privacy authorizations are required to utilize personal identifiers for registry purposes; Chapter 6 discusses the legal requirements for including patient identifiers. Systems and processes must be in place to manage security and confidentiality of these data. Confidentiality can be enhanced by assigning a registry-specific identifier via a crosswalk algorithm, as discussed below. Demographics, such as date of birth (to calculate age at any time point), gender, and ethnicity, are typically collected and may be used to stratify the registry population.

Disease/condition—Disease or condition data include those related to the disease or condition of focus for the registry and may incorporate comorbidities. Elements of interest related to the confirmation of a diagnosis or condition could be date of diagnosis and the specific diagnostic results that were used to make the diagnosis, depending on the purpose of the registry. Disease or condition is often a primary eligibility or outcome variable in

registries, whether the intent is to answer specified treatment questions (e.g., measure effectiveness or safety) or to describe the natural history. This information may also be collected in constructing a medical history for a patient. In addition to "yes" or "no" to indicate presence or absence of the diagnosis, it may be important to capture responses such as "missing" or "unknown."

Treatment/therapy—Treatment or therapy data include specific identifying information for the primary treatment (e.g., drug name or code, biologic, device product or component parts, or surgical intervention, such as organ transplant or coronary artery bypass graft) and may include information on concomitant treatments. Dosage (or parameters for devices), route of administration, and prescribed exposure time, such as daily or three times weekly for 4 weeks, should be collected. Pharmacy data may include dispensing information, such as the primary date of dispensation and subsequent refill dates. Data in device registries can include the initial date of dispensation or implantation and subsequent dates and specifics of required evaluations or modifications. Compliance data may also be collected if pharmacy representatives or clinic personnel are engaged to conduct and report pill counts or volume measurements on refill visits or return visits for device evaluations and modifications.

Laboratory/procedures—Laboratory data include a broad range of testing, such as blood, tissue, catheterization, and radiology. Specific test results, units of measure, and laboratory reference ranges or parameters are typically collected. Laboratory databases are becoming increasingly accessible for electronic transfer of data, whether through a system-wide institutional database or a private laboratory database. Diagnostic testing or evaluation may include procedures such as psychological or behavioral assessments. Results of these procedures and physician exam procedures may be difficult to obtain through data sources other than the patient medical record.

Health care provider characteristics—Information on the health care provider (e.g., physician, nurse, or pharmacist) may be collected, depending on the purpose of the registry. Training, education, or specialization may account for differences in care patterns. Geographic location has also been used as an indicator of differences in care or medical practice.

Hospital/clinic/health plans—System interactions include office visits, outpatient clinic visits, emergency room visits, inpatient hospitalizations, procedures, and pharmacy visits, as well as associated dates. Data on all procedures as defined by the registry protocol or plan (e.g., physical exam, psychological evaluation, chest x-ray, CAT scan), including measurements, results, and units of measure where applicable, should be collected. Cost accounting data may also be available to match these interactions and procedures. Descriptive information related to the points of care may be useful in capturing differences in care patterns and can also be used to track patterns of referral of care (e.g., outpatient clinic, inpatient hospital, academic center, emergency room, pharmacy).

Insurance—The insurance system or payer claims data can provide useful information on interactions with the health care system, including visits, procedures, inpatient stays, and costs associated with these events.

Data Sources

Data sources are classified as primary or secondary based on the relationship of the data to the registry purpose. Primary data sources incorporate data collected for direct purposes of the registry (i.e., primarily for the registry). Primary data sources are typically used when the data of interest are not available or, if available, are unlikely to be of sufficient accuracy and reliability for the planned analyses and uses. Primary data collection increases the probability of completeness, validity, and reliability (see Chapter 4) because the registry drives the methods of measurement and data collection. These data are prospectively planned and collected under the direction of a protocol or study plan, using common procedures and the same format across all registry sites and patients. The data are readily integrated for tracking and analyses. Since

the data entered can be traced to the individual who collected them, primary data sources are more readily reviewed through automated checks or followup queries from a data manager than is possible with many secondary data sources.

Secondary data sources are comprised of data originally collected for purposes other than the registry under consideration (e.g., standard medical care, insurance claims processing). Data that are collected as primary data for one registry would be considered secondary data from the perspective of a second registry if matching were done. These data are often stored in electronic format and may be available with appropriate permissions and systems consideration for transfer and import into the registry databases. Health professionals are accustomed to entering the data for defined purposes, and additional training and support for data collection are not required. Often, these data are not constrained by a data collection protocol and represent the diversity observed in real-world practice. However, there may be increased probability of errors and underreporting because of inconsistencies in measurement, reporting, and collection. There may also be increased costs for matching the data from the secondary source to the primary source and dealing with any potential duplicate or unmatched patients.

Sufficient identifiers are necessary to accurately match data between the secondary sources and registry patients. The potential for mismatch errors and duplications must be managed. (See Case Example 12.) The complexity and obligations inherent in the collection and handling of personal identifiers have previously been mentioned (e.g., obligations for informed consent, appropriate data privacy, and confidentiality procedures).

Some of the secondary data sources do not collect information at a specific patient level but are anonymous and intended to reflect group or population estimates. For example, census tract or ZIP-Code-level data are available from the Census Bureau and can be merged with registry data. These data can be used as "ecological variables" to support analyses of income or education when such socioeconomic data are missing from registry

75

Case Example 12: Integrating Data From Multiple Sources With Patient ID Matching	
Description	KIDSNET is Rhode Island's computerized registry to track children's use of preventive health services. The program collects data from multiple sources and uses those data to help providers and public health professionals identify children in need of services. The purpose of the program is to ensure that all children in the State receive the appropriate preventive care measures in a timely manner.
Sponsor	State of Rhode Island, Centers for Disease Control and Prevention, and others
Year Started	1997
Year Ended	Ongoing
No. of Sites	130 participating practices plus other authorized users
No. of Patients	193,036

Challenge

In the 1990s, the Rhode Island Department of Health recognized that its data on children's health were fragmented and program specific. The State had many children's health initiatives, such as programs for hearing assessment and lead prevention, but these programs collected data separately and did not attempt to link the information. This type of fragmented structure is common in public health agencies, as many programs receive funding to fulfill a specific need but no funding to link that information with other programs. This type of linkage would benefit the department's activities, as children who are at risk for one health issue are often at risk for other health issues. By integrating the data, the department would be able to better integrate services and provide better service.

To integrate the data from these multiple sources and to allow new data to be entered directly into the program, the department implemented a computerized registry. The registry consolidates data from 11 different sources to provide an overall picture of a child's use of preventive health care services. The sources include newborn developmental risk screening; the immunization registry; lead screening; hearing assessment; Women, Infants, and Children (WIC); home visiting; early intervention; blood spot screening; foster care; birth defects; and vital records data. The goals of the registry are to monitor the use of preventive health services, proactively promote referrals when services are needed, provide a lead screening reminder and recall directly to parents, and give providers reporting capacity to identify children who are behind in services.

After launching in 1997, the registry began accumulating data on children who were born in the State or receiving preventive health care services in the State. Some of the 11 data sources entered data directly into the registry, and some of the data sources sent data from another database to the registry. The registry then consolidated data from these 11 sources into a single patient record for each child by matching the records using simple deterministic logic. As the registry began importing records, the system held some records as questionable matches, since it could not determine if the record was new or a match to an existing record. These records required manual review to resolve the issue, which was time consuming, at approximately 3 minutes per record.

Without resources to devote to the manual review, the number of records held as questionable matches increased to 48,685 by 2004. The time to resolve these records manually was estimated at 17 months, and the registry did not have the resources to devote to that task. However, the incomplete data resulting from so many held records made the registry less successful at tracking children's health and less utilized by providers.

(continued)

76

Case Example 12: Integrating Data From Multiple Sources With Patient ID Matching (continued)

Proposed Solution

To resolve the issue of patient matching, the sponsor implemented an automated solution to the matching problem after evaluating several options, including probabilistic and deterministic matching strategies and commercial and open-source options for matching software. Since the State had limited funds for the project, an open-source product, Febrl, was selected.

A set of rules to process incoming records was developed, and an interface was created for the manual review of questionable records. Using the rules, the software determines the probability of a match for each record. The registry then sets probability thresholds above which a record is considered a certain match and below which a record is considered a new record. All of the records that fall into the middle ground require manual review.

Results

After considerable testing, the new system launched in spring 2004. Immediately upon implementation, 95 percent of the held records were processed and removed from the holding category, resulting in the addition of approximately 11,000 new patient records to the registry. The new interface for manual review reduced the time to resolve an error from 3 minutes to 40 seconds. With these improvements, the registry now imports 95 percent of the data sent to the database and is able to process the questionable records through the improved interface.

Key Point

Many strategies and products exist to deal with matching patients from multiple data sources. Once a product has been selected, careful consideration must be given to the probability thresholds for establishing a match. Setting the threshold for matches too high may result in an unmanageable burden of manual review. However, setting the threshold too low could affect data quality, as records may be merged inappropriately. A careful balance must be found between resources and data quality in order for matching software to help the registry.

For More Information

Wild EL, Hastings TM, Gubernick R et al. Key elements for successful integrated health information systems: lessons learned from the states. J Public Health Manag Pract 2004 Nov 10 Suppl:S36-S47.

77

primary data collection. The intended use of the data elements will determine whether patient-level information is required.

The potential for data completeness, variation, and specificity must be evaluated in the context of the registry and intended use of the data. It is advisable to have a solid understanding of the original purpose of the secondary data collection, including processes for collection and submission, and verification and validation practices. Questions to ask include: Is data collection passive or active? Are standard definitions or codes used in reporting data? Are standard measurement criteria or instruments utilized (e.g., diagnoses, symptoms, quality of life)? The existence and completeness of claims data, for example, will depend on insurance company coverage policies. One company may cover many preventive services, whereas another may have more restricted coverage. Also, coverage policies can change over time. These variations must be known and carefully documented so as not to misinterpret use rates. Additionally, secondary data may not all be collected in the format required for registry purposes (e.g., units of measure) and may require transformation for integration and analyses.

An overview of secondary data sources that may be used for registries is given below. Table 7 identifies some key strengths and limitations of the identified data sources.

Medical chart abstraction—Medical charts primarily contain information collected as a part of routine medical care. These data reflect the practice of medicine or health care in general and at a specific level (e.g., geographical, by specialty care provider). Charts also reflect uncontrolled patient behavior (e.g., noncompliance). Collection of standard medical practice data is useful in looking at treatments and outcomes in the real world, including all of the confounders that impact the measurement of effectiveness (vs. efficacy) and safety outside of the controlled conditions of a clinical trial. Chart documentation is often much poorer than one might expect, and there may be more than one patient-specific medical record (e.g., hospital and clinical records). A pilot collection is recommended for this labor-intensive method of data collection to explore the availability and reproducibility of the data of interest. It is important to recognize that physicians and other clinicians do not generally use standardized data definitions in entering information into medical charts, meaning that one clinician's documented diagnosis of "chronic sinusitis" or "osteoarthritis" or description of "pedal edema" may differ from that of another clinician.

Electronic medical records.—The use of electronic medical records (EMRs) is increasing. EMRs have an advantage over paper medical records because the data in some EMRs can be readily searched and integrated with other information (e.g., laboratory data). The ease with which this is accomplished depends on whether the information is in a relational database or exists as scanned documents. An additional challenge relates to terminology and relationships. For example, including the term "fit" in a search for patients with epilepsy can yield a record for someone who was noted as "fit," as in healthy. Relationships can also be difficult to identify through searches (e.g., patient had breast cancer vs. patient's mother had breast cancer). The quality of the information has the same limitations as described in the paragraph above.

Institutional or organizational databases— Institutional or organizational databases may be evaluated as a potential source of a wide variety of data. System-wide institutional or hospital databases are central data repositories, or data warehouses, that are highly variable from institution to institution. They may include a portion of everything from admission, discharge, and transfer information to data reflecting diagnoses and treatment, pharmacy prescriptions, and specific laboratory tests. The latter might be chemistry or histology laboratory data, including patient identifiers with associated dates of specimen collection and measurement, results, and standard "normal" or reference ranges. Catheterization laboratory data for cardiac registries may be accessible and may include details on the coronary anatomy and percutaneous coronary intervention. Other organizational examples are pharmacies, blood banks, and radiology departments.

Table 7: Key Data Sources—Strengths and Limitations

Data source	Strengths and uses	Limitations
Direct patient reports	• Patient and/or caregiver outcomes. • Unique perspective. • Obtaining information on treatments not necessarily prescribed by clinicians (e.g., over-the-counter drugs, herbal medications). • Obtaining intended compliance information. • Useful when timing of followup may not be concordant with timing of clinical encounter.	• Literacy, language, or other barriers that may lead to underenrollment of some subgroups. • Validated data collection instruments may need to be developed. • Loss to followup or refusal to continue participation. • Limited confidence in reporting clinical information and utilization information.
Direct clinician reports	• More specific information than available from coded data or medical record.	• Clinicians are highly sensitive to burden. • Consistency in capture of patient signs, symptoms, use of nonprescribed therapy.
Medical chart abstraction	• Information on routine medical care and practice, with more clinical context than coded claims. • Potential for comprehensive view of patient medical and clinical history. • Use of abstraction and strict coding standards (including handling of missing data) increases the quality and interpretation of data abstracted.	• The underlying information is not collected in a systematic way. For example, a diagnosis of bacterial pneumonia by one physician may be based on a physical exam and patient report of symptoms, while another physician may record the diagnosis only in the presence of a confirmed laboratory test. • It is difficult to interpret missing data. For example, does absence of a specific symptom in the visit record indicate that the symptom was not present or that the physician did not actively inquire about this specific symptom or set of symptoms? • Data abstraction is resource intensive. • Complete medical and clinical history may not be available (e.g., new patient to clinic).

(continued)

Table 7: Key Data Sources—Strengths and Limitations (continued)

Data source	Strengths and uses	Limitations
Electronic medical records (EMRs)	• Information on routine medical care and practice, with more clinical context than coded claims. • Potential for comprehensive view of patient medical and clinical history. • Efficient access to medical and clinical data. • Use of data transfer and coding standards (including handling of missing data) will increase the quality of data abstracted.	• Underlying information from physicians was not collected using uniform decision rules. (See example under "Medical chart abstraction.") • Consistency of data quality and breadth of data collected varies across sites. • Difficult to handle information uploaded as text files into the EMRs (e.g., scanned physician reports) vs. direct entry into data fields. • Historical data capture may require manual chart abstraction prior to implementation date of medical records system. • Complete medical and clinical history may not be available (e.g., new patient to clinic). • EMR systems vary widely. If data come from multiple systems, the registry should plan to work with each system individually to understand the requirements of the transfer.
Institutional or organizational databases	• Diagnostic and treatment information (e.g., pharmacy, laboratory, blood bank, radiology). • Resource utilization (e.g., days in hospital). • May incorporate cost data (e.g., billed and/or paid amounts from insurance claims submissions).	• Important to be knowledgeable on coding systems used in entering data into the original systems. • Institutional or organizational databases vary widely. The registry should plan to work with each system individually to understand the requirements of the transfer.
Administrative databases	• Useful for tracking health care utilization and cost-related information. • Range of data includes anything that is reimbursed by health insurance (generally including visits to physicians and allied health providers, most prescription drugs, many devices, hospitalization, if a lab test was performed, and in some cases, actual lab test results for selected tests (e.g., blood test results for cholesterol, diabetes). • In some cases, demographic information (e.g., gender, date of birth from billing files) can be uploaded.	• Represents clinical cost drivers vs. complete clinical diagnostic and treatment information. • Important to be knowledgeable on the process and standards used in claims submission. For example, only primary diagnosis may be coded and secondary diagnoses not captured. In other situations, value-laden claims may not be used (e.g., an event may be coded as a "nonspecific gynecologic infection" rather than a "sexually transmitted disease").

(continued)

80

Table 7: Key Data Sources—Strengths and Limitations (continued)

Data source	Strengths and uses	Limitations
Administrative databases (continued)	• Potential for efficient capture of large populations.	• Important to be knowledgeable on data handling and coding systems used when incorporating the claims data into the administrative systems. • Can be difficult to gain the cooperation of partner groups, particularly in regard to receiving the submissions in a timely manner.
Death indexes	• Completeness—death reporting is mandated by law in the United States. • Strong backup source for mortality tracking (e.g., patient lost to followup). • National Death Index (NDI)—centralized database of death records from State vital statistics offices, database updated annually. • NDI causes of death relatively reliable (93-96 percent) compared with State death certificates. • Social Security Administration's (SSA) Death Master File—database of deaths reported to SSA, database updated weekly.	• Time delay—indexes depend on information from other data sources (e.g., State vital statistics offices), with delays of 12 to 18 months or longer. It is important to understand the frequency of updates of specific indexes that may be utilized. • Absence of information in death indexes does not necessarily indicate "alive" status at a given point in time.
U.S. Census Bureau databases	• Population data. • Core census survey conducted every decade. • Wide range in specificity of information from U.S. population down to neighborhood and household level. • Useful in determining population estimates (e.g., numbers, age, family size, education, employment status).	• Targets participants via survey sampling methodology and estimates. • Does not provide subject-level data.
Existing registries	• Can be merged with another data source to answer additional questions not considered in the original registry protocol or plan. • May include specific data not generally collected in routine medical practice. • Can provide historical comparison data. • Reduces data collection burden for sites, thereby encouraging participation.	• Important to understand the existing registry protocol or plan to evaluate data collected for element definitions, timing, format. • Creates a reliance on the other registry. • Other registry may end. • Other registry may change data elements (which highlights the need for regular communication). • Some sites may not participate in both. • Must rely on the data quality of the other registry.

82

Administrative databases—Private and public medical insurers collect a wealth of information in the process of tracking health care, evaluating coverage, and managing billing and payment. Information in the databases includes patient-specific information (e.g., insurance coverage and copays; identifiers such as name, demographics, Social Security Numbers, or plan numbers; and dates of birth) and health care provider descriptive data (e.g., identifiers, specialty characteristics, locations). Typically, private insurance companies organize health care data by physician care (e.g., physician office visits) and hospital care (e.g., emergency room visits, hospital stays). Data include procedures and associated dates, as well as costs charged by the provider and paid by the insurers. Amounts paid by insurers are often considered proprietary and unavailable. Standard coding conventions are utilized in the reporting of diagnoses, procedures, and other information. Coding conventions include the Current Procedure Terminology (CPT) for physician services and International Classification of Diseases (ICD) for diagnoses. The databases serve the primary function of managing and implementing insurance coverage, processing, and payment.

Research identifiable data files (RIFs) maintained by the Centers for Medicare & Medicaid Services (CMS) are good examples of accessible administrative databases. The RIFs contain person-specific data on providers, beneficiaries, and recipients, including individual identifiers that would permit the identity of a beneficiary or physician to be deduced. Data with personal identifiers are clearly subject to privacy rules and regulations. As such, the information is confidential and is to be used only for reasons compatible with the purpose(s) for which the data are collected. The Research Data Assistance Center (ResDAC), a CMS contractor, provides free assistance to academic, government, and nonprofit researchers interested in using Medicare and/or Medicaid data for their research.[103]

Death and birth records—Death indexes are national databases tracking population death data (e.g., NDI[104] and the Death Master File [DMF] of the Social Security Administration [SSA][105]). Data include patient identifiers, date of death, and attributed causes of death. These indexes are populated through a variety of sources. For example, the DMF includes death information on individuals who had an SSN and had their death reported to the SSA. Reports may come in to the SSA by different paths, including from survivors or family members requesting benefits or from funeral homes. However, because of the importance of tracking Social Security benefits, all States, nursing homes, and mortuaries are required to report all deaths to the SSA, thus ensuring virtually 100-percent complete mortality ascertainment for those eligible for SSA benefits. The NDI is updated annually with computer death records submitted by State vital statistics offices and has all or nearly all deaths in the United States. The NDI can be used to provide both fact of death and cause of death, as recorded on the death certificate. Cause-of-death data in the NDI are relatively reliable (93-96 percent) compared with death certificates.[106,107] Time delays in death reporting should be considered when using these sources, and vital status should not be assumed to be alive by the absence of information at a recent point in time. These indexes are a valuable source of data for death tracking. Of course, mortality data can be accessed directly through queries of State vital statistics offices and health departments when targeting information on a specific patient or within a State. Likewise, birth certificates are available through State departments and may be useful in registries of children or births.

Census databases—U.S. Census Bureau databases[108] provide population-level data utilizing survey sampling methodology. The Census Bureau conducts many different surveys, the main one being the population census conducted every 10 years. The primary use of the data is to determine the number of seats assigned to each State in the House of Representatives, although the data are used for many other purposes. These surveys calculate estimates through statistical processing of the sampled data. Estimates can be provided with a broad range of granularity, from population numbers for large regions (e.g., specific States), to ZIP Codes, all the way down to a household level (e.g., neighborhoods identified by street addresses). Information collected includes demographic, gender, age, education, economic, housing, and work data. The data are not collected at an individual level but may serve other registry purposes, such as understanding population numbers in a specific region or by specific demographics.

Existing registry databases—There are numerous national and regional registry databases that may be leveraged for incorporation into other registries (e.g., disease-specific registries managed by nonprofit organizations, professional societies, or other entities). An example is the National Marrow Donor Program (NMDP),[109] a global database of cord blood units and volunteers who have consented to donate marrow and blood cells. Databases maintained by the NMDP include identifiers and locators in addition to information on the transplants, such as samples from the donor and recipient, histocompatibility, and outcomes. NMDP actively encourages research and utilization of registry data through a data application process and submission of research proposals. In accessing data from one registry for the purposes of another, it is important to recognize that data may have changed during the course of the source registry, and this may or may not have been well documented by the providers of the data. For example, in the United States Renal Data System (USRDS),[110] a vital part of personal identification is CMS 2728, an enrollment form that identifies the incident data for each patient as well as other pertinent information, such as the cause of renal failure, initial therapy, and comorbid conditions. Originally created in 1973, this form is in its third version, having been revised in 1995 and again in 2005. Consequently, there are data elements that exist in some versions and not others. The coding for some variables has changed over time. For example, race has been redefined to correspond with Office of Management and Budget

directives and Census categories. Further, in the early years of the registry, this form was optional, so until 1983, it was only filled out for about one-half of the subjects. Since 1995 it has been mandatory for all persons with end-stage renal disease. These changes in form content, data coding, and completeness would not be evident to most researchers trying to access the data.

Other Considerations for Secondary Data Sources

The discussion below focuses on logistical and data issues to consider when incorporating data from other sources. Chapter 8 fully explores data collection, management, and quality assurance for registries.

The importance of patient identifiers for linking to secondary data sources cannot be overstated. Multiple patient identifiers should be used, and primary data for these identifiers should not be entered into the registry unless the identifying information is complete and clear. While an SSN is very useful, high quality probabilistic linkages can be made to secondary data sources using various combinations of such information as name (last, middle initial, and first), date of birth, and gender. For example, the NDI will make possible matches based on any of seven conditions. As noted earlier, the various types of data (e.g., personal history, adverse events, hospitalization, drug use) have to be linked through a common identifier. It is common in clinical trials to embed some intelligence into that identifier, such as SSN, initials, or site identifiers. While this may make sense for a closed system, it raises privacy concerns. (Privacy issues are covered in detail in Chapter 6.) The best identifier is one that not only is unique but has no embedded personal identification, unless that information is scrambled and the key for unscrambling is stored remotely and securely. The group operating the registry should have a process by which each new entry to the registry is assigned a unique code and there is a crosswalk file(s) to enable the system to append this identifier to all new data as they are accrued. The crosswalk file should not be

83

accessible by persons or entities outside the management group.

In addition, consideration should be given to the fact that a registry may need to accept and link data sets from more than one outside organization. Each institution contributing data to the registry will have unique requirements for patient data, access, privacy, and duration of use. While having identical agreements with all institutions would be ideal, this may not always be possible from a practical perspective. Yet all registries have resource constraints, and decisions about including certain institutions have to be determined based on the resources available to negotiate specialized agreements or to maintain specialized requirements. To the extent that some variability is allowed, agreements should be coordinated as much as possible so that the function of the registry is not greatly impaired. All organizations participating in the registry should have a common understanding of the rules regarding access to the data. Although exceptions can be made, it should be agreed that access to data will be based on independent assessment of research protocols and that participating organizations will not have veto power over access.

When data from secondary sources are utilized, agreements should specify ownership of the source data and clearly permit data use by the recipient registry. The agreements should also specify the roles of each institution, its legal responsibilities, and any oversight issues. It is critical that these issues and agreements be put in place before data are transferred so that there are no ambiguities or unforeseen restrictions on the recipient registry later on.

When incorporating other data sources, consideration should also be given to the registry update schedule. (See Case Example 13.) A mature registry will usually have a mix of data update schedules. The registry may receive an annual update of large amounts of data, or there could be monthly, weekly, or even daily transfers of data. Regardless of the schedule of data transfer, routine data checks should be in place to ensure proper transfer of data. These should include simple counts of records as well as predefined distributions of key variables. Conference calls or even routine meetings to go over recent transfers will help avoid mistakes that might not otherwise be picked up until much later. An example of the need for regular communication is a situation that arose with the United Network for Organ Sharing (UNOS) data a few years ago. UNOS changed the coding for donor type in their transplant records. This resulted in an apparent 100-percent loss of living donors in a calendar year. This was not conveyed to USRDS and was not detected by USRDS staff. Standard analysis files that had been sent to researchers with the errors had to be replaced.

Summary

In summary, a registry is not a static enterprise. The management of registry data sources requires attention to detail, constant feedback to all participants, and a willingness to make adjustments to the operation as dictated by changing times.

Case Example 13: Incorporating Data From Multiple Sources

Description	The Registry of Liver Diseases provides a repository of patients with the most common liver diseases. The registry was initially designed to facilitate clinical research by providing information on the availability of clinical subjects and to help identify and recruit subjects. As the Registry has gathered data, it has expanded its purpose to include providing a natural history of the diseases.
Sponsor	Roche Pharmaceutical (seed funding)
Year Started	2004
Year Ended	Ongoing
No. of Sites	5 academic centers
No. of Records	47,000

Challenge

The registry began as an outgrowth of a homegrown system created by a gastroenterologist. After seeing the possibilities for improving patient care and supporting research, the Liver Institute took on the project of creating a registry that would include data from multiple centers. The project team began by developing a database that was scalable and included privacy protections for the patients. They then assembled an advisory board, which selected the 12 liver diseases to include. The board decided that the registry would collect basic data on all patients, plus specific data on each disease. The registry collects data on patients at multiple visits, creating a picture of the treatment of these chronic diseases over time.

The five centers that were participating in the registry each collected these data already, but they were stored in various systems, and the registry team did not want to ask the sites to re-enter those data in another database. The registry team also wanted to include data from lab reports and images, and they wanted the registry to be a useful tool for participating sites. To meet these various needs, the registry team needed to find a way to integrate data from multiple sources.

Proposed Solution

The team decided to upload data from various systems into the database, thereby creating patient records without asking sites to re-enter data. The initial data uploads included mostly demographic data, and the data came from various sources, ranging from electronic medical record systems to Excel spreadsheets. Once the registry was launched, the team worked with sites to set up regular data uploads. The uploads occur nightly, importing all new data on all patients into the database. While the data stored locally include all patient identifiers, the identifiers are stripped during the upload process, so only de-identified data are in the registry database.

After setting up the upload system for the sites, the team worked on uploading lab data for the patients. The lab data were more challenging, as the Health Level 7 (HL7) format for lab data is complicated. The data were also coming from hospitals, and the team had to coordinate with the hospitals' information technology (IT) departments to set up the data transfers. When the lab data are uploaded to the database, the database compares the header of the lab data file to the records in the database and fills in all data that match. If lab reports come in for a patient who is not in the database, the database creates a record for that patient, assuming that the patient has been referred to the center and the data will be useful.

The team simplified the data transfers from the lab by opting to receive batches on a regular basis. This approach also minimized the IT resources necessary on the hospital side, which made it easier to gain the cooperation of the hospital IT teams.

85

(continued)

Case Example 13: Incorporating Data From Multiple Sources (continued)

Results

The registry has successfully incorporated data from multiple databases on the site level and imported data from five hospital labs to create a registry database of 47,000 records. The database has been used to identify patients for clinical trials, and the team plans to use it for research on the natural history of liver diseases.

Key Point

Incorporating data from existing electronic sources can reduce the burden of data entry on sites and increase the completeness of patient records. However, integrating multiple data sources is a complex task that requires extensive planning, with technical resources and detailed workflow discussions with registry participants. Without national standards for all required data transfers, these efforts may be more achievable in registries with fewer sites.

Chapter 6. Principles of Registry Ethics, Data Ownership, and Privacy

This chapter covers the ethical and legal considerations that should accompany the development and use of all health information registries, including patient registries as defined in this document, for the purposes of public health activities, governmental health program oversight, quality improvement/assurance, and research. These considerations apply generally accepted ethical principles for scientific research involving human subjects to health information registries. Related topics include issues of transparency in the operation of registries, oversight of registry activities, and property rights in health care information and registries. The purpose of this chapter is solely to provide information that will help readers understand the issues, not to provide specific legal opinion or regulatory advice. Legal advisors should always be consulted to address specific issues and to ensure that all applicable Federal, State, and local laws are followed.

In the context of this chapter, "health information" is broadly construed to include any individual patient information created or used by health care providers and insurance plans that relates to a health condition, the provision of health care services, or payment for health care services.[111] As a result, health information may include demographic information and personal characteristics, such as socioeconomic and marital status, the extent of formal education, developmental disability, cognitive capacities, emotional stability, as well as gender, age, and race, all of which may affect health status or health risks. Health information as defined here should be regarded as intimately connected to individual identity, and thus intrinsically private. Typically, health information includes information about family members, so it also can have an impact on the privacy of third parties. Patients widely regard health information as a confidential communication to a health care provider and expect confidentiality to be maintained.

Serious ethical concerns have led to Federal legal requirements for prospective review of registry projects and specific permissions to use health information for research purposes. The creation and use of patient registries for a research purpose ordinarily constitute "research involving human subjects" as defined by regulations applicable to research activities funded by the U.S. Department of Health and Human Services[112] (HHS) and certain other Federal agencies. Moreover, Federal privacy regulations resulting from the Health Insurance Portability and Accountability Act of 1996 (HIPAA)[113] specifically apply to the use and disclosure of certain individually identifiable health information for research purposes.

The term "human subjects" is used throughout this chapter for consistency with applicable Federal law. Some may prefer the term "research participants."

This chapter provides a general guide to Federal legal requirements in the United States. (Legal requirements in other countries may also be relevant and may be different from those in this country, but even a general discussion of the international situation is beyond the scope of this document.) These legal requirements may influence registry decisions involving the selection of data elements and data verification procedures, as well as affect subsequent uses of registry data for secondary research purposes. State laws also may apply to the use of health information for research purposes. The purpose of a registry, the status of its developer, and the extent to which registry data are identifiable largely determine applicable regulatory requirements. Table 8, included at the end of this chapter, provides an overview of the applicable regulatory requirements based on the type of registry developer and the extent to which registry data are identifiable. This chapter reviews the most common of these interactions. The complexity and sophistication of registry structures and operations vary widely, with equally variable processes for obtaining data. Nonetheless, common ethical and legal principles are associated with the creation and use of registries; these commonalities are the focus of this chapter.

Ethical concerns about the conduct of biomedical research, especially research involving the interaction of the clinical research community with their patients and commercial funding agencies, have produced an impetus to make financial and other arrangements more public. The discussion of transparency in this chapter includes recommendations for the public disclosure of registry operations as a means of maintaining public trust and confidence in the use of health information. Reliance on a standing advisory committee is recommended to registry developers as a way to provide expert technical guidance for registry operations and firmly establish the independence of the registry from committed or conflicted interests, as described in Chapter 2. This discussion of transparency in methods is not intended to discourage private investments in registries that produce proprietary information in some circumstances. Neither the funding source nor the generation of proprietary information from a registry determines whether a registry achieves the good practices described in this handbook.

Registry developers are likely to encounter licensing requirements, including processing and use fees, in obtaining health and claims information. Health care providers and plans have plausible claims of ownership to health and claims information, although the public response to these claims has not been tested. Registry developers should anticipate negotiating access to health and claims information, especially when it is maintained in electronic form. The processes for use of registry datasets, especially in multiple analyses by different investigators, should be publicly disclosed if the confidentiality protections required for health information are to remain credible.

The next section of this chapter discusses the ethical concerns and considerations involved with the uses of confidential health information in registries. The transformation of ethical concerns into the legal regulation of human subjects research and

individually identifiable health information is then described. After that, an overview is presented of these regulatory requirements and their interactions specifically as they relate to registries. Next, recommendations are made about registry transparency and oversight, based on the need to ensure the independence, integrity, and credibility of biomedical research, while preserving and improving the utility of registry data. In addition, this section discusses property rights in health information and registries.

Ethical Concerns Relating to Health Information Registries

Application of Ethical Principles

The Belmont Report[114] is a summary of the basic principles and guidelines developed to assist in resolving ethical problems in the conduct of research with human subjects. It was the work product of the National Commission for the Protection of Human Subjects of Biomedical and Behavioral Research, which was created by the National Research Act of 1974.[115]

The Belmont Report identifies three fundamental principles for the ethical conduct of scientific research that involves human subjects. These principles are *respect for persons* (as autonomous agents; self-determination), *beneficence* (do good; do no harm; protect from harm), and *justice* (fairness; equitable distribution of benefits and burdens; equal treatment). Together they provide a foundation for the ethical analysis of human subjects research, including the use of health information in registries developed for scientific purposes with a prospect of producing social benefits. These principles are substantively the same as those identified by the Council for International Organizations of Medical Sciences (CIOMS) in its international guidelines for the ethical review of epidemiologic studies.[116] Nevertheless, the application of these principles to specific research activities can result in different conclusions about what comprises the ethical design and conduct of the research in question. These different conclusions frequently occur because the principles are assigned different values and relative importance by the person performing the ethical analysis. In most of these situations, however, a generally supported, consensus position on the ethical design and conduct of the research is a desirable and achievable goal. This goal does not preclude reanalysis as social norms or concerns about research activities change over time in response to new technologies or persistent ethical questioning.

The ethical principle of *respect for persons* supports the practice of obtaining individuals' consent to the use of their health information for research purposes that are unrelated to the clinical and insurance reasons for creating it. In connection with research registries, consent may have multiple components: (1) consent to registry creation by the compilation of patient information; (2) consent to the initial research purpose and uses of registry data; and (3) consent to subsequent use of registry data by the registry developer or others for the same or different research purposes. The consent process should adequately describe registry purposes and operations to inform potential subjects' decisions about participation in a research registry. In some defined circumstances, the principle of *respect for persons* may be subordinate to other ethical principles and values, with the result that an explicit consent process for participation in the registry may not be necessary. A waiver of informed consent requirements may apply to the registry and be ethically acceptable. (See discussion of waivers of informed consent requirements in this chapter's section "Potential for Individual Patient Identification.") In these situations, alternatives to an explicit consent process for each individual contributing health information to the registry may be adequate (e.g., readily accessible, publicly available information about registry activities).

A general ethical requirement for consent clearly implies that human subjects voluntarily permit the use of their health information in a registry unless a specific exception to voluntary participation applies to the registry. One such exception is a legally mandated, public health justification for the

compilation of health information (e.g., certain infectious disease reporting). Voluntary agreement to the use of health information in a registry necessarily allows a subsequent decision to discontinue participation. Any inability to withdraw information from the registry (e.g., once incorporation into aggregated data has occurred) should be clearly communicated in the consent process as a condition of initial participation. The consent process should also include instructions about the procedures for withdrawal at any time from participation in the registry unless a waiver of consent applies to the registry. Incentives for registry use of health information (e.g., insurance coverage of payments for health care services) should be carefully evaluated for undue influence on both the individuals whose health information is sought for registry projects and the health care providers of those services.[117,118]

Conflicts of interest may also result in undue influence on patients and compromise voluntary participation. One potential source of conflict widely identified with clinical research is the use of recruitment incentives paid by funding agencies to health care providers.[119] Some professional societies and research organizations have developed positions on recruitment incentives. Many entities have characterized incentives that are significantly beyond fair market value for the work performed by the health care provider as unethical; others require disclosure to research subjects of any conflicting interest, financial or otherwise.[120] Research organizations, particularly grantees of Federal research funding, may have systematic processes that registry developers can rely on for managing employee conflicts of interest. Nonetheless, in their planning, registry developers should specify and implement recruitment practices that protect patients against inappropriate influences.

Further considerations in applying the principle of *respect for persons* to the research use of health information generate ethical concerns about preserving the privacy and dignity of patients and about protecting the confidentiality of health information. These concerns have intensified as health care services, third-party payment, and health information systems have become more complex. Legal standards for the use and disclosure of health information have replaced professional and cultural norms for handling individually identifiable health information. Nonetheless, depending on the particular health condition or population of interest, safeguards for the confidentiality of registry data beyond applicable legal requirements may be ethically necessary to protect the privacy and dignity of those individuals contributing health information to the registry.

The principle of *beneficence* ethically obligates developers of health information registries for research purposes to minimize potential harms to the individuals or groups[121] whose health information is included in the registry. There are usually no apparent benefits for offsetting harms to individuals or groups whose health information is used in the registry. Exceptions to this arise when the registry is designed to provide benefits to the human subjects, ranging from longitudinal reports on treatment effects or health status to quality-of-care reports. Risks to privacy and dignity are minimized by conscientious protection of the confidentiality of the health information included in the registry[122] through the use of appropriate physical, technical, and administrative safeguards for data in the operations of the registry. These safeguards should also control access to registry data, including access to individual identifiers that may be included in registry data. Minimization of risks also requires a precise determination of what information is necessary for the research purposes of the registry.

In an analysis applying the principle of *beneficence*, research involving human subjects that is unlikely to produce valid scientific information is unethical. This conclusion is based on the lack of social benefit to offset even minimal risks imposed by the research on participating individuals. Health information registries should incorporate an appropriate design (including, where appropriate, calculation of the patient sample as described in Chapter 3) and data elements, written operating procedures, and documented methodologies, as necessary, to assure the achievement of their scientific purpose.[123]

Certain populations of patients may be vulnerable to social, economic, or psychological harms as a result of a stigmatizing health condition. Developers of registries compiling this health information must make special efforts to protect the identities of the human subjects contributing data to the registry. Pediatric and adolescent populations generate particular ethical concern because of a potential for lifelong discrimination that may effectively exclude them from educational opportunities and other social benefits (e.g., health care insurance).[124]

An ethical analysis employing the principle of *justice* also yields candid recognition of the potential risks to those who contribute health information to a registry and the probable lack of benefit to those individuals (except in the cases where registries are specifically constructed to provide benefit to those individuals). The imbalance of burden and benefit to individuals, which is an issue of distributive justice, emphasizes the need to minimize the risks from registry use of health information. Reasonably precise and well-developed scientific reasons for inclusion (or exclusion) of defined health information in a registry contribute to making the research participation burden fair.

The above analysis refers to research activities. However, the ethical concerns expressed also may apply to other activities that use the health information of individuals in scientific methodologies solely for nonresearch purposes. Public health, oversight of the delivery of health care services through government programs, and quality improvement/assurance (I/A) activities all can invoke the same set of ethical concerns as research activities about the protection of patient self-determination, privacy, and dignity; maintaining the confidentiality of individually identifiable health information to avoid potential socioeconomic harms; and imposing a risk of harm on some individuals to the benefit of others not at risk. In the past, different assignments of social value to these activities and different potential for the social benefits and harms they produce created different levels of social acceptance and formal oversight for these activities than for research. Nonetheless, these activities may include a research component in

90

addition to their ostensible and customary objectives, which reinforces the ethical concerns discussed above and produces additional concerns about compliance with the legal requirements for research activities. Registry developers should give careful prospective scrutiny to the proposed purposes for and activities of a registry in consultation with appropriate institutional officials to avoid both ethical and compliance issues that may undermine achievement of the registry's objectives.

Registry developers must also consider confidentiality protections for the identity of the health care providers, at the level of both individual professionals and institutions, and the health care insurance plans from which they obtain registry data. Information about health care providers and insurance plans can also identify certain patient populations and, in rare circumstances, individual patients. Moreover, the objectives of any registry, broadly speaking, are to enhance the value of the health care services received, not to undermine the credibility and thus the effectiveness of health care providers and insurance plans in their communities. Developers of registries created for public health investigations, health system oversight activities, and quality I/A initiatives to monitor compliance with recognized clinical standards must consider and implement confidentiality safeguards for the identity of service professionals and institutions.

Transformation of Ethical Concerns Into Legal Requirements

Important ethical concerns about the creation, maintenance, and use of patient registries for research purposes involve risks of harm to the human subjects from inappropriate access to registry data and inappropriate use of the compiled health information. These concerns recognize public expectations of confidentiality for health information and the importance of that confidentiality in preserving the privacy and dignity of individual patients.

Over the last decade, two rapid technological developments intensified these ethical concerns. One of these advances was DNA sequencing, replication, recombination, and the concomitant application of this technology to biomedical research activities in human genetics. The other advance was the rapid development of electronic information processing as applied to the management of health information. Widespread anticipation of potential social benefits produced by biomedical research as a result of these technologies was accompanied by ethical concerns about the potential for dignity, economic, social, or psychological harms to the individuals or related third parties.

In addition to specific ethical concerns about the effect of technological advances in biomedical research, general social concerns about the privacy of patient information accompanied the advance of health information systems technology and communications. These social concerns produced legal protections, first in Europe and later in the United States. The discussion below about legal protections for the privacy of health information focuses solely on U.S. law. Health information is also legally protected in European and some other countries by distinctly different and even more complex rules, none of which are discussed in this chapter. If registry developers intend to obtain health information from outside of the United States, they should consult legal counsel early in the registry planning process for the necessary assistance.

The Common Rule. The analysis in the Belmont Report on the ethical conduct of human subjects research eventually resulted in a uniform set of regulations from the Federal agencies that fund such research known as the "Common Rule."[125,126] The legal requirements of the Common Rule apply to research involving human subjects that is conducted or supported by the 17 Federal departments and agencies that adopted it. (Some of these agencies may require additional legal protections for human subjects. The Department of Health and Human Services regulations will be used for all following references to the Common Rule.) Among these requirements is a formal, written agreement from each institution engaged in such research to comply with the Common Rule. For human subjects research conducted or supported by most of the

Federal entities that apply the Common Rule, the required agreement is called a Federalwide Assurance (FWA).[127] Research institutions may opt in their FWA to apply Common Rule requirements to all human subjects research activities conducted within their facilities or by their employees and agents, regardless of the source of funding. The application of Common Rule requirements to a particular registry depends on the institutional context of the registry developer, relevant institutional policies, and whether the health information contributed to the registry maintains patient identifiers.

The Office for Human Research Protections (OHRP) administers the regulation of human subjects research conducted or supported by HHS. Guidance published by OHRP discusses research use of identifiable health information. This guidance makes clear that OHRP considers the creation of health information registries for research purposes containing individually identifiable private information to be human subjects research for the institutions subject to its jurisdiction.[128] In "Research Transparency, Oversight, and Ownership," the applicability of the Common Rule to research registries is discussed in more detail.

Regulations for human subjects protection require prospective review and approval of the research by an institutional review board (IRB) and the informed consent (usually written) of each of the human subjects involved in the research unless an IRB expressly grants a waiver of informed consent requirements.[129] (See Case Example 14.) A research project must satisfy certain regulatory conditions to obtain IRB approval of a waiver of the informed consent requirements. (See "Potential for Individual Patient Identification" for discussion of waivers of informed consent requirements.) A registry plan is the research "protocol" reviewed by the IRB. At a minimum, the protocol should identify (1) the research purpose of a health information registry, (2) detailed arrangements for obtaining informed consent or detailed justifications for not obtaining informed consent to collect health information, and (3) appropriate safeguards for protecting the confidentiality of registry data, in addition to any

---

Case Example 14: Considering the Institutional Review Board Process During Registry Design

Description	The National Oncologic PET Registry (NOPR) collects data to assess the impact of positron emission tomography with F-18 fluorodeoxyglucose (PET) on cancer patient management. The registry was designed to meet the Centers for Medicare & Medicaid Services (CMS) data submission requirements for expanded coverage for new indications and additional cancers.
Sponsor	Academy of Molecular Imaging (AMI), managed by American College of Radiology (ACR) through the American College of Radiology Imaging Network (ACRIN)
Year Started	2006
Year Ended	Ongoing
No. of Sites	Began accepting registrations in late 2005
No. of Patients	Began accepting patients in 2006

Challenge

The NOPR is one of the first examples of CMS's new coverage with evidence development (CED) approach. For the expanded coverage of PET for cancer, the agency required the collection of prospective clinical and demographic data. From the beginning, the organizations developing the registry understood the need to define the requirements for institutional review board (IRB) approval and informed consent. They were uncertain, however, about how Department of Health and Human Services (HHS) regulations for the protection of human research subjects, including IRB requirements, would apply to the planned registry. Implementing NOPR required ACR and AMI, in conjunction with CMS and

(continued)

Case Example 14: Considering the Institutional Review Board Process During Registry Design (continued)

HHS's Office for Human Research Protections (OHRP), to resolve these issues.

Based on their initial assessment of the registry, as well as discussions with CMS, the sponsors believed that the registry was not subject to IRB approval because it was "conducted by or subject to the approval of Department or Agency heads" for the purpose of evaluating a "public benefits or services program." The ACR IRB likewise judged upon review of the proposal that the registry qualified for the "public benefits" exemption. Several IRBs at institutions planning to participate in the registry reached the same conclusion. Accordingly, the registry's original design did not include a provision for obtaining IRB approval or patient consent. However, 1 week before the registry was to begin operation, registry investigators and CMS staff received an email from OHRP rejecting that interpretation on the grounds that the purpose of the registry was not only to evaluate Medicare coverage policy but also to generate clinical data that would potentially affect patient management. OHRP's decision raised the prospect that each of the hundreds of participating hospitals and freestanding PET facilities would be required to obtain approval from its own IRB (or a commercial IRB)—a process that would have been administratively cumbersome, expensive, and very time consuming. The registry investigators suspended the launch and, in consultation with several IRB Chairs, CMS, and other HHS staff, sought to develop an alternative approach.

Proposed Solution

The issue was ultimately resolved only when registry investigators and IRB Chairs from Duke University, Washington University, and ACR spoke directly with OHRP. The parties reached consensus that ACR, the institution operating the registry, was the only entity engaged in research, and that the registry therefore needed to be approved only by a single IRB designated under ACR's Federalwide Assurance (FWA). This plan reflects guidance under development at OHRP, and likely could not have been devised without the help of that agency.

The ACR IRB has since approved the use of data collected by the registry for research purposes based on this model.

Results

Under this approach, individual PET facilities and referring physicians do not have to obtain IRB approval in order to submit data to the registry, thus avoiding the waste and redundancy of requiring parallel action by hundreds of individual IRBs. Both patients and referring physicians are considered research subjects, however, and must therefore provide informed consent before their data can be used for research. With the guidance of OHRP, registry investigators also developed a rationale for waiver of written consent. Either before or upon arrival at a PET facility, each patient receives a standard registry information document, describing the registry and requesting that the patient provide oral consent for the use of his or her identified data for research purposes. Consent from the referring physician, who also receives a standard registry information sheet, is recorded on one of the two data collection forms the physician must complete. If either the patient or the referring physician withholds consent, the identified data are still collected by the PET facility, sent electronically to the registry, and then submitted to CMS for the purpose of determining payment; however, the data will not be used for research. In such cases, CMS nevertheless pays for the PET scan.

Key Point

Even when the primary purpose of a medical data registry is to evaluate Medicare payment policy, its implementation necessarily involves a host of issues related to protecting the subjects whose data will be used. It is essential to address these issues early, so that appropriate systems and procedures can be incorporated into the design of the registry. Additionally, if the institution operating the registry is the only entity engaged in research, then the registry needs to be approved only by a single IRB designated under that institution's FWA.

other information required by the IRB on the risks and benefits of the research.[130]

As noted previously, for human subjects research conducted or supported by most Federal departments and agencies that have adopted the Common Rule, an FWA satisfies the requirement for an approved assurance of compliance. Some research organizations extend the application of their FWA to all research, regardless of the funding source. Under these circumstances, any patient information registry created and maintained within the organization may be subject to the Common Rule. In addition, some research organizations have explicit institutional policies and procedures that require IRB review and approval of all human subjects research.

The Privacy Rule. In the United States, the Health Insurance Portability and Accountability Act of 1996 and its implementing regulations[131] (here collectively called the Privacy Rule) created legal protections for the privacy of individually identifiable health information created and maintained by so-called "covered entities." Covered entities are health care providers that engage in certain financial and administrative health care transactions electronically, health plans, and health care clearinghouses.[132] For the purposes of this chapter, the relevant entities are covered health care providers and health care insurance plans, which may include individual health care providers (e.g., a physician, pharmacist, or physical therapist). The discussion in this chapter *assumes* the data sources for registries are "covered entities" to which the Privacy Rule applies. In the unlikely event a registry developer intends to collect and use data from sources that are *not* covered entities under the Privacy Rule, these sources are subject only to applicable State law and accreditation requirements, if any, for patient information.

Although data sources are assumed to be subject to the Privacy Rule, registry developers and the associated institutions where the registry will reside may not be. Notably, the Privacy Rule does *not apply* to registries that reside outside of a covered entity. Within academic medical centers, for example, registry developers may be associated with units that are outside of the institutional health care component to which the Privacy Rule applies, such as a biostatistics or economics department. But because many, if not virtually all, data sources for registries are covered entities, registry developers are likely to find themselves deeply enmeshed in the Privacy Rule. This involvement may occur with noncovered entities as well—for instance, as a result of business practices developed in response to the Privacy Rule. In addition, the formal agreements required by the Privacy Rule in certain circumstances in order to access, process, manage, and use certain forms of patient information impose continuing conditions of use that are legally enforceable by data sources under contract law. Therefore, registry developers should become cognizant of the patient privacy considerations confronting their likely data sources and should consider following certain Privacy Rule procedures, necessary or not, for reasons of solidarity with those data sources.

In general, the Privacy Rule defines the circumstances under which health care providers and insurance plans (covered entities) may use and disclose patient information for a variety of purposes, including research. Existing State laws protecting the confidentiality of health information that are contrary to the Privacy Rule are preempted unless the State law is more protective (which it may be).[133] The Privacy Rule regulates the use of identifiable patient information within health care providers and insurance plans and the *disclosure* of patient information to others outside of the institution that creates and maintains the information.[134] The initial collection of registry data from covered entities is subject to specific Privacy Rule procedures, depending on the registry's purpose, whether the registry resides within a covered entity or outside of a covered entity, and the extent to which the patient information identifies individuals. The health care providers or insurance plans that create, use, and disclose patient information for clinical use or business purposes are subject to civil and criminal liability for violations of the Privacy Rule.

94

Registry developers should be sufficiently knowledgeable about the Privacy Rule to facilitate the necessary processes for their data sources. They should expect this assistance to involve interactions with clinicians, the Privacy Officer, the IRB or Privacy Board staff, health information system representatives, legal counsel, compliance officials, and contracting personnel.

Subsequent use and sharing of registry data may be affected by the regulatory conditions that apply to initial collection, as well as by new ethical concerns and legal issues. The Privacy Rule created multiple pathways by which registries can compile and use patient information. To use or share compiled registry data for research purposes, a registry developer may need to employ several of these pathways sequentially and satisfy the regulatory requirements of each pathway. For instance, a registry within a covered entity may arrange to obtain written documentation of an authorization required by the Privacy Rule from each patient contributing identifiable information to a registry for a particular research project, such as the relationship between hypertension and Alzheimer's disease. If the registry then seeks to make a subsequent use of the data for another research purpose, it may do so if it uses another permission in the Privacy Rule—for example, by obtaining additional patient authorizations or first de-identifying the data to Privacy Rule standards.

The authors recommend that registry developers plan a detailed tracking system, based on the extent to which registry data remain identifiable for individual patients, for the collection, uses, and disclosures of registry data. The tracking system should produce comprehensive documentation of compliance with both Privacy Rule requirements and legally binding contractual obligations to data sources.

The Privacy Rule defines research as "a systematic investigation, including research development, testing, and evaluation, designed to develop or contribute to generalizable knowledge."[135] Commentary by HHS to the Privacy Rule explicitly includes the development (building and maintenance) of a repository or database for future

research purposes within this definition of research.[136] The definition of "research" in the Privacy Rule partially restates the definition of research in the preexisting Common Rule for the protection of human subjects of the HHS and other Federal agencies.[137] Some implications of this partial restatement of the definition of research are discussed later in this chapter.

Guidance published by the National Institutes of Health (NIH) discusses how the Privacy Rule impacts health services research and research databases and repositories. The NIH guidance identifies the options available to investigators under the Privacy Rule for access to the health information held by health care providers and insurance plans.[138]

In addition to provisions for the use or disclosure of identifiable patient information for research, the Privacy Rule permits health care providers and insurance plans to use or disclose patient information for certain defined public health activities.[139] (See Case Example 15.) The Privacy Rule defines a public health authority as "an agency or authority of the United States, a State, a territory, a political subdivision of a State or territory, or an Indian tribe, or a person or entity acting under a grant of authority from or contract with such public agency . . . that is responsible for public health matters as part of its official mandate."[140] The Centers for Disease Control and Prevention (CDC) and HHS have jointly published specific guidance on the Privacy Rule for public health activities.[141]

Other Privacy Rule provisions permit the use or disclosure of patient health information as required by other laws.[142]

The privacy protections for patient information created by the Privacy Rule that are generally relevant to registries developed for research purposes include explicit individual patient authorization for the use or disclosure of identifiable information,[143] legally binding agreements for the release of "limited data sets" between health information sources and users,[144] the removal of specified identifiers or statistical certification to achieve de-identification of health information,[145] and an accounting of disclosures to be made

Case Example 15: Using Registries for Public Health Activities	
Description	Immunization registries collect data on vaccinations within a geographic area. The registries consolidate records from multiple sources, provide vaccination reminders, and support public health entities in improving and sustaining high vaccination rates. Many State and local public health agencies use immunization registries to improve and track vaccination rates in their area. The Michigan Childhood Immunization Registry, San Diego Regional Immunization Registry, and Utah Statewide Immunization Information System are three examples of such registries.
Sponsor	Michigan: Healthy Michigan Fund and Medicaid match dollars San Diego: Centers for Disease Control and Prevention (CDC), State of California, County of San Diego Utah: Health plans, Medicaid, State of Utah, CDC
Year Started	Michigan: 1996 San Diego: 1996 Utah: 1995
Year Ended	Michigan: Ongoing San Diego: Ongoing Utah: Ongoing
No. of Sites	Michigan: 2,600 San Diego: 151 Utah: 203
No. of Records	Michigan: 3.3 million San Diego: 560,000 Utah: 1.6 million

Challenge

Children often receive vaccinations from different providers. Because these data are then stored in different locations, it is difficult for new providers to assess a child's vaccination history in order to understand what vaccinations may be needed. This lack of consolidated information impacts both the child's health and, potentially, the health of the community at large, as vaccinations support public health.

Proposed Solution and Results

Immunization registries consolidate vaccination data from multiple caregivers into one central database. From this database, other providers can check the status of a child's vaccinations. Schools can also confirm vaccination records before enrolling a child. With data on what vaccinations a child has received and what shots may be due, the registry can issue reminders to providers. These functions serve the public health purpose of monitoring vaccination status and increasing the number of children who are up to date on all of their vaccinations.

The importance of these public health goals is underscored by the national health objective regarding immunization registries. The objective for 2010 is to increase the proportion of children under the age of 6 who are enrolled in immunization registries to 95 percent. To meet this goal, 37 States have implemented registries that target their entire State. Seven other States have registries that focus on regions within the State.

Three examples of these immunization registries are the Michigan Childhood Immunization Registry (MCIR), the San Diego Regional Immunization Registry (SDIR), and the Utah Statewide Immunization Information System (USIIS). Each of these registries meets the basic needs outlined above. In addition, each registry focuses on a unique challenge in providing vaccinations and uses the registry data and framework to address those issues. The MCIR focuses on integrating health plan data into the registry to create a smooth flow of information.

(continued)

Case Example 15: Using Registries for Public Health Activities (continued)

The SDIR implemented new procedures to improve the quality of vaccinations by identifying potential errors through the registry data. The USIIS has identified and addressed geographic vagaries using the registry data.

The purpose of the MCIR is standard for an immunization registry: to protect communities from vaccine-preventable diseases and to assure that all children in Michigan are appropriately immunized. Data from the registry indicated room for improvement in the area of Medicaid recipient children. To address this gap, the registry added a field for the Medicaid ID number. The Medicaid ID number is updated on a monthly basis, along with information on the child's health plan enrollment. Coverage reports are generated on a monthly basis; children who do not have complete immunization records are identified and lists are distributed to health plans.

Integrating the MCIR with the Medicaid ID number is a key strategy for addressing these deficiencies in child immunization records. It allows providers to verify the age-appropriate immunization status of all Medicaid recipient children, and it allows qualified health plans to more accurately assess their population coverage levels as required for HEDIS (Health plan Employer Data and Information Set) reporting. This integration has enabled the registry to provide clinicians with health plan enrollment data. As a result, providers save time by knowing to which plan to bill the immunizations. The health plan benefits from having a central repository of immunization data for HEDIS reporting. The child benefits from having up-to-date vaccinations.

In San Diego, the registry team focused on a different aspect of immunizations: not only is it important to vaccinate all children, but it is critical to provide the vaccinations on the right schedule. The registry team used the data from the registry to evaluate immunization procedures and identify probable errors. These errors included giving influenza vaccines to infants under 6 months of age, giving PPV23 doses to children under 1 year of age, and giving the Hib vaccine to children 5 and over. By developing and implementing a data quality plan, the registry team was able to identify these types of issues. The team then used registry liaisons to deliver this information to the health care providers.

The SDIR experience demonstrated that reviewing registry data for less than optimal immunization practices is critical to ensuring the adequate immunization coverage of the public. Generating regular reports from the registry is an efficient method of quality assurance review that can quickly identify problem areas to focus on in other quality improvement programs.

Utah also used the data in its registry to identify issues with the immunization practices in the State. In this case, the National Immunization Survey, a yearly assessment of immunization rates for children ages 19-35 months conducted by CDC, indicated that immunization rates had declined significantly in Utah from 2003 to 2004. The rates dropped from 80.4 percent to 75.4 percent. To better understand the drop, Utah turned to the data in USIIS.

The USIIS program developed a strategy to identify where the lowest immunization rates were within the State by utilizing the immunization registry, Geographic Information System software, and digital maps provided by the Utah Automated Geographic Reference Center. Analyses were conducted for each of the 12 local health districts. The results of the analyses showed that the rates of adequately immunized children ranged from 82 percent to 39 percent. Using these data, local health departments determined to focus their efforts and resources on the areas that needed the most improvement.

Key Point

Immunization registries are an example of how a registry can be used to consolidate data from multiple caregivers to achieve a national health objective.

available to patients at their request.[146] In addition, if certain criteria required by the Privacy Rule are satisfied, an IRB or Privacy Board can grant a waiver of individual patient authorization for the use or disclosure of health information in research.[147]

FDA regulations. U.S. Food and Drug Administration (FDA) regulatory requirements for research supporting an application for FDA approval of a product also include protections for human subjects, including specific criteria for protection of privacy and maintaining the confidentiality of research data.[148]

Applicability of regulations to research; multiple-purpose registries. At many institutions, the IRB or the office that provides administrative support for the IRB is the final arbitrator of the activities that constitute human subjects research and thus may itself require IRB review. A registry developer is strongly encouraged to consult his or her organization's IRB early in the registry planning process to avoid delays and revision of documentation for the IRB. Distinctions between research and other activities that apply scientific methodologies are frequently unclear. Such other activities include both public health practice[149] and quality-related investigations.[150] Both the ostensible and secondary purposes of an activity are factors in the determination of whether registry activities constitute research subject to the Common Rule. As interpreted by OHRP, if any secondary purpose of an activity is research, then the activity should be considered research.[151] This OHRP interpretation of research purpose differs from that of the Privacy Rule where quality-related studies performed by health care providers and insurance plans are concerned. Under the Privacy Rule, only if the *primary* purpose of a quality-related activity is to obtain generalizable knowledge do the research provisions of the Privacy Rule apply; otherwise, the Privacy Rule defines the activity as a "health care operation."[152]

Registry developers should rely on their Privacy Officer's and IRB's experience and resources in defining research and other activities for their institutions and determining which activities require IRB review as research. In response to accreditation standards, inpatient facilities typically maintain standing departmental (e.g., pediatrics) or service (e.g., pharmacy or nursing) committees to direct, review, and analyze quality-related activities. Some physician groups also establish and maintain quality-related programs, because good clinical practice includes ongoing evaluation of any substantive changes to the standard of care. These institutional quality committees can provide guidance on the activities that usually fall within their purview. Similarly, public health agencies typically maintain systematic review processes for identifying the activities that fit within their legal authority.

As briefly mentioned previously, use of registry data for multiple research purposes may entail obtaining additional permissions from patients or satisfying different regulatory requirements for each research purpose. Standard confidentiality protections for registry data include requirements for physical, technical, and administrative safeguards to be incorporated into plans for a registry. In some instances, an IRB may not consider legally required protections for the research use of patient information sufficient to address relevant ethical concerns, including the protections of the Privacy Rule that may be applicable to registries created and maintained within health care providers and insurance plans as covered entities. For example, information about certain conditions (such as alcoholism or HIV-positive status) and certain populations (such as children) may present an unusual potential for harm from social stigma and discrimination. Under these circumstances, the IRB can make its approval of a registry plan contingent on additional safeguards that it determines are necessary to minimize the risks to individuals contributing health information to the registry.

98

Applicable Regulations

This section describes the specific applicability of the Common Rule[153] and the Privacy Rule[154] to the creation and use of health information registries.

The discussion in this chapter assumes three general models for health information registries. One model is the creation of a registry containing the contact, demographic, and diagnostic or exposure information of potential research subjects who will be individually notified about projects in which they may be eligible to participate. The notification process permits the registry to shield registry participants from an inordinate number of invitations to participate in research projects, as well as to protect privacy. This model is particularly applicable to patients with unusual conditions, patients who constitute a vulnerable population,[155] or both (e.g., children with a rare condition). A second model is the creation of a registry and all subsequent research use of registry data by the same group of investigators. No disclosures of registry data will occur and all research activities have the same scientific purpose. This model applies in general to quality-related investigations of a clinical procedure or service. A third model is the creation of a registry for an initial, specific purpose by a group of investigators with the express intent to use registry data themselves, as well as to disclose registry data to other investigators for additional related or unrelated scientific purposes. An example of this last model is a registry of health information from patients diagnosed with a condition that has multiple known comorbidities to which registry data can be applied. This third model is most directly applicable to industry-sponsored registries. The American College of Epidemiology encourages the data sharing contemplated in this last registry model.[156] Data sharing enhances the scientific utility of registry data and diminishes the costs of compilation.

A registry developer should try to evaluate how the regulations apply to each of these models. Registry developers are strongly encouraged to consult with their organization's Privacy Officer and IRB or Privacy Board early in the planning process to clarify applicable regulatory requirements and the probable effect of those requirements on considerations of registry design and development.

Public Health, Health Oversight, FDA-Regulated Products

When Federal, State, or municipal public health agencies create registries in the course of public health practice, specific legislation typically authorizes the creation of the registries and regulates data acquisition, maintenance, security, use, and disclosures of registry data for research. Ethical considerations and concerns about maintaining the confidentiality of patient information used by public health authorities are similar to those for research use, but they are explicitly balanced against potential social benefits during the legislative process. Nonetheless, if the registry supports research activities as well as its public health purposes, Common Rule requirements for IRB review may apply to the creation of the registry.

Cancer registries performing public health surveillance activities mandated by State law are well-known exceptions to Common Rule regulation. Secondary uses of public health registry data for research and the creation of registries funded by public health agencies such as the CDC and the Agency for Healthcare Research and Quality (AHRQ) as sponsored research activities may be subject to the Common Rule. The Common Rule's definitions of human subjects research[157] may encompass these activities, which are discussed in the next subsections of this chapter. Not all cancer registries support public health practice alone, even though the registries are the result of governmental programs. For example, the Surveillance Epidemiology and End Results (SEER) program, funded by the National Cancer Institute, operates and maintains a population-based cancer reporting system of multiple registries, including public use data sets with public domain software. SEER program data are used for many research purposes in addition to aiding public health practices.[158]

Disclosures of health information by health care providers and insurance plans for certain defined public health activities are expressly recognized as an exception to Privacy Rule requirements for patient authorization.[159] An example of a public health activity is the practice of surveillance, which monitors and disseminates the distributions and trends of designated risk factors, injuries, or diseases in populations.[160] Health care providers or insurance plans are likely to demand documentation of public health authority for legal review before making any disclosures of health information. Registry developers should obtain this documentation from the agency that funds or enters into a contract for the registry and present it to the health care provider or insurance plan well in advance of data collection efforts.

The Privacy Rule permits uses and disclosures by health care providers and insurance plans for "health oversight activities" authorized by law.[161] These activities include audits and investigations involving the "health care system" and other entities subject to government regulatory programs for which health information is relevant to determining compliance with program standards.[162] The collection of patient information, such as occurrences of decubitus ulceration, from nursing homes that are operating under a compliance agreement with a Federal or State health care program is an example of a health oversight activity.

The Privacy Rule characterizes responsibilities related to the quality, safety, or effectiveness of a product or activity regulated by FDA as public health activities. This public health exception for uses and disclosures of patient information in connection with FDA-regulated products or activities includes adverse event reporting; product tracking; product recalls, repairs, replacement, or look-back; and postmarketing surveillance (e.g., as part of a risk management program that is a condition for approval of an FDA-regulated product).[163]

Research Purpose of Registry

The Common Rule defines "research," and that definition is partially restated in the Privacy Rule. These regulatory definitions affect how the regulatory requirements of each rule are applied to research activities.[164]

In the Common Rule:

> Research means a systematic investigation, including research development, testing and evaluation, designed to develop or contribute to generalizable knowledge. Activities which meet this definition constitute research for purposes of this policy, whether or not they are conducted or supported under a program which is considered research for other purposes. For example, some demonstration and service programs may include research activities.[165]

OHRP interprets the Common Rule definition of research to include activities having *any* research purpose, no matter what the ostensible objective of the activity may be. Compliance with Common Rule requirements depends on the nature of the organization where the registry resides. If an organization receives Federal funding for research, then it is likely that Common Rule requirements apply.

The Privacy Rule's definition of research[166] restates the first sentence of the Common Rule definition. However, the Privacy Rule distinguishes between research and quality improvement/assurance activities conducted by covered entities,[167] which are defined as "health care operations."[168] As a result, if the *primary* purpose of a quality-related registry maintained by a covered entity is to support a research activity (i.e., to create generalizable knowledge), Privacy Rule requirements for research apply to the use or disclosure of the patient information to create the registry and to subsequent research use of registry data. If, however, the primary purpose is other than to create generalizable knowledge, the study is considered a health care operation of the covered entity and is not subject to Privacy Rule requirements for research activities or patient authorization.

As noted earlier, both public health practice and quality I/A activities can be difficult to distinguish from research activities.[169] The determination of whether a particular registry should be considered as or include a research activity depends on a number of factors, including the nature of the organization where the registry will reside; the employment duties of the people performing the activities associated with the registry; the source of funding for the registry; the original, intended purpose of the registry; the sources of registry data; and whether subsequent uses or disclosures of registry data are likely.

Quality I/A activities entail many of the same ethical concerns about protecting the confidentiality of health information as research activities do. Express consent to quality I/A activities is not the usual practice; instead, the professional and cultural norms of health care providers, both individual and institutional, regulate these activities. Registry developers should consider whether the ethical concerns associated with a proposed quality I/A registry require independent review and the use of special procedures, such as notice to patients. Registry advisory committee members, quality I/A literature,[170] hospital ethics committees, IRB members, and clinical ethicists can make valuable contributions to these decisions.

To avoid surprises and delays, the decision about the nature of the activity that the registry is intended to support should be made prospectively, in consultation with appropriate officials of the funding agency and officials of the organization where the registry will reside. Some research institutions may have policies that either require IRB review for quality I/A activities, especially if publication of the activity is likely, or exclude them from IRB review. Most frequently, IRBs make this determination on a case-by-case basis.

Potential for Individual Patient Identification

The specific regulatory requirements applicable to the use or disclosure of patient information for the creation of a registry to support research depend in part on the extent to which patient information received and maintained by the registry can be attributed to a particular person. Various categories of information, each with a variable potential for identifying individuals, are distinguished in the Privacy Rule: individually identifiable health information, "de-identified" information, and a "limited data set" of information.[171] The latter two categories of information may or may not include a code linked to identifiers.

If applicable, Common Rule requirements affect all research involving patient information that is individually identifiable and obtained by the investigator conducting the research. The definition of "human subject" in the Common Rule is "a living individual about whom an investigator (whether professional or student) conducting research obtains (1) data through intervention or interaction with the individual, or (2) identifiable private information." This regulatory definition further explains:

> Private information includes . . . information which has been provided for specific purposes by an individual and which the individual can reasonably expect will not be made public (for example, a medical record). Private information must be individually identifiable (i.e., the identity of the subject is or may readily be ascertained by the investigator or associated with the information) in order for obtaining the information to constitute research involving human subjects.[172]

In short, the Common Rule definition of "human subject" makes all research use of identifiable patient information subject to its requirements; if the identity of the patients whose information is used for research purposes is *not* readily ascertainable to the investigator, the research is *not* human subjects research to which the Common Rule applies. Moreover, research involving the collection of information from existing records is exempted from the Common Rule if the information is recorded by the investigator in such a manner that subjects cannot be identified, directly or through identifiers (coded link), to the subjects. Registry developers should consult the IRB early in the process of selecting data elements to obtain guidance about whether registry activities constitute human subjects research or may be exempt from Common Rule requirements.

Also among the criteria specified by the Common Rule for IRB approval of research involving human subjects are provisions to protect the privacy of subjects and to maintain the confidentiality of data.[173] In addition, the consent process for research subjects should include explicit information about confidentiality protections for the use of records containing identifiers.[174]

Data collection frequently requires patient identifiers, especially in prospective registries with ongoing data collection, revision, and updates. Secondary or subsequent research use by outside investigators (i.e., those not involved in the original data collection) of patient information containing direct identifiers is complicated, however, because ethical principles for the conduct of human subjects research require that risks, including risks to confidentiality of patient information, be minimized. In addition, the Privacy Rule requires an authorization to specifically describe the purpose of the use or disclosure of patient information. Unless the registry developer sufficiently anticipates the purposes of secondary research, the authorization may not be valid for the use of identifiable registry data for secondary research purposes. The Privacy Rule provides options for the collection and use of health information that is identifiable to a greater or lesser extent; it also contains standards for de-identifying information and creating limited data sets.[175] Nonetheless, use of identifiable health information may be essential to population-based studies and to achieve certain scientific and public health goals.

Direct identifiers generally include a patient's name, initials, contact information, medical record number, and Social Security Number, alone or in combination with other information. As described by the Privacy Rule standard, a limited data set of patient information does not include specified direct identifiers of the patient or the patient's relatives, employer, or household members.[176]

In an electronic environment, masking individual identities is a complex task. Data suppression limits the utility of the information from the registry, and linkage or even triangulation of information can re-identify individuals. A technical assessment of electronic records for their uniqueness within any data set is necessary to minimize the potential for re-identification. In aggregated published data, standard practice assumes that a subgroup size of less than six may also be identifiable, depending on the nature of the data. An evaluation for uniqueness should ensure that the electronic format does not produce a potential for identification greater than this standard practice, even when the information is triangulated within a record or linked with other data files.

If a registry for research, public health, or other purposes will use any of the categories of health information discussed below, a registry developer should consult the IRB, the Privacy Officer, and the institutional policies developed specifically in response to the Privacy Rule early in his or her planning. These consultations should establish the purpose of the registry, the applicability of the Common Rule requirements to registry activities, and the applicability of the Privacy Rule to the collection and use of registry data. In addition, the registry developer should consult a representative of the Information Technology or Health Information System office of *each* health care provider or insurance plan that will be a source of data for the registry to obtain feasibility estimates of data availability and formats, as well as a representative of the IRB or Privacy Board, for *each* data source.

De-identified patient information. The Privacy Rule describes two methods for de-identifying health information.[177] One method requires the removal of certain data elements. The other method requires a qualified statistician to certify that the potential for identifying an individual from the data elements is negligible. A qualified statistician should have "appropriate knowledge of and experience with generally accepted statistical and scientific principles and methods for rendering information not individually identifiable" in order to make this determination.[178] De-identified information may include a code permitting re-identification of the original record by the data source (covered entity).[179] The code may not be derived from information about an individual and should resist translation. In addition, the decoding key must remain solely with the health care provider or plan that is the source of the patient information.[180]

102

Research on existing data in which individual patients cannot be identified directly or indirectly through linked identifiers, does not involve human subjects, as defined by the Common Rule, and thus is not subject to the requirements of the Common Rule.[181] Refer to the discussion later in this chapter.

As a prudent business practice, each health care provider or insurance plan that is a source of de-identified information is likely to require an enforceable legal agreement with the registry developer. It should be signed by an appropriate institutional official on behalf of the registry developer. At a minimum, this agreement will likely contain the following terms, some of which may be negotiable: the identification of the content of the data and the medium for the data; a requirement that the data recipient, and perhaps the health care provider or insurance plan providing the data, make no attempt to identify individual patients; the setting of fees for data processing and data use; limitations on disclosure or further use of the data, if any; and an allocation of the risks of legal liability for any improper use of the data.

Limited data sets of health information. De-identified health information may not suffice to carry out the purposes of a registry, especially if the registry will receive followup information through the monitoring of patients over time or information from multiple sources to compile complete information on a health event (e.g., cancer incidence). Dates of service and geographic location may be crucial to the scientific purposes of the registry or to the integrity and use of the data. Health information provided to the registry without direct identifiers may constitute a limited data set as defined by the Privacy Rule.[182] A health care provider or insurance plan may disclose a limited data set of health information by entering into a data use agreement (DUA) with the recipient. The terms of the DUA should satisfy specific Privacy Rule requirements.[183] Institutional officials for both the data source and the registry developer should sign the DUA so a legal contract results. The DUA establishes the uses of the limited data set permitted by the registry developer (i.e., the creation of the registry and subsequent use of registry data for specified research purposes). The DUA may not authorize the registry developer to use or disclose information in a way that would violate the Privacy Rule if done by the data source.[184]

An investigator who works within a health care provider or insurance plan to which the Privacy Rule applies and that is the source of the health information for a registry may use a limited data set to develop a registry for a research purpose. In these circumstances, the Privacy Rule still requires a DUA that satisfies the requirements of the Privacy Rule between the health care provider or insurance plan and the investigator. This agreement may be in the form of a written confidentiality agreement.[185]

A registry developer may assist a health care provider or insurance plan by creating the limited data set. In some situations, this assistance may be crucial to data access and availability for the registry. In order for the registry developer to create a limited data set on behalf of a data source, the Privacy Rule requires the data source (the covered entity) to enter into a business associate agreement with the registry developer (the business associate) that satisfies certain regulatory criteria.[186] The business associate agreement is a binding legal arrangement that should be signed by appropriate institutional officials on behalf of the data source and registry developer. This agreement contains terms for managing health information that are required by the Privacy Rule and that become a legally binding contract between the data source and data recipient.[187] Most health care providers have developed a standard business associate agreement in response to the Privacy Rule and will likely insist on using it, although it may require some negotiated modifications for the production of registry data.

The registry populated with a limited data set may include a coded link that connects the data back to patient records, provided the link does not replicate part of a direct identifier.[188] The key to the code may allow health information obtained from monitoring patients over time to supplement existing registry data or allow the combination of information from multiple sources.

103

The DUA for a limited data set of health information requires the data recipient to warrant that no attempt will be made to identify the health information with individual patients or contact those patients.[189]

If the registry data obtained by investigators constitute a limited data set and do not contain a coded link to identifiers, then the research would not involve human subjects, as defined by HHS regulations at 45 Code of Federal Regulations (CFR) 46.102(f), and the Common Rule requirements would not apply to the registry.[190] An IRB or an institutional official knowledgeable about the Common Rule requirements should make the determination of whether a research registry involves human subjects; frequently, a special form for this purpose is available from the IRB. The IRB (or institutional official) should provide documentation of its decision to the registry developer.

Direct identifiers: authorization and consent. The Privacy Rule permits the use or disclosure of patient information for research with a valid, written authorization from each patient whose information is disclosed.[191] The Privacy Rule specifies the content of this authorization, which gives permission for a specified use or disclosure of the health information.[192] Health care providers and insurance plans frequently insist on use of the specific authorization form they develop to avoid legal review and potential liability from the use of other forms.

One exception to the requirement for an authorization occurs when a health care provider or insurance plan creates a registry to support its "health care operations."[193] Health care operations specifically include quality I/A activities, outcomes evaluation, and the development of clinical guidelines; however, the Privacy Rule definition of health care operations clearly *excludes* research activities.[194] For example, a hospital registry created to track its patient outcomes against a recognized clinical care standard as a quality improvement initiative has a health care operations purpose. The hospital would not have to obtain an authorization for use of the health information from the patients it tracks in this registry.

Research use of health information containing identifiers constitutes human subjects research as defined by the Common Rule.[195] In general, the Common Rule requires documented, legally effective, voluntary, and informed consent of each research subject.[196]

Documentation of the consent process required by the Common Rule may be combined with the authorization required by the Privacy Rule for disclosure and use of health information.[197] A health care provider or insurance plan may not immediately accept the combination of these forms as a valid authorization; it may insist on legal review of the combination form before permitting disclosure of any health information.

Authorizations for the use or disclosure of health information under the Privacy Rule and informed consent to research participation under the Common Rule should be legally effective—i.e., patients must be legally competent to provide these permissions. Adults, defined in most States as 18 years and over, are presumed legally competent in the absence of a judicially approved guardianship. Children under 18 years old are presumed legally incompetent; a biological, adoptive, or custodial parent or guardian must provide permission on the child's behalf. Registry developers should consult legal counsel about situations in which these presumptions seem inapplicable, such as a registry created to investigate contraceptive drug and device use by adolescents, and to which State law exceptions may exist. (See Case Example 16.)

In addition to being voluntary and legally effective, consent should be informed about the research, including what activities are involved, as well as the expected risks and potential benefits from participation. The Common Rule requires the consent process to include specific elements of information.[198] Registry developers should plan to provide non-English-speaking patients with appropriate resources to assure that the communication of these elements during the consent process is comprehensible. All written information for patients should be translated, or alternatively, arrangements should be made for qualified translators to attend the consent process.

Case Example 16: Issues With Obtaining Informed Consent	
Description	The Registry of the Canadian Stroke Network (RCSN) is a prospective, national registry of stroke patients in Canada. The registry, currently in Phase III, is a non-consent-based registry that collects detailed clinical data on the acute stroke event, from the onset of symptoms, emergency medical service transport, and emergency department care to hospital discharge status. The purposes of the registry are to monitor stroke care delivery, to evaluate the Ontario Stroke System, and to provide a rich clinical database for research.
Sponsor	Canadian Stroke Network, Networks of Centres of Excellence, and Ministry of Health and Long Term Care of Ontario
Year Started	2001
Year Ended	Ongoing
No. of Sites	12 in Phase III (21 sites in Phases 1 and II)
No. of Records	23,886

Challenge

The registry began in 2001 with Phase I, which gathered data from 21 hospitals in Canada. All patients admitted to the hospital or seen in the emergency department with symptoms of acute stroke within 14 days of onset or transient ischemic attack (TIA), as well as those with acute in-hospital stroke, were included in this phase. Research nurse coordinators identified eligible patients through daily reviews of emergency and admission patient lists and approached these patients for consent. Informed patient consent was required for full data collection, linkages to administrative data, and 6-month followup interviews.

Despite the need for informed consent for full data collection, consent was obtained for only 39 percent of eligible patients. Subsequent analyses showed that patients who consented to participate were not representative of the overall stroke population, as they were less likely to have severe or fatal stroke, and also less likely to have minor stroke or TIA.

Phase II of the registry began in 2002, with 21 hospitals and 4 Ontario Telestroke sites. In this phase, all patients admitted to the hospital or seen in the emergency department with symptoms of acute stroke within 14 days of onset or TIA were included. Patients with in-hospital stroke were no longer recruited. In order to standardize workload across the country, a random sample of eligible patients was selected to be approached for consent for full data collection. Consent was obtained on 50 percent of eligible patients.

After obtaining consent of only 39 percent and 50 percent of patients in Phases I and II, the team realized that obtaining written patient consent for participation in the registry on a representative sample of stroke patients was impractical and costly. Patient enrollment threatened the viability and generalizability of the stroke registry. The registry team published these findings in the *New England Journal of Medicine* in April 2004.

Proposed Solution

The registry team approached the Ontario Information and Privacy Commissioner to discuss a non-consent-based registry for Phase III. Because of these discussions, the registry was "prescribed" by the Privacy Commissioner under the Personal Health Information Protection Act, 2004, which allowed the registry to collect data legally on stroke patients without written consent.

(continued)

> **Case Example 16: Issues With Obtaining Informed Consent (continued)**
>
> **Results**
>
> Phase III of the registry includes all patients presenting to emergency departments of the 11 Stroke Centres in Ontario and 1 Stroke Centre in Nova Scotia with a diagnosis of acute stroke or TIA within 14 days of onset. Nurse coordinators identify eligible patients through daily reviews of emergency and admission patient lists. Patients are identified prospectively with retrospective chart review without consent. No followup interviews are done. Because informed consent is not required, the data collected over the past 3 years provide a representative sample of stroke patients in Canada, making the data more viable for use in research and in developing initiatives to improve quality of care.
>
> **Key Point**
>
> The impact of obtaining informed consent should be considered in developing a registry. Requiring that registries obtain the consent of patients with acute medical conditions such as stroke may result in limited selective participation, as it is not possible to obtain consent on all patients. For example, patients who die in the emergency department and patients who have brief hospital visits may be missed. Mechanisms such as obtaining a waiver of informed consent or using the approach outlined in this case may be alternatives.
>
> **For More Information**
>
> Tu JV, Willison DJ, Silver FL et al. The impracticability of obtaining informed consent in the Registry of the Canadian Stroke Network. N Engl J Med 2004 Apr; 350:1414-21.

IRBs may approve waivers for both authorization (for disclosure of patient information for registry use) and consent (to registry participation), provided the research use of health information satisfies certain regulatory conditions. In addition, the Privacy Rule created Privacy Boards specifically to approve waivers of authorization for the research use of health information in organizations without an IRB.[199] Waivers are discussed in detail below.

An important distinction exists between the Common Rule and Privacy Rule concerning the scope of permission to use health information for research purposes. Under the Common Rule, consent for participation in future, unspecified research may be obtained, provided potential subjects receive clear notice during the consent process that this research is intended to occur. For an authorization to be valid under the Privacy Rule, however, the authorization should describe *each* purpose of the use or disclosure of health information.[200]

In certain limited circumstances, research subjects can consent to future unspecified research using their identifiable patient information. The Common Rule permits an IRB-approved consent process to be broader than a specific research project[201] and to include information about research that may be done in the future. In its review of such future research, an IRB subsequently can determine that the previously obtained consent (1) satisfies the regulatory requirements for informed consent or (2) does not satisfy the regulatory requirements for informed consent. If it does not satisfy the regulatory requirement for informed consent, it requires an additional consent process; alternatively, the IRB may grant a waiver of consent, provided the regulatory criteria for waiver are satisfied.

For example, an IRB-approved consent process for the creation of a research registry should include a description of the specific types of research to be conducted using registry data. For any future research that involves identifiable information maintained by the registry, the IRB may determine that the original consent process (for the creation of the research registry) satisfies the applicable regulatory requirements, because the prospect of future research and future research projects were adequately described. The specific details of that future research on registry data may have been unknown when data were collected to create the registry, but the future research may have been sufficiently anticipated and described to satisfy the regulatory requirements for informed consent. For consent to be informed as demanded by the ethical principle of *respect for persons*, however, any description of the nature and purposes of the research should be as specific as possible.

If a registry developer anticipates subsequent research use of identifiable registry data, he or she should request an assessment by the IRB of the description of the research used in the consent process for potential subjects at the time the data are initially collected. Nonetheless, in its review of any subsequent research, an IRB may find it appropriate to require an additional consent process for each research subject or to grant a waiver for obtaining further consent.

The commentary accompanying the publication of the Privacy Rule clearly rejected broadening the description of purpose in authorizations to include future, unspecified research.[202] As a result, the research purpose stated in an original authorization for a registry limits the use of registry data to that purpose.[203] Subsequent use of registry data maintained within a health care provider or insurance plan for a different research purpose requires a new authorization from each individual whose registry data would be involved or an approved waiver of authorization. Alternatively, the use or disclosure of a limited data set or de-identified registry data can occur, provided regulatory criteria are satisfied. Registries maintained by organizations to which the Privacy Rule does *not* apply (e.g., funding agencies for research that are *not* health care providers or insurance plans, professional societies, or non-health-care components of hybrid entities such as universities) are not legally bound by the limited purpose of the original authorization. However, data sources subject to the Privacy Rule are likely to be unwilling to provide patient information without a written agreement with the registry developer that

includes legally enforceable protections against redisclosure of identifiable patient information. A valid authorization contains a warning to patients that their health information may not be protected by Privacy Rule protections in recipient organizations.[204]

Registry developers can request that patients obtain and share copies of their own records from their health care provider or insurance plan. This strategy can be useful for mobile populations, such as elderly retirees who occupy different residences in winter and summer. A Federal privacy law[205] protects the health records of children held by schools from disclosure without explicit parental consent; thus, parents can often obtain copies of these records more easily than investigators. Alternatively, individuals can simply volunteer health information in response to an interview or survey. These collection strategies do not require obtaining a Privacy Rule authorization from each subject; however, IRB review and other requirements of the Common Rule, including careful protections of the confidentiality of registry data, may nonetheless apply to a registry project with a research purpose. Moreover, a registry developer may encounter Privacy Rule requirements for the use or disclosure of patient information by a health care provider or insurance plan for recruitment purposes. For example, a patient authorization or waiver of authorization (discussed below) may be necessary for the disclosure of patient contact information by a health care provider or insurance plan (covered entity) to a registry developer.

Certificates of confidentiality and other privacy protections. Certificates of confidentiality granted by the National Institutes of Health permanently protect identifiable information about research subjects from legally compelled disclosure. Federal law authorizes the Secretary of HHS (whose authority is delegated to NIH) to provide this privacy protection for subjects of biomedical, behavioral, clinical, and other research.[206] Federal funding for the research is not a precondition for obtaining a certificate of confidentiality.[207] An investigator whose research project has been granted a certificate of confidentiality may refuse to disclose identifying information collected for that research even though a valid subpoena exists for the information in a civil, criminal, administrative, or legislative proceeding at the Federal, State, or local level. The protection provided by a certificate of confidentiality is intended to prevent the disclosure of personal information that could result in adverse effects on the social, economic, employment, or insurance status of a research subject.[208] Detailed information about certificates of confidentiality is available on the NIH Web site.[209]

The grant of a certificate of confidentiality to a research project, however, is not intended to affect State laws requiring health care and other professionals to report certain conditions to State officials, such as designated communicable diseases, neglect and abuse of children and the elderly, or threatened violent harm. If investigators are mandatory reporters under State law, in general they continue to have a legal obligation to make these reports.[210] In addition, other legal limitations to the privacy protection provided by certificates of confidentiality exist and may be relevant to particular research projects. Information on the NIH Web site describes some of these other legal limitations.[211]

Registry developers should also be aware that Federal law provides specific confidentiality protections for the identifiable information of patients in drug abuse and alcoholism treatment programs that receive Federal funding.[212] These programs may disclose identifiable information about their patients for research activities only with the documented approval of the program director.[213] The basis for the director's approval is receipt of written assurances about the qualifications of the investigator to conduct the research, the confidentiality safeguards incorporated into the research protocol, and no further disclosure of identifying information by the investigator. Moreover, an independent review of the research project should determine and verify in writing that the protocol provides adequate protection of the rights and welfare of the patients and that the benefits of the research outweigh any risks to

patients.[214] Prior to submitting proposed consent documentation to an IRB, registry developers should consult legal counsel for important information about the limitations of these confidentiality protections.

As a condition of approval, IRBs frequently require investigators to obtain a certificate of confidentiality for research involving information about substance abuse or other illegal activities (e.g., underage purchase of tobacco products), sexual attitudes and practices, and genetic information. Registry developers should consult legal counsel to determine if and how the limitations of a certificate of confidentiality may affect privacy protection planning for registry data. In all circumstances, the consent process should communicate clear notice to research subjects about the extent of privacy protections they may expect for their health information when it is incorporated into a registry.

In the absence of a certificate of confidentiality, a valid subpoena or court order for registry data will usually compel disclosure of the data unless State law specifically protects the confidentiality of data. For example, Louisiana's laws specifically protect the collection of information on tobacco use from subpoena.[215] On the other hand, a subpoena or court order may supersede State law confidentiality protections. These legal instruments can be challenged in the court having jurisdiction for the underlying legal proceeding. In some circumstances, research institutions may be willing to pursue such a challenge. The remote yet definite possibility of this sort of disclosure should be clearly communicated to research subjects as a limitation on confidentiality protections during the consent process and in an authorization for use or disclosure of patient information.

State law may assure the confidentiality of certain quality I/A activities performed by health care providers as peer review activities.[216] When State law protects the confidentiality of peer review activities, generally it is implementing public policy that encourages internal activities and initiatives by health care providers to improve health care services by reducing the risks of medical errors and systematic failures. Protection by peer review statutes may limit the use of data generated by quality I/A activities for any other purposes.

Waivers and alterations of authorization and consent. As mentioned above, the Privacy Rule authorizes Privacy Boards and IRBs to sometimes waive or alter authorizations by individual patients for the disclosure or use of health information for research purposes. In addition, the Common Rule authorizes IRBs to waive or alter the consent process. The Privacy Rule and the Common Rule each specify the criteria under which waivers or alterations of authorization and the consent process are permitted.[217] The potential risks to patients participating in the registry resulting from these waivers of permission differ. A waiver of authorization potentially imposes the risk of a loss of confidentiality and consequent invasion of privacy. A waiver of consent potentially imposes risks of harm from the loss of self-determination, dignity, and privacy expected under the ethical principles of *respect for persons* and *beneficence*. Acknowledging these potential risks, regulatory criteria for waiver and alterations require an IRB or Privacy Board to determine that risks are minimal. This determination is a necessary condition for approval of an investigator's request for a waiver or alteration of these permissions.

The following discussion refers only to waivers; registry developers should note that Privacy Boards and IRBs may approve alterations to authorizations or the consent process, provided a requested alteration satisfies *all* the same criteria required for a waiver by the Privacy Rule or Common Rule. Alterations are generally preferable to waivers in an ethical analysis based on the principle of *respect for persons*, because they acknowledge the importance of self-determination. In requesting alterations to an authorization or to the consent process, registry developers should be prepared to justify each proposed change or elimination of required elements. Plausible justifications include a registry to which a specific element does not apply or a registry in which one element contradicts other required information in the authorization or consent documentation. The justifications for alterations

should relate as specifically and directly as possible to the regulatory criteria for IRB or Privacy Board approval of waivers and alterations.

The Privacy Rule authorizes an IRB or Privacy Board to approve a waiver of authorization if the following criteria are met: (1) the use or disclosure involves no more than minimal risk to the privacy of individuals; (2) the research cannot be practicably conducted without the waiver; and (3) the research cannot be practicably conducted without access to and use of health information. The determination of minimal risk to privacy includes several elements: an adequate plan to protect identifiers from improper use or disclosure; an adequate plan to destroy identifiers, unless a health or research justification exists to retain them; and adequate written assurances that the health information will not be reused or disclosed to others, except as required by law, as necessary for oversight of the research, or as permitted by the Privacy Rule for other research.[218] The Privacy Board or IRB should provide detailed documentation of its decision for presentation to the health care provider or insurance plan (covered entity) that is the source of the health information for registry data.[219] The documentation should clearly communicate that each of the criteria for a waiver required by the Privacy Rule has been satisfied.[220] The Privacy Board or IRB documentation should also provide a description of the health information it determined necessary to the conduct of the research and the procedure it used to approve the waiver.[221] A health care provider or insurance plan may insist on legal review of this documentation before permitting the disclosure of any health information.

The criteria for a waiver of consent in the Common Rule are similar to those for a waiver of authorization under the Privacy Rule. An IRB should determine that: (1) the research involves no more than minimal risk to subjects; (2) the waiver will not adversely affect the rights and welfare of subjects; (3) the research cannot practicably be carried out without a waiver; and (4) whenever appropriate, subjects will be provided with additional information after participation.[222] The criterion for additional information can be satisfied at least in part by public disclosure of the purposes, procedures, and operations of a registry, as discussed later in "Registry Transparency."

Some IRBs produce guidance about what justifications constitute "not practicable" and the circumstances in which these justifications apply. For population-based research projects, registry developers may also present the scientific justification of avoiding selection bias. A waiver permits the registry to include the health information of all patients who are eligible. An IRB may also agree to consider requests for a limited waiver of consent that applies only to those individuals who decline use of their health information in a registry project. This limited waiver of consent most often permits the collection of de-identified and specified information sufficient to characterize this particular population.

An important difference between the Common Rule and FDA regulations for the protection of human subjects involves consent to research participation. The FDA regulations require consent, except for emergency treatment or research, and do not permit the waiver or alteration of informed consent.[223] If registry data are intended to support the labeling of an FDA-regulated product, a registry developer should plan to obtain the documented, legally effective, voluntary, and informed consent of each individual whose health information is included in the registry.

The Privacy Rule creates a legal right for patients, by request, to receive an accounting of certain disclosures of their health information that are made by health care providers and insurance plans.[224] The accounting must include disclosures that occur with a waiver of authorization approved by a Privacy Board or IRB. The Privacy Rule specifies the information that an accounting should contain[225] and requires it to cover a 6-year period or any requested shorter period of time.[226] If multiple disclosures are made to the same recipient for a single purpose, including a research purpose, a summary of these disclosures may be made. In addition, because most waivers of authorization cover records of many individuals, and thus an individualized accounting in such circumstances may be burdensome, the Privacy

Rule provides that if the covered entity has disclosed the records of 50 or more individuals for a particular research purpose, the covered entity may provide to the requestor a more general accounting, which lists the research protocols for which the requestor's information may have been disclosed, among other items.[227]

The Common Rule permits an IRB to waive documentation of the consent process under two different sets of regulatory criteria. The first set of conditions for approval of this limited waiver require that the only record linking an individual subject to the research is the consent document; the principal risk to subjects is the potential harm from a breach of confidentiality; *and* each subject individually determines whether his or her consent should be documented.[228] Alternatively, an IRB can waive documentation of consent if the research involves no more than minimal risk of harm to subjects *and* no procedures for which written consent is normally obtained outside of a research context.[229] For either set of regulatory criteria, the IRB may require the investigator to provide subjects with written information about the research activities in which they participate.[230] The written information may be as simple as a statement of research purposes and activities or more elaborate, such as a Web site for regularly updated information describing progress on the research project.

Summary of Regulatory Requirements

The use and disclosure of health information by health care providers and insurance plans for research purposes, including registries, *are assumed* by the authors of this chapter to be subject to regulation under the Privacy Rule and *may be* subject to the Common Rule.

In general, the Privacy Rule permits the use or disclosure of patient information for a registry, subject to specific conditions, in the following circumstances: (1) registries serving public health activities, including registries developed in connection with FDA-regulated products; (2) registries developed for the health care operations of health care providers and insurance plans (covered entities), such as quality I/A; (3) registries created by health oversight authorities for health system oversight activities authorized by law; (4) registries using de-identified health information; (5) registries using a "limited data set" of patient information that lacks specified direct identifiers; (6) registries using information obtained with patient authorizations; or (7) registries using information obtained with a waiver of authorization.

The Common Rule will apply to the creation and use of registry data if (1) the organization where the registry resides is subject to Common Rule requirements and has an FWA that encompasses the registry project; *and* (2) the creation of the registry and subsequent research use of the registry data constitute human subject research as defined by the Common Rule and are not exempt from Common Rule requirements; *and* (3) registry activities include a research purpose, which may be in addition to the main purpose of the registry. Registry developers are strongly encouraged to consult the IRB, not only about the applicability of the Common Rule, but also about the selection of data elements, the content of the consent process or the regulatory criteria for waiver, and any anticipated future research involving identifiable registry data.

State laws regulate public health activities and also may apply in various ways to the research use of health information. NIH can issue certificates of confidentiality to particular research projects for the protection of identifiable personal information from most legally compelled disclosures. Federal law provides specific privacy protections to the health information of patients in substance abuse programs that receive Federal funding. The institutional policies of health care providers and insurance plans may also affect the use and disclosure of the health information from their patient and insured populations.

Legal requirements applying to use or disclosures of health information for research can significantly influence the planning decisions of registry developers and investigators. Early and frequent consultation with institutional privacy officers, Privacy Board or IRB staff and members,

information system representatives of health care providers and insurance plans—plus technology transfer representatives and legal counsel, as necessary—is prudent.

Registry Transparency, Oversight, and Data Ownership

Registry Transparency

Efforts to make registry operations transparent (i.e., making information about registry operations public and readily accessible to anyone who is interested) are desirable. Such efforts may be crucial to realizing the potential benefits of research using health information. Registry transparency can also educate about scientific processes. Transparency contributes to public and professional confidence in the scientific integrity and validity of registry processes, and therefore in the conclusions produced by registry activities. Public information about registry operations may also increase the scientific utility of registry data by promoting inquiries from scientists with interests to which registry data may apply.

Registry developers can achieve transparency by making the registry's scientific objectives, governance, eligibility criteria, sampling and recruitment strategies, general operating protocol, and sources of data available to anyone who is interested. Proprietary interests by funding agencies, contractual conditions, and licensing terms for the use of patient or claims information may limit to some extent the information about the registry that is available to the public. It is important to stress that, while transparency and access to information are values to be encouraged, investments in patient registries that produce proprietary information are not intended to be discouraged or criticized. Neither the funding source nor the generation of proprietary information from a registry determines whether a registry achieves the good practices described in this handbook. Funding agencies, health care providers, and insurance plans, however, also have an important stake in maintaining public confidence in health information management. The extent of registry transparency should be prospectively negotiated with these entities.

Creating a Web site of information about registry objectives and operations is one method of achieving transparency; ideally, registry information should be available in various media. An IRB may require registry transparency as a condition of approval to satisfy one of the regulatory criteria for granting a waiver of consent. The regulatory requirement is to provide "additional pertinent information after participation."[231] Currently, an international transplant registry maintains a Web site that provides a useful model of registry transparency.[232]

Registry Oversight

Registry governance must reflect the nature and extent of registry operations. As described in Chapter 2, possible governing structures can vary widely, from the registry developer as a sole decisionmaker to committee(s) comprising representatives of all stakeholders in the registry, including investigators, the funding agency, patients, clinicians, biostatisticians, information technology specialists, and government agencies.

Registry developers should also consider appointing an independent advisory board to provide oversight of registry operations. An advisory board can assist registry operations in two important areas: providing guidance for the technical aspects of the registry operations and establishing the scientific independence of the registry. The latter function can be valuable when dealing with controversies, especially those about patient safety and treatment, or actions by a regulatory agency. Advisory board members collectively should have relevant technical expertise but include appropriate representatives of other registry stakeholders, including patients. Advisory board oversight should be limited to making recommendations to the ultimate decisionmaker, whether that is an executive committee or the registry developer.

Registry developers may also appoint other types of

oversight committees to resolve specific recurring problems, such as verifying diagnoses of patient conditions or adjudicating data inconsistencies.

Data Ownership

Health information ownership in general. Multiple entities are positioned to assert ownership claims to health information in various forms. Certain States have enacted laws that assign ownership to health records.[233] The Privacy Rule was not intended to affect existing laws governing the ownership of health records.[234] At the current time, such claims of ownership are plausible, but none is known to be legally tested or recognized, with the exception of copyright. The entities potentially claiming ownership include health care providers and insurance plans, funding agencies for registry projects, research institutions, and government agencies. Individuals may also assert ownership claims to health information, including patients, registry developers, and investigators. The basis for these claims is control of the tangible expression of and access to the health information. There is no legal basis for assertions of ownership for facts or ideas; in fact, established public policy supports the free exchange of ideas and wide dissemination of facts as fundamental to innovation and social progress.[235] As health information moves from its creation as a tangible expression to various forms in the control of successive entities, rights of ownership may be transferred (assigned), shared, or maintained, with use of the information licensed (i.e., a limited transfer of rights for use on specific terms and conditions). Currently, in each of these transactions, the rights of ownership will be negotiated on a case-by-case basis and formalized in written private agreements. The funding agency for a registry may also assert claims to ownership as a matter of contract law in their sponsorship agreements with research organizations.

Many health care providers are currently installing systems for electronic health records at great expense. Many are also contemplating an assertion of ownership in their health records, which may include ownership of copyright. The claim to ownership by health care providers may be an overture to commercialization of their health care information in aggregate form.[236] Public knowledge of and response to such assertions of ownership are uncertain at this time. A licensing program for the use of health information may permit health care providers to recoup some of their investment in electronic health records and the infrastructure, including full-time technicians, required to maintain them. In the near future, research use of health information for a registry may require licensing in addition to the terms and conditions in data use agreements and, if necessary, in business associate agreements required by Privacy Rule regulations. Subsequent research use of the registry data will likely depend on the terms of the original license for use.

Publication rights are an important component of intellectual property rights in data for academic institutions. Formal institutional policies may address publication rights resulting from faculty educational and research activities. Moreover, the social utility and benefit of any registry is evaluated on the basis of its publicly known findings and any conclusions based on them. The authors strongly encourage registry developers to maximize public communication of registry findings through the customary channels of scientific conferences and peer-reviewed journals. The goals of public communication for scientific findings and conclusions apply equally to registries operated outside of academic institutions (i.e., directly by industry or professional societies). For further discussion of developing data access and publication policies for a registry, see Chapter 2.

The concept of ownership does not fit health information comfortably, because it largely fails to acknowledge individual patient privacy interests in health information. An inescapable personal nexus exists between individuals and information about their health. A similar failure that occurred recently with regard to patient interests in residual tissue from clinical procedures resulted in widely publicized litigation.[237] Alternatively, the legal concept of custody may be useful. Custodians have legal rights and responsibilities; for instance, those that a guardian has for a ward or parents have for

their children. Custody also has a protective function, which supports public expectations of confidentiality for health information that preserves the privacy and dignity of individual patients. Custody and its associated legal rights and responsibilities are also transferable from one custodian to another. The concept of custody can support health care provider investments in information systems and the licensed use of health information for multiple, socially beneficial purposes without denying patient interests in their health information.

The sharing of registry data subsequent to their collection currently presents special ethical challenges and legal issues.[238] The arrangements that will determine the essential conditions for shared use include applicable Federal or State law and regulatory requirements under which the health information was originally obtained. These legal and regulatory requirements, as well as processing and licensing fees, claims of property rights, and concerns about legal liability are likely to result in formal written agreements for each use of registry data. To educate patients and to establish the scientific independence of their registry, registry developers should make transparent the criteria under which uses of data occur.

In short, no widely accepted social or legal standards currently govern property rights in health information, with the possible exception of copyright, which is discussed below. At this time, agreements between health information sources and other users privately manage access and control. The Privacy Rule regulates the use and disclosure of health information by covered entities (certain health care providers and insurance plans), plus certain third parties working on behalf of covered entities, but does not affect current laws regarding property rights in health information, when they exist.

Copyright protection for health information registries. In theory, a health information registry is likely to satisfy the statutory definition of a compilation[239] and reflect independent creativity by its developer.[240] Thus, copyright law may provide certain protections for a health information registry

113

existing in any medium, including electronic digital media. The "facts" compiled in a health information registry, however, do not correlate closely to other compilations protected by copyright, such as telephone books or even genetic databases.[241] Instead registry data constitute legally protected, confidential information about individual patients to which independent and varied legal protections apply. Copyright protections may marginally enhance, but do not diminish, other legal restrictions on access to and use of health information and registry data. For more information on copyright law, see Appendix B.

Conclusions

Ethical considerations are involved in many of the essential aspects of planning and operating a registry. These considerations can affect the scientific, logistical, and regulatory components of registry development, as well as claims of property rights in health information and the registry. The guiding ethical principles for these considerations are *respect for persons*, *beneficence*, and *justice*.

At the most fundamental level, investigations that involve human subjects and are not capable of achieving their scientific purpose are unethical. The risk-benefit ratio of such studies is unacceptable in an analysis based on the principle of *beneficence*, which obligates investigators to avoid harming subjects, as well as maximizing the benefits and minimizing the harms of research projects. Ethical scientific design must be robust, be based on an important question, and incorporate sufficient statistical power, precise eligibility criteria, appropriately selected data elements, and adequately documented operating procedures and methodologies.

In addition, an ethical obligation to minimize harms involves planning adequate protections for the confidentiality of the health information disclosed to a registry. Such planning should include devising physical, technical, and administrative safeguards for access to and use of registry data. Reducing the potential harms from the use of health information in a registry is particularly important, because

ordinarily no offsetting benefit from participation in a registry accrues to individuals whose health information is used in the registry. In an analysis applying the principle of *justice*, research activities that produce a significant imbalance of potential risks and benefits to participating individuals are unethical.

Protection of the confidentiality of the health information used to populate a registry reflects the ethical principle of *respect for persons*. Health information intimately engages the privacy and dignity of patients. Registry developers should acknowledge public expectations of protection for patient privacy and dignity with clear and consistent communications to patients about protections against inappropriate access to and use of registry data.

The regulatory requirements of the Privacy Rule and Common Rule have deep connections to past ethical concerns about research involving human subjects, to general social anxiety about privacy associated with rapid advances in health information systems technology and communications, and to current biomedical developments in human genetics. Compliance with these regulatory requirements not only is a cost of doing business for a registry project but also demonstrates recognition of the ethical considerations accompanying use of health information for scientific purposes. Compliance efforts by registry developers also acknowledge the important public relations and liability concerns of health care providers and insurance plans, public health agencies, health oversight agencies, and research organizations. Regulatory compliance contributes to and generally supports the credibility of scientific research activities and research organizations, as well as that of particular projects. Public confidence is crucial to the continuing support of health care institutions, to which society entrusts the sick, and to academic institutions, to which society entrusts its children and its hopes for the future.

Other Federal and State privacy laws may affect registry development, especially registries created for public health purposes. These laws express an explicit, legislatively determined balance of

114

individual patient interests in health information against the potential social benefits from various uses of health information, including research. Consultation with legal counsel is strongly recommended to determine the possible effect of these laws on a particular registry project.

Ethical considerations also affect the operational aspects of registries, including governance, transparency, and data ownership. Registry governance, discussed in Chapter 2, should reflect both appropriate expertise and representation of stakeholders, including patients. Advisory committee recommendations can provide useful guidance in dealing with controversial issues. Transparency involves making information about registry governance and operations publicly available. Registry transparency improves both public and professional credibility for the scientific endeavors of a registry, the confidential use of health information for scientific purposes, and the results produced from analyses of registry data. In short, registry transparency promotes public trust.

Claims of "ownership" for health information and registries are feasible, but have not yet been legally tested. In addition, public response to such claims is uncertain. On their face, such claims do not seem to acknowledge patient interests in health information. Nonetheless, in theory, copyright protections for compilations may be applied to the patient information held by health care providers and insurance plans, as well as to registries. In general, claims of property rights in health information are likely to be negotiated privately as additions to the regulatory terms and conditions in formal agreements between registry developers, funding agencies, and health care providers or insurance plans. As a practical matter, "ownership" implies operational control of registry data and publication rights.

In summary, careful attention to the ethical considerations related to the design and operation of a registry, as well as the applicable legal requirements, will contribute to the success of registry projects and ensure the realization of their social and scientific benefits.

Summary of Privacy Rule and Common Rule Requirements

In Table 8, which summarizes Privacy Rule and common Rule requirements, it is generally assumed that the Privacy Rule applies to the data source—i.e., that the data source is a "covered entity." The exception is Category 8, registry developers that use data not subject to the Privacy Rule. The information in the table is merely a summary that is subject to change by other applicable law and may be amplified by institutional policies. Reference to this table is not a substitute for consultation with appropriate institutional officials about the regulatory requirements that may apply to a particular registry project.

115

Table 8: Summary of Privacy Rule and Common Rule Requirements				
Registry developer or purpose of registry	**Extent an individual may be identified from health information**			**Waiver of authorization, documentation of consent, or consent process**
	Health information is de-identified[a]	**Health information excludes direct identifiers**	**Health information includes direct identifiers**	
1A. Federal or State public health agency: Registry for *public health practice within agency's legal authority* **not** *involving research*	No requirements.	The Privacy Rule permits use or disclosure to a public health authority for public health activities. The Common Rule is not applicable.	The Privacy Rule permits use or disclosure to a public health authority for public health activities. The Common Rule is not applicable.	Waivers are not applicable.
1B. Federal or State public health agency: Registry as agency *research project*	No requirements. If the Common Rule applies,[b] it permits an Institutional Review Board (IRB) grant of exemption from review unless a re-identification code is used.	The Privacy Rule permits the use or disclosure of limited data set, provided the data source and registry developer enter into a data use agreement. If the Common Rule applies,[b] it permits an IRB grant of exemption unless a re-identification code is used.	The Privacy Rule permits use or disclosure with patient authorization or IRB or Privacy Board waiver of authorization. If the Common Rule applies,[b] IRB review and documented consent are required, unless an IRB grants a waiver of documentation or waiver for the consent process.	Privacy Board or IRB approval of a waiver of authorization depends on satisfaction of specific regulatory criteria. If the Common Rule applies,[b] IRB approval of a waiver of consent documentation or process depends on satisfaction of specific regulatory criteria.
2. Registry producing evidence in support of labeling for an *FDA-regulated product.*	No requirements.	The Privacy Rule permits use or disclosure to a person responsible for an FDA-regulated product.	The Privacy Rule permits use or disclosure to a person responsible for an FDA-regulated product. FDA regulations, and Common Rule, if applicable,[b] require IRB review, a documented consent process, and protection of confidentiality of research data.	Waivers are not applicable.

(continued)

Table 8: Summary of Privacy Rule and Common Rule Requirements (continued)

Registry developer or purpose of registry	Extent an individual may be identified from health information			Waiver of authorization, documentation of consent, or consent process
	Health information is de-identified	Health information excludes direct identifiers	Health information includes direct identifiers	
3. Health oversight agency registry to perform *a health oversight activity* **not** *involving research*	No requirements.	The Privacy Rule permits use or disclosure for health oversight activities authorized by law. The Common Rule is not applicable.	The Privacy Rule permits use or disclosure for health oversight activities authorized by law. Institutional policy may apply the Common Rule or require IRB review.	Waiver of authorization is not applicable. If institutional policy applies the Common Rule, IRB approval of a waiver of consent documentation or process depends on satisfaction of specific regulatory criteria.
4. Registry *required by law*; Common Rule may apply[b] if registry *involves research*	No requirements.	The Privacy Rule permits use or disclosure required by other law. If the Common Rule applies,[b] it permits an IRB grant of exemption, unless a re-identification code is used.	The Privacy Rule permits use or disclosure required by other law. Institutional policy may apply the Common Rule or require IRB review whether or not a research purpose is involved.	Waiver of authorization is not applicable. If the Common Rule applies,[b] IRB approval of a waiver of consent documentation or process depends on satisfaction of specific regulatory criteria.
5. *Quality improvement or assurance registry* **not** *involving research*	No requirements.	The Privacy Rule permits the use or disclosure of a limited data set, provided the data source and registry developer enter into a data use agreement. The Common Rule is not applicable.	The Privacy Rule permits use or disclosure for the "health care operations" of the data source and, in certain circumstances, of another covered entity. The Common Rule is not applicable.	Waivers are not applicable.
6. Research registry residing in organization to which Common Rule applies[b]	No requirements. Not human subjects research under Common Rule definitions unless a re-identification code is used.	The Privacy Rule permits the use or disclosure of a limited data set for research, provided the data source and registry developer enter into a data use agreement. *(continued)*	The Privacy Rule permits use or disclosure for research with individual patient authorization or an IRB or Privacy Board waiver of authorization. *(continued)*	IRB or Privacy Board approval depends on satisfaction of specific regulatory criteria.

(continued)

Table 8: Summary of Privacy Rule and Common Rule Requirements (continued)				
Registry developer or purpose of registry	Extent an individual may be identified from health information			Waiver of authorization, documentation of consent, or consent process
	Health information is de-identified	Health information excludes direct identifiers	Health information includes direct identifiers	
(continued) 6. Research registry residing in organization to which Common Rule applies[b]		(continued) The Common Rule permits an IRB grant of exemption from review unless a re-identification code is used.	(continued) The Common Rule requires IRB review and documented consent unless the IRB grants a waiver of documentation of consent or a waiver for the consent process.	
7. *Research registry* developed by organization that is **not** a health care provider or insurance plan and is **not** subject to the Common Rule, using health information obtained from a health care provider or insurance plan	No requirements.	The Privacy Rule permits the disclosure of a limited data set, provided the data source and registry developer enter into a data use agreement.	The Privacy Rule permits use or disclosure for research with individual patient authorization or waiver of authorization.	Privacy Board approval of a waiver of authorization depends on satisfaction of specific regulatory criteria.
8. *Research registry* developed by organization that is **not** a health care provider or insurance plan and is **not** subject to the Common Rule, using health information collected from entities **not** subject to the Privacy Rule.	No requirements.	No requirements.	No requirements.	Waivers are not applicable.

[a] Information lacks the data elements specified in the Privacy Rule standard for de-identification.

[b] The Common Rule likely applies if: (1) Federal funding is involved with the registry project, (2) the organization within which the registry will reside has agreed in its Federal-wide Assurance (FWA) to apply the Common Rule to all research activities conducted in its facilities or by its employees, or (3) institutional policy applies the Common Rule.

Note: FDA = U.S. Food and Drug Administration. IRB = Institutional Review Board.

Section II.
Operating Registries

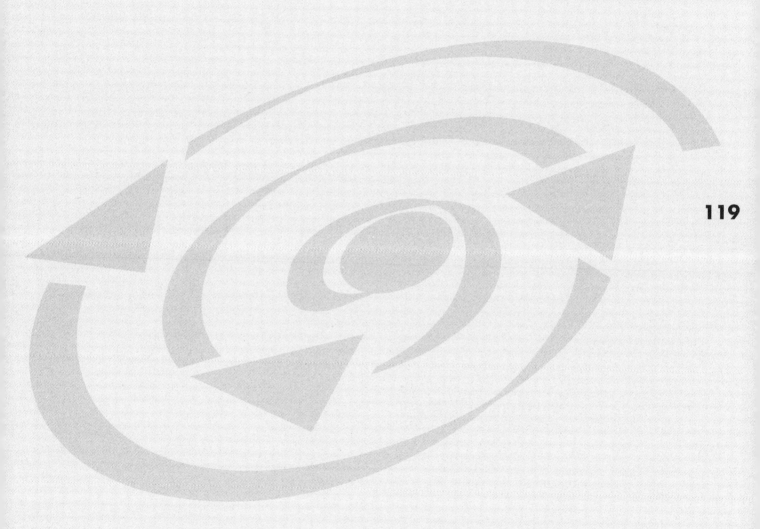

Chapter 7. Patient and Provider Recruitment and Management

Recruitment and retention of providers and patients are essential elements in the design and operation of a registry. The problems commonly described for clinical studies in general, such as difficulties with patient enrollment, losses to followup, and certain sites contributing the majority of patients, can have profound negative consequences on registry validity because the registry patients that are enrolled are not randomized. When registry patients are not representative of the target population, the results obtained are not meaningful. For policy determinations, the enrolled sites or providers must be representative of the types of sites and providers to which the policy determination would apply for the results of the registry to be generalizable. Differences in how effectively sites enroll or follow patients can skew results and overly reflect the sites with the most data. This oversampling within a particular site or location must also be considered in sample size calculations. If the sample size of a key unit of analysis is not sufficient to detect a clinically important difference, the validity of the entire registry is weakened. (See Chapters 3 and 10.)

Well-planned strategies for enrollment and retention are critical to avoiding these types of concerns about registry validity. Because registries typically operate with limited resources and with voluntary rather than mandatory participation by both providers and patients, it is particularly important to keep an appropriate balance between participation burden and reward. The term "voluntary" in this context is intended to mean that participation in the registry by either providers or patients is not mandated (e.g., by the U.S. Food and Drug Administration), nor is participation required as a necessary condition for a patient to gain access to a health care product or for a provider to be eligible for payment for a health care service. Registries that are not voluntary have different drivers for participation. In general, the burden of participation should be kept as low as possible while the relative rewards, particularly nonmonetary rewards, should

be maximized. As described in Chapters 2 and 4, minimizing burden typically starts with focusing on the key goals of the registry.

Building participation incentives into a registry should also be included in the planning phase. A broad range of incentives, spanning a spectrum from recognition, to monetary incentives, to useful data and reports, can and have been used in registries and are described further in this chapter. Many registries incorporate multiple types of incentives, even when they pay for participation. Monetary incentives can be very helpful in recruiting sites. However, because the payments should not exceed fair market value for work performed, registries cannot solely rely on these incentives. A number of nonmandated registries have achieved success in recruitment and retention by providing a combination of ethical incentives that are tailored to and aligned with the specific groups of sites, providers, and patients that are asked to participate. (See Case Examples 17, 18, and 19.)

Recruitment

Depending on the purpose of a registry, recruitment may occur at any of three levels: facility (e.g., hospital, practice, pharmacy), provider, or patient. While frequently these levels are a means to accrue patients for sample size purposes, such as for a safety registry, they may also constitute potential units of analysis. As an example, a registry focused on systems of care that is examining both hospital system processes and patient outcomes might need to consider characteristics of the individual patients, the providers, and/or the places where they practice (i.e., clusters). If the question is about the practices of orthopedic surgeons in the United States, the registry will be strengthened by describing the number and characteristics (e.g., age, gender, and geographic distribution) of U.S. orthopedic surgeons, perhaps by citing membership data from the American Academy of Orthopedic Surgeons.

Case Example 17: Building Value as a Means To Recruit Hospitals	
Description	Get With The Guidelines^{SM} (GWTG) is the flagship program for in-hospital quality improvement of the American Heart Association (AHA) and American Stroke Association (ASA). The program uses the experience of the AHA and ASA to ensure the care that hospitals provide for coronary artery disease, heart failure, and stroke is aligned with the latest evidence-based guidelines.
Sponsor	American Heart Association and American Stroke Association
Year Started	2000
Year Ended	Ongoing
No. of Sites	1,331
No. of Records	804,071

122

Challenge

Recruiting hospitals for registries or quality improvement (QI) programs can be arduous. Human and financial capital is constrained. Accreditation and reimbursement programs, such as those of The Joint Commission (formerly the Joint Commission on Accreditation of Healthcare Organizations, or JCAHO) and Centers for Medicare & Medicaid Services (CMS), contend for the same valuable human and financial capital. As a result, in the absence of specific benefits, many hospitals defer the data collection and report utilization required for successful QI execution.

Like most registries and QI programs, the sponsor's program faced barriers to data entry. Unlike other registries, GWTG offered no reimbursements for data entry and entered a market characterized by significant competition.

The registry team wanted to motivate resource-strapped hospitals to consistently and proactively enter data and analyze improvement.

Proposed Solution

The team began by listening to the customer through indepth interviews designed to understand the motivations and deterrents underlying behavior. Interviews were conducted with hospital decisionmakers at all levels (nurses, QI professionals, administrators/chief executive officers, and physicians).

Based on the research findings, the team developed strategies that differentiated and built value for the program. Some of the more noteworthy strategies included the following:

- Systems were designed to allow data transmission from and to Joint Commission and CMS vendors, enabling hospitals to reduce the burden of duplicate data entry while still participating in other programs.

- A new tag line, Turning Guidelines into Lifelines^{SM}, linked the brand's value proposition to the brand name and logo. Key messages for each target audience were included in marketing communications.

- A newly designed national recognition program motivated participation and advancement and received the attention of hospital decisionmakers.

- Return-on-investment studies for the program demonstrated the value of participation.

- Product innovations/enhancements created additional incentives to participate. Immediate, point-of-care flags highlighted variances from guidelines. Benchmarking filters/reports empowered decisionmakers to benchmark performance with national averages and similar institutions. Customizable notes explaining diseases, tests, and medications can be sent to both the referring physician and patient.

(continued)

Case Example 17: Building Value as a Means To Recruit Hospitals (continued)

Results

By providing a mix of innovative, nonfinancial incentives, the program increased both enrollment and advancement by about one-third in 12 months. Currently, more than 1,300 hospitals participate in the program. The database includes over 800,000 patient records and is considered by many to be the most robust database for coronary artery disease, heart failure, and stroke. In 2004, the program received the Innovation in Prevention Award from the Department of Health and Human Services.

Key Point

Nonfinancial incentives that meet the needs of decisionmakers can assist in site recruitment. When creating such incentives, consider both tangible and nontangible benefits.

For More Information

http://www.americanheart.org/getwiththeguidelines

This will allow documentation of the similarities and differences in the characteristics of the surgeons participating in the registry compared with the target population. (See Chapter 3.)

Hospital Recruitment

A hospital or health system may choose to participate in a patient registry for many reasons, including the research interest of a particular investigator or champion, the ability for the hospital to achieve other goals through the registry (such as requirements for reimbursement, certification, or recognition), or the general interest of the particular institution in the disease area (e.g., specialty hospitals). Increasingly, external mandates to document compliance with practice standards provide an incentive for hospitals to participate in registries that collect and report mandatory hospital performance or quality-of-care data. For example, a number of registries allow hospitals to document their performance to meet the Joint Commission (formerly JCAHO) requirements for hospital accreditation.[242] Hospitals in the United States must submit these data to maintain accreditation. Therefore, hospital administrators may be willing to supply the staff time to collect these data without the need for any additional financial incentives from the registry sponsor, provided that registry participation allows the hospital to meet external quality-of-care mandates. In other cases, participation in a quality monitoring or health system surveillance registry may be required by payers or governments for differential payments or patient referrals under various programs, ranging from the Centers for Medicare & Medicaid Services public reporting initiative, to centers of excellence programs, to pay-for-performance programs.

The presence of quality assurance departments in U.S. hospitals provides a natural foundation for recruiting and supporting cooperative, hospital-based outcomes and performance registries. In addition, the American Hospital Association database provides a valuable resource for identifying hospitals by key characteristics, including hospital ownership, number of beds, and the presence of an intensive care unit.

123

Case Example 18: Using Registry Tools To Recruit Sites	
Description	The objective of the OPTIMIZE-HF (Organized Program to Initiate Lifesaving Treatment in Hospitalized Patients with Heart Failure) registry was to improve quality of care and promote evidence-based therapies in heart failure. The registry provided a comprehensive process-of-care improvement program and gathered data that allowed hospitals to track their improvement over time.
Sponsor	GlaxoSmithKline
Year Started	2003
Year Ended	2005
No. of Sites	270 hospitals
No. of Patients	Over 50,000

Challenge

The registry was designed to help hospitals improve care for patients hospitalized with heart failure. The objective was to accelerate the adoption of evidence-based guidelines and increase the use of the guideline-recommended therapies, thereby improving both short-term and long-term clinical outcomes for heart failure patients.

Proposed Solution

To increase compliance with guidelines, the registry team promoted the implementation of a process-of-care improvement component and the use of comprehensive patient education materials. They combined these materials into a hospital toolkit, which included evidence-based practice algorithms, critical pathways, standardized orders, discharge checklists, pocket cards, and chart stickers. The toolkit also included algorithms and dosing guides for the guideline-recommended therapies and a comprehensive set of patient education materials. The team engaged the steering committee in designing the toolkit to ensure that the materials reflected both the guideline-recommended interventions and the practical aspects of hospital processes.

In addition to the toolkit, the registry offered point-of-care tools, such as referral notes and patient letters that could be customized for each patient based on data entered into the registry. The registry also included real-time performance reports that hospitals could use to assess their improvement on a set of standardized measures based on the guidelines.

Results

The hospital toolkit was a key component of the marketing campaign for the registry. Hospitals could view the toolkit at recruitment meetings, but they did not receive their own copy until they joined the program. The toolkit gained credibility among hospitals because its creators included some of the most prominent members of the heart failure community. Hospitals also actively used the reports to track their improvement over time and identify areas for additional work. Overall, the registry recruited 270 hospitals and met its patient accrual goal 6 months ahead of schedule.

Key Point

Nonfinancial incentives, such as patient education materials, toolkits, and reports, can encourage sites to join a registry. Incentives that also add value for the site by improving their processes or providing materials that they use frequently can aid retention.

For More Information

Fonarow GG, Abraham WT, Albert NM et al. Organized Program to Initiate Lifesaving Treatment in Hospitalized Patients with Heart Failure (OPTMIZE-HF): rationale and design. Am Heart J 2004 July;148(1):43-51.

Case Example 19: Using Proactive Awareness Activities To Recruit Patients for a Pregnancy Exposure Registry	
Description	The Ribavirin Pregnancy Registry is a component of the Ribavirin Risk Management Program. It was designed to evaluate the association between ribavirin and birth defects occurring in the offspring of female patients exposed to ribavirin during pregnancy or the 6 months prior to conception, as well as female partners of male patients exposed to ribavirin during the same time period. The registry collects prospective, observational data on pregnancies and outcomes following pregnancy exposure to ribavirin.
Sponsor	Hoffmann-La Roche Inc.; Sandoz Pharmaccuticals Inc.; Schering-Plough Corp.; Teva Pharmaceuticals USA, Inc.; Three Rivers Pharmaceuticals, LLC; Zydus Pharmaceuticals (USA) Inc.
Year Started	2003
Year Ended	Ongoing
No. of Sites	N/A (population-based)
No. of Records	Approximately 100

Challenge

Ribavirin is used in combination with interferon alfa or pegylated interferon alfa for the treatment of hepatitis C. Chronic hepatitis C presents a serious health concern for approximately three million Americans, as the infection, if left untreated, can lead to end-stage liver disease, primary liver cancer, and death. When used as part of a combination therapy, ribavirin can significantly increase both viral clearance and liver biopsy improvement for hepatitis C patients. However, ribavirin showed teratogenic properties in all animal models tested, making pregnancy exposure a concern. There are minimal data on ribavirin exposure in human pregnancies. Thus the U.S. Food and Drug Administration (FDA) designated ribavirin as a Pregnancy Category X product based on the animal data, and ribavirin carries product label warnings against becoming pregnant.

Despite the product warnings, pregnancies are likely to occur during ribavirin use because the incidence of hepatitis C is highest among people with reproductive potential (25-45 years of age). Health care professionals have insufficient data on the teratogenic properties of ribavirin in humans to counsel pregnant women exposed to ribavirin either during pregnancy or in the 6 months prior to conception. The registry was established to gather prospective data on ribavirin exposure in pregnancy and pregnancy outcomes in order to better understand the actual risk.

The registry collects data on direct exposures through the pregnant female and indirect exposures through her male sexual partner. Health care providers, pregnant patients, or pregnant patients' male sexual partners may submit data to the registry. The registry collects minimal, targeted data at each trimester and at the outcome of the pregnancy through the obstetric health care providers. For live births, the registry collects data at 6 months and 12 months after the birth by contacting the pediatric health care provider.

To gather data on these patients, the registry needed to develop proactive awareness activities to make patients and providers aware of the program and encourage enrollment without promoting ribavirin use during pregnancy.

Proposed Solution

The registry team developed a multipronged approach to recruiting patients. First, the team developed a comprehensive Web site with information for patients and providers. The Web

125

(continued)

Case Example 19: Using Proactive Awareness Activities To Recruit Patients for a Pregnancy Exposure Registry (continued)

site contains fact sheets, data forms, information on how to participate, and contact information. The site also contains a complete slide set that health care providers can use for teaching activities. While the site contains detailed information on the scientific reasons for the registry, the tone and content of the Web site are patient friendly, making it a good resource for both potential patients and providers.

Next, the team began targeting professional service groups whose members might treat patients with ribavirin exposure during pregnancy. The groups included hepatologists, gastroenterologists, obstetricians, and pediatricians. By contacting the groups' leadership and sending individualized mailings to members, the team hoped to raise awareness across a broad spectrum of providers. The team also talked to nursing groups, including a nursing group specifically focused on hepatitis and liver disease, with the goal of utilizing the nurse's role as a patient educator. As a result of these efforts, the American Gastroenterological Association placed a link for the registry Web site on its Web site, and the American Association for the Study of Liver Diseases posted an expert opinion piece written by the registry advisory board chair on its Web site.

The registry team also raised awareness among professional groups by attending conferences. In 2005, the team presented a poster about the registry, including some information on demographics and program objectives, at the Centers for Disease Control and Prevention (CDC) National Viral Hepatitis Prevention Conference.

To raise awareness among patients, the team talked to hepatitis C patient advocacy groups. The registry gained exposure with patients when one patient group wrote an article about the registry for its newsletter and included the registry phone number on its fact sheet. This effort led to many patient-initiated enrollments, despite the lack of patient incentives. In working with patients, the registry has found that emphasizing the goal of

gathering information to help future patients make better decisions resonates with patients. Most patients submit data to the registry over the phone, and the rapport that the interviewers have developed with patients has helped to reduce the number of patients who are lost to followup.

In addition to targeting providers and patients directly, the team enlisted the help of public health agencies, since the registry has a strong public health purpose. CDC agreed to include a link on its Web site to the registry Web site, and the registry team is now targeting other public health agencies in hopes of posting information on their Web sites.

The team also reviewed the registry process to identify any potential barriers to enrollment. Under the initial rules for giving informed consent, the registry call center contacted patients and asked them if they were interested in participating. If patients agreed to participate over the phone, the call center sent a package of information through the mail, including an informed consent document, which the patients needed to sign and return before they could enroll. While many patients agreed to participate over the phone, a much smaller number actually returned the informed consent document. The team identified the process of obtaining written informed consent as a key barrier to enrollment.

After discussions with FDA, the registry team and FDA approached the study Institutional Review Board (IRB) about receiving a waiver of written informed consent because of the public health importance of the registry. The IRB agreed that oral consent over the phone would be sufficient for this study. Now, the call center can complete the enrollment process in a single step, as they can obtain oral consent over the phone and then proceed with the interview. This change improved and streamlined the enrollment process and significantly increased the number of participants in the registry.

(continued)

126

Case Example 19: Using Proactive Awareness Activities To Recruit Patients for a Pregnancy Exposure Registry (continued)

Throughout all of these recruitment activities, the registry team has emphasized that the purpose of the registry is to answer important safety questions for the benefit of future patients and providers. By focusing on the public health purpose of the registry, the team has been able to encourage participation from both patients and providers. The team has also found that a key element of their recruitment strategy is their detailed awareness plan, which calls for completing awareness activities every month or two. Because the leadership and membership of professional groups change and new patients begin taking ribavirin, the team has found that continual awareness activities are important for keeping patients and providers aware of the registry.

Results

Through proactive awareness activities, the registry team has generated interest in the project and enrolled approximately 100 exposed pregnancies with outcome information to date. The streamlined oral consent process has proven successful in this registry, and other pregnancy registries have begun adopting it as a way to increase enrollments.

Key Point

Recruitment activities may include working with professional groups, contacting patient groups, targeting public health agencies, and using a Web site to share information. Once recruitment and enrollment have begun, the registry team may need to re-evaluate the process to identify any potential barriers to enrollment, if enrollment is not proceeding as planned. If a registry has an ongoing enrollment process, a plan to continually raise awareness about the registry is an important part of the recruitment plan.

Table 9 describes characteristics of registries that can be critical for success in recruiting hospitals and lists methods that might be used for recruiting hospitals. While programs need not incorporate all of these characteristics or use all of these methods, successful programs typically incorporate several.

Physician Recruitment

There are many reasons why a physician practice may or may not choose to participate in a voluntary registry. As with hospitals, these reasons can include the research interests of the physician and the ability of the practice to achieve other goals through the registry (such as reimbursement or recognition). When deciding to participate, physicians often focus on several concerns:

- *Relevance*: Does the registry have meaning for the practice and patients?

- *Trust*: Are the goals clearly stated? Is the registry transparent?

- *Risks*: Will confidentiality be maintained? Are patient records secure?

- *Effort*: Will the amount of effort expended be properly compensated?

- *Disruption*: Will participation disrupt the activity of the staff?

Physicians who manage only a few patients per year with the disease that is the subject of the registry are less likely to be interested in enrolling their patients than physicians who see many such patients unless the disease is rare or extremely rare, in which case the registry may be of great interest.

Because most registries are voluntary and physicians in nonacademic practice settings may have less infrastructure and staff available to enroll their patients, recruitment of representative physicians is a major challenge for registries that aim to compare physician practices across a full spectrum of practice settings. In general, community-based physicians are less well equipped to collect data for research

127

Table 9. Hospital Recruitment	
Keys to hospital recruitment	• The condition being studied satisfies one of the hospital's quality assurance mandates. • Sufficient funds, data, or other benefits will be realized to justify the effort required to participate. • The confidentiality of the hospital's performance data is ensured. • Clinically relevant, credible, timely, actionable self-assessment data—ideally data that are risk adjusted and benchmarked—are provided back to the hospital to help it identify opportunities for enhancing patient care outcomes. • High-profile hospitals (regional or national) are participating in the registry. • Participation assists the hospital in meeting coverage and reimbursement mandates, gaining recognition as a center of excellence, or meeting requirements for pay-for-performance initiatives.
Methods of hospital recruitment	• Identify eligible hospitals from the American Hospital Association database. • Utilize stakeholder representatives to identify potentially interested hospitals. • Enroll hospitals through physicians who work there and are interested in the registry. • Use invitation letters or cold calls to directors of quality assurance or chiefs of the clinical department responsible for the condition that is the target of the registry. • If the registry has a physician advisory board, ask the board members to network with their colleagues in other hospitals. • Reach out to physician contacts or hospital administrators through relevant professional societies or hospital associations. • Leverage mandates by external stakeholders, including third-party payers, health plans, or government agencies.

studies because they work in busy practices that are geared to routine clinical care rather than research. To increase recruitment of nonacademic physicians, it can be helpful to clearly explain the purpose and objectives of the registry, how registry data will be used and specifically that individual results will not be shared or published and that registry outcomes data will be released only in large aggregates that protect the identities of individual hospitals, physicians, and patients.

Table 10 describes some considerations that might improve success in recruiting physicians to participate in patient registries and outlines several methods of physician recruitment that are employed in different registries. Some registries use more than one approach.

Vetting Potential Hospital and Physician Participants

Once potential hospital or physician participants have been identified, it is important to vet them to ensure that the registry is gathering the appropriate mix of data. Issues to consider when vetting potential participants include:

• Representativeness.

• Hospital characteristics (e.g., bed size, geographic location).

• Physician characteristics (e.g., specialty training).

• Practice setting (health maintenance organization [HMO], private practice).

• Ability to recruit patients.

• Volume of target cases per year.

128

Table 10. Physician Recruitment	
Keys to physician recruitment	• The condition being studied is part of the physician's specialty. • The registry is viewed as a scientific endeavor. • The registry is led by respected physician opinion leaders. • The registry is endorsed by leading medical, government, or patient advocacy organization(s). • The effort needed to recruit patients and collect and submit data is perceived as reasonable. • Useful self-assessment data are provided to physicians. • The registry meets other physician data needs, such as maintenance of certification requirements, credentialing requirements, or quality-based differential reimbursement payment programs (pay-for-performance).
Methods of physician recruitment	• Purchase mailing lists from physician specialty organizations. • Ask opinion leaders in the field to suggest interested colleagues. • Partner with local medical societies or large physician hospital organizations. • Use stakeholder representatives to identify interested physicians. • Recruit and raise awareness at conferences. • Advertise using e-mail and Web.

- Internal resources.
- Availability of a study coordinator on local physician or hospital staff.
- Availability of computer facilities (Internet connectivity) for studies with electronic data capture.

Patient Recruitment

Patients may be recruited based on the judgment of the physician who provides their care; the diagnosis of a disease; receipt of a procedure, operation, device, or pharmaceutical; membership in a health insurance plan; or being a member of a group of individuals who have a particular exposure. Recruitment of patients by the physician who is providing their care is one of the most successful strategies. The direct involvement in and support of the registry by their personal physicians is an important factor for patients. Since registries should not modify the usual care that physicians provide to their patients, there should be little or no conflict between the role of the physician as the patient's doctor and the role of the physician as a scientist in a research program (See Chapter 6.) In addition,

patients may see participation in the registry as an opportunity to increase their communication with their doctor. Another incentive for many patients is the feeling that they are contributing to the knowledge base of sometimes poorly understood and undertreated conditions.

Recruitment of patients presents different challenges, depending on the nature of the condition being studied. In general, patient recruitment plans should address the following questions:

- Does the plan understand the needs and interests of potential participants?
- Does the plan address patient recruitment issues and procedural challenges, including informed consent and explanation of risks?
- What are the patient retention goals? What is a reasonable followup period? What is a reasonable followup rate? When does retention compromise validity?
- What, if any, patient incentives are offered, including different types of incentives and the ethical, legal, or study validity issues to be considered with patient incentives?

129

- What are the costs of patient recruitment and retention?

Table 11 describes several keys to patient recruitment and outlines methods of recruitment, grouped by the basic categories of patients at the time of recruitment.

Partnerships as Recruitment Tools

Many agencies/organizations can assist in the recruitment of physicians and patients. These partners may have access to patients or their families and physicians who treat the condition, and they may lend credibility to the effort. These agencies/organizations include:

- Government agencies.
- Physician professional associations or State medical associations.
- Patient advocacy groups (e.g., Muscular Dystrophy Association).
- Nonprofit foundations (e.g., Robert Wood Johnson Foundation).
- Industry (e.g., pharmaceutical companies).
- HMOs and other third-party insurance providers.

Procedural Considerations Related to Recruitment

When developing a recruitment plan for a registry, consideration should be given to the procedural concerns that may be factored into potential participants' decisions. These concerns include the clarity of the contract, the process for institutional review board (IRB) approval, and confidentiality. The first step in recruiting participants is usually the development of a generic contract that can be presented to hospitals or physicians. This contract should clearly state the roles and responsibilities of the participants, the data coordinating center, and the sponsor. If monetary remuneration is being offered, the amount and requirements that need to be fulfilled before payments are made should be stated. It is often worthwhile to explain to sites the concept of fair market value. There is no specific formula (such as whether to separate startup payments from

per-patient payments), but total remuneration must reflect work effort and should be determined based on the facts in each registry. Some individual factors, ranging from location to specialty, may have a bearing on fair market value. It is also important to spell out which body will have ownership of the data and how the data will be used.

The contract should clearly explain the registry policy regarding any necessary approvals. Generic templates can be offered to participants to assist them in obtaining ethical and IRB approval. Because the costs of obtaining IRB approval are often substantial, it is essential that the contract with the participants clearly indicates which party is responsible for bearing this cost.

Lastly, confidentiality is a key requirement. Methods of ensuring institutional, physician, and patient confidentiality need to be clearly elucidated in all registry-related documentation. Case-report forms and patient logs must be designed to minimize patient identification (such as by transmitting limited data sets rather than more identifiable information if such information is not required to meet a registry objective).

Retention

Once hospitals and physicians are recruited into registries, maintaining their participation becomes a key to success. All of the factors identified as important for recruitment are important for retention as well. A critical factor in retention is ensuring that promises made during recruitment (e.g., that the burden of participation is low) prove to be true during site implementation. By carefully pilot testing all aspects of the registry prior to full recruitment, there is less likelihood that problems will arise that threaten the reputation of the registry. Registries with an advisory board or steering committee can use this resource to help with retention. The advisory board adds transparency and credibility, sets appropriate expectations among its peers on what to expect from a registry (e.g., compared with a clinical trial), ensures that the burden of the registry is minimized (or at least never outweighs its value to participants), and maintains

130

Table 11. Patient Recruitment	
Keys to patient recruitment	• Recruit through a physician who is caring for the patient. • Communicate to the patient that registry participation may help to improve care for all future patients with the target condition. • Write all patient materials (brochures, consent forms) in a manner that is easily understandable by the lay public. • Keep the survey forms short and simple. • Provide incentives—nonmonetary (such as newsletters, reports) and in some cases, monetary (if approved by the Institutional Review Board).

Methods of patient recruitment	• Noninstitutionalized residents of the general U.S. population:
	  • Recruit via letter survey or by telephone.
	  • Recruit during well-patient visits to outpatient clinics.
	• Outpatients attending the clinic of a physician who is participating in the registry:
	  • Recruit through the patient's physician.
	  • Recruit via brochures placed in physician's office.
	• Hospital inpatients who are hospitalized for treatment of a condition that is the subject of the registry:
	  • Recruit through the patient's physician.
	  • Recruit through hospitalists or consultant specialists.
	  • Recruit through a hospital research nurse.
	• Residents of nursing homes and similar long-term care facilities:
	  • Establish a relationship with the nursing home and staff.

131

the relevancy and currency of the registry for the investigators. Ideally, advisory board members serve as ambassadors for the program. The level of credibility, engagement, practicality, and enthusiasm of the advisory board can significantly affect provider recruitment and retention. For example, an advisory board whose clinical members are not themselves participating in the registry will have greater difficulty addressing the concerns of participating practices that invariably arise over the course of the registry.

Throughout the registry, communication from the data coordinating center and the advisors, as well as community building, are important for strong retention. Early and continued engagement of the site champions or principal investigators can help tremendously. Some registries utilize a small number of face-to-face meetings of all site principal investigators. While this is not always economically feasible, online meetings can be performed with similar effect. Visibility of the registry at relevant national meetings can help maintain clinician awareness and sense of community, and regular presentations and publications reinforce the credibility of the registry to its participants. As the data set grows, so too does the value of the registry for all participants, and regular updates on the registry growth can be important. Finally, enhancing site value through nonfinancial rewards can be particularly useful in retention, and the registry should continually seek to bring value to the participants in creative and useful ways. Participation retention tools include:

• Web sites.

• Newsletters.

• Telephone help lines.

• Instruction manuals.

• Training meetings.

• Site audit/retraining visits.

• Customer satisfaction/opinion surveys.

- Regular data reports to stakeholders.
- Presentations at conferences.
- Regular reports to registry participants on registry growth and publications.

Pitfalls in Recruitment and Retention

Pitfalls abound in recruitment and retention. The most important is the risk of bias. Targeting hospital- or academic-based physicians to the exclusion of community-based physicians is tempting because the former are often more accessible and are frequently more open to involvement in and more experienced in research projects. If an advisory board or committee is used to help design the registry and aid in recruitment, there may be a tendency for advisors to recruit known colleagues or target disease experts, when a wider range of participants may be necessary to provide the appropriate data to meet the research goals.

Biases in patient recruitment can also occur. For example, older and more seriously ill patients may be excluded because of challenges in enrollment and followup. From the outset, physicians involved in recruitment efforts need to be aware of the potential for bias, and they must understand the importance of adhering to well-delineated inclusion and exclusion criteria. They must also adhere to the registry's enrollment strategy, which is typically designed to reduce this bias (e.g., consecutive or randomized enrollment). In addition, overly demanding followup schedules can affect retention. The schedule should be designed to obtain relevant data in a timely fashion without overtaxing the resources of patients and providers.

Another major pitfall is confusing terminology. This can be a major problem when the registry is international. When designing training materials, instruction manuals, and questionnaires, it is critical that the language and terminology are clear and concise. Materials that are translated into other languages must undergo strict quality assurance measures to ensure that terms are translated properly.

Proposed Model for Registry Site Recruitment and Management

The model presented here describes the five basic steps of site participation in a registry. Each site may go through Steps 1 and/or 2 to establish interest in the registry and determine the feasibility of participation. Participating sites then go through Steps 3 through 5.

Step 1. Prerecruitment considerations:

- Does a site/organization meet the inclusion criteria for the registry? (See "Vetting Potential Hospitals and Physicians.")
- Does the site have an adequate population of cases?
- Does it have the necessary resources to support insertion of data into the registry (personnel or electronic data transfer structures)?
- Are there barriers to contracts or IRB issues that are so significant as to impede a reasonable timeframe to recruit a site?

Step 2. During this phase, all points in "Procedural Considerations Related to Recruitment" need to be reviewed as part of the feasibility assessment and final agreement to participate in the registry.

Step 3. Issues raised in "Retention" need to be addressed. Retention could include, but is not limited to, instruction manuals (paper/online) and training meetings.

Step 4. Is the site delivering quality data? Sites that do not deliver quality data may need to be decommissioned.

Step 5. At the conclusion of a registry, it is desirable to share the results with the sites.

132

Chapter 8. Data Collection and Quality Assurance

This chapter focuses on data collection procedures and quality assurance principles for patient registries. The integrated system for collecting, cleaning, storing, monitoring, reviewing, and reporting on registry data determines the utility of the data for meeting the goals of the registry. Quality assurance, on the other hand, aims to assure that the data were in fact collected in accordance with these procedures and that the data stored in the registry database meet the requisite standards of quality, which are generally defined based on the intended purposes. In this chapter, the term "registry coordinating activities" is used to refer to the centralized procedures performed for a registry and the term "registry coordinating center" refers to the entity or entities that performs these procedures and oversees the registry activities at the site and patient levels.

Because the range of registry purposes can be broad, a similar range of data collection procedures may be acceptable, but only certain methodologies may be suitable for particular purposes. Furthermore, certain end users of the data may require that data collection or validation be performed in accordance with their own guidelines or standards. For example, a registry that collects data electronically and intends for those data to be used by the U.S. Food and Drug Administration (FDA) should meet the systems validation requirements of that end user of the data, such as 21 Code of Federal Regulations Part 11 (21 CFR Part 11). Such requirements may have a substantial effect on the registry procedures. Similarly, registries may be subject to specific processes depending on the type of data collected, the types of authorization obtained, and the governmental regulations.

Requirements for data collection and quality assurance should be defined during the registry inception and creation phases. Certain requirements may have significant cost implications, and these should be assessed on a cost-to-benefit basis in the context of the intended purposes of the registry.

This chapter describes a broad range of centralized and distributed data collection and quality assurance activities that are currently in use or expected to become more commonly used in patient registries.

Data Management

Database Requirements or Case Report Forms

Chapter 1 defined a key characteristic of patient registries for evaluating patient outcomes as the use of highly structured data. As in randomized controlled trials, the case report form (CRF) is the paradigm for this structure. A CRF is a formatted listing of data elements that can be presented in paper or electronic formats. More importantly, a CRF is a representation of the patient-level fields and data entry options in the registry database; it could also be described as the database requirements. Defining the registry CRFs or database requirements is the first step in data collection. Chapter 4 describes the selection of data elements for a registry.

Two related documents should also be considered part of the database requirements: the data dictionary (including data definitions) and the data validation parameters or edits. The data dictionary and definitions describe both the data elements and how those data elements are interpreted. The data dictionary contains a detailed description of each variable used by the registry, including the source of the variable, coding information if used, and normal ranges if relevant. For example, the term "current smoker" should be defined as to whether "smoker" refers to tobacco or other substances and whether "current" refers to active or within a recent time period. Several cardiovascular registries, such as the Get With The Guidelines℠ Coronary Artery Disease program,[243] define "current smoker" as someone who smoked tobacco within the last year.

Data validation parameters refer to the logical checks on data entered into the database against predefined rules for either value ranges (e.g., systolic blood pressure less than 300 mmHg) or logical consistency with respect to other data fields for the same patient; these are described more fully under "Cleaning Data," below. While neither registry database structures nor database requirements are standardized, the Clinical Data Interchange Standards Consortium[244] is actively working on representative models for data interchange and portability using standardized concepts and formats. Chapter 4 further discusses these models, which are applicable to registries as well as clinical trials.

Data Collection: Procedures, Personnel, and Data Sources

Data collection procedures need to be carefully considered in planning the operations of a registry. Successful registries depend on a sustainable workflow model that can be integrated into the day-to-day clinical practice of active physicians, nurses, pharmacists, and patients with minimal disruption. (See Chapter 7.) Programs can benefit tremendously from preliminary input from health care workers or study coordinators who are likely to be participants.

Pilot testing. One method of gathering input from likely participants before the full launch of a registry is pilot testing. Whereas feasibility testing, which is discussed in Chapter 2, focuses on whether a registry should be implemented, pilot testing focuses on how it should be implemented. Piloting can range from testing a subset of the procedures, CRFs, or data capture systems to a full launch of the registry in a limited subset of sites and patients.

The key to effective pilot testing is to conduct it at a point where the results of the pilot can still be used to modify how the registry will be implemented. Through pilot testing, one can assess comprehension, acceptance, feasibility, and other factors that influence how readily the patient registry processes will fit into patient lifestyles and the normal practices of the health care provider. Chapter 4 discusses pilot testing in more detail.

Documentation of procedures. The data collection procedures for each registry should be clearly defined and described in a detailed manual. The term "manual" here refers to the reference information in any appropriate form, including hard copy, electronic, or via interactive Web or software-based systems. Although the detail of this manual may vary from registry to registry depending on the intended purpose, the required information generally includes protocols, policies, and procedures, as well as the data collection instrument and a listing of all the data elements and their full definitions. If the registry has optional fields (i.e., fields that do not have to be completed on every patient), these should be clearly specified. In addition to patient inclusion and exclusion criteria, the screening process should be specified, as should any documentation to be retained at the site level and any plans for monitoring or auditing of screening practices. If sampling is to be performed, the method or systems used should be explained, and tools should be provided to simplify this process for the sites. The manual should clearly explain how patient identification numbers are created or assigned and how duplicate records should be prevented. Any required training for data collectors should also be described.

If paper CRFs are utilized, the manual should describe specifically how the paper CRFs are used and which parts of the forms (e.g., two-part or three-part no-carbon-required forms) should be retained, copied, submitted, or archived. If electronic CRFs are utilized, clear user manuals and instructions should be available. These procedures are an important resource for all personnel involved in the registry (and for external auditors who might be asked to assure the quality of the registry).

The importance of standardizing procedures to ensure that the registry uses uniform and systematic methods for collecting data cannot be overstated. At the same time, some level of customization of data entry methods may be required or permitted to enable the participation of particular sites or subgroups of patients within some practices. As discussed in Chapter 7, if the registry provides payments to sites for participation, then the specific requirements for site payments should be clearly documented, and this information should be provided with the registry documents.

Personnel. All personnel involved in data collection should be identified, and their job descriptions and respective roles in data collection and processing should be described. Examples of such "roles" include patient, physician, data entry personnel, site coordinator, help desk, data manager, and monitor. The necessary documentation or qualification required for any role should be specified in the registry documentation. As an example, some registries require personnel documentation such as a curriculum vitae, protocol signoff, attestation of intent to follow registry procedures, or confirmation of completion of specified training.

Data sources. The sources of data for a registry may include new information collected from the patient, new or existing information reported by or derived from the clinician and the medical record, and ancillary stores of patient information such as laboratories. Since registries for evaluating patient outcomes should employ uniform and systematic methods of data collection, all data-related procedures—including the permitted sources of data; the data elements and their definitions; and the validity, reliability, or other quality requirements for the data collected from each source—should be predetermined and defined for all collectors of data. As described under "Quality Assurance," data quality is dependent on the entire chain of data collection and processing. Therefore, the validity and quality of the registry data as a whole ultimately derive from the least rigorous link, not the most.

In Chapter 5, data sources are classified as primary or secondary based on the relationship of the data to the registry purpose and protocol. Primary data sources incorporate data collected for direct purposes of the registry (i.e., primarily for the registry). Secondary data sources are comprised of data originally collected for purposes other than the registry (e.g., standard medical care, insurance claims processing). The data are abstracted for registry purposes. The section below incorporates and expands on these definitions.

Patient-reported data. Patient-reported data are data specifically collected from the patient for the purposes of the registry rather than interpreted through a clinician or an indirect data source (e.g., laboratory value, pharmacy records). Such data may range from basic demographic information to validated scales of patient-reported outcomes. From an operational perspective, a wide range of issues should be considered in obtaining data directly from patients. These range from presentation (e.g., font size, language, reading level) to technologies (e.g., paper-and-pencil questionnaires, computer inputs, telephone or voice inputs, or hand-held patient diaries). Mistakes at this level can inadvertently bias patient selection, invalidate certain outcomes, or significantly affect cost. Limiting the patient-reported data to particular languages or technologies may limit participation. Patients with specific diagnoses may have difficulties with specific technologies (e.g., small font size for visually impaired, paper and pencil for those with rheumatoid arthritis). Other choices, such as providing a patient-reported outcomes instrument in a format or method of delivery that differs from how it was validated (e.g., questionnaire rather than interview), may invalidate the results. (See Case Example 20.)

Clinician-reported data. Clinician-reported or -derived data can also be divided into primary and secondary. As an example, specific clinician rating scales (e.g., National Institutes of Health Stroke Scale)[245] may be required for the registry but not routinely captured in clinical encounters. Some variables might be collected directly by the clinician for the registry or obtained from the medical record. Data elements that must be collected directly by the clinician (e.g., because of a particular definition or need to assess a specific comorbidity that may or may not routinely be in the medical record) should be specified. These designations are important because they determine who can collect the data for a particular registry or what changes must be made in the procedures that the clinician follows in recording a medical record for a patient in a registry. Furthermore, the types of error that arise in registries (discussed under "Quality Assurance")

135

Case Example 20: Developing Data-Collection Tools and Systems for Patient-Reported Data

Description	The Patient-Centered Diabetes Registry provides support for evidence-based diabetes care in several primary care practices in Colorado. The registry uses its database to send diabetes summary reports to patients and provides information to providers to be used at the point of care. The goal of the registry is to evaluate and improve diabetes care.
Sponsor	Agency for Healthcare Research and Quality (AHRQ)
Year Started	Planning began in 2004, with registry launch in late 2006
Year Ended	To be determined
No. of Sites	6
No. of Records	Registry is in initial launch phases

Challenge

The registry works with six physician office practices to gather data on type 2 diabetes patients. These clinical data are extracted from electronic systems, including billing, laboratory, and pharmacy systems, and do not require any direct data entry on the part of clinicians or staff. The registry matches the clinical data with patient-reported data, which are gathered over the phone, by Web, or on paper. The registry uses the clinical and patient-reported data to produce patient care reports that summarize the patient's diabetes care and self-management. These reports are sent to the patient and the provider in order to improve patient self-management and guideline-concordant care.

During the registry planning phase, the registry team worked with its information technology (IT) department to develop data transfer systems to upload the clinical data from the practices' electronic systems. Once the clinical data were in place, the registry team needed to develop data collection tools and systems that the patients would find easy to use and accessible to collect the patient-reported data.

Proposed Solution

The team planned to offer telephone, Web-based, and paper data entry options for patients. While they wanted to push the telephone and Web-based options, they did not want to eliminate any potential patients because of type of data collection. To develop user-friendly systems, the team completed extensive rounds of user acceptance testing before the registry launch. Most of the user acceptance testing focused on the telephone and Web-based systems.

While the technology was being built, the team completed a round of mock telephone testing and Web testing using screenshots and mock-ups. This allowed the team to make critical changes before the technology development was finished. Next, the team did a round of real-time "walk-throughs" with volunteers. This round generated more feedback for the IT team, but the registry team found it difficult at times to convey the issues to the IT team. To address this communication gap, the registry team included an IT team member in the user testing.

Once the team had completed the user acceptance testing in English, it completed another round of testing in Spanish to make sure that all of the changes were appropriate for the Spanish-language systems and forms. To encourage participation in user testing, the team used incentives.

Results

Most of the participants in the user testing were able to use and liked both the Web and telephone systems. Project staff hoped that the telephone would be viewed as a helpful replacement to paper entry. Patients can call the system, and the system

(continued)

136

Case Example 20: Developing Data-Collection Tools and Systems for Patient-Reported Data (continued)

also places outgoing calls to prompt patients to enter information on diabetes care, exercise, weight management, and tobacco use. The registry populates the database with this information and matches it to the clinical data from the practices to produce short but detailed diabetes summary reports. These reports are available on the Web and by mail for patients, and they are sent to the practices. The system also places outgoing calls as reminders for upcoming visits.

The registry was initially scheduled to launch in 2005, but the launch was delayed because of technology issues and changes that were made as a result of the user testing. The registry is currently in its launch phase, and while it is too soon to measure its success, the initial response to the patient recruitment efforts has been positive.

Key Point

User acceptance testing can provide valuable information on how the registry procedures and data collection tools will be perceived by potential users. In cases where patient-reported data are collected, user acceptance testing can be an important way to determine if the registry is patient friendly and if there are any procedures that could lead to selection bias in patient enrollment.

will differ by the degree of primary and secondary sources, as well as other factors. As an example, registries that utilize medical chart abstracters, as discussed below, may be subject to more interpretive errors.[246]

Data abstraction. Data abstraction is the process by which a data collector other than the clinician interacting with the patient extracts clinician-reported data. While physical exam findings, such as height and weight, or laboratory findings, such as white blood cell counts, are straightforward, abstraction usually involves varying degrees of judgment and interpretation.

Clarity of description and standardization of definitions are paramount to the assurance of data quality and to the prevention of interpretive errors when using data abstraction. Knowledgeable registry personnel should be designated as resources for the data collectors in the field, and processes should be put in place to allow the data collectors in the field continuous access to these designated registry personnel for questions on specific definitions and clinical situations. Registries that span long periods, such as those intended for surveillance, may be well served by a structure that allows for the review of definitions on a periodic basis to ensure the timeliness and completeness of data elements and definitions and to add new data elements and definitions. A new product or procedure introduced after the start of a registry is a common reason for such an update.

Abstracting data from unformatted hard copy (e.g., a hospital chart) is often an arduous and tedious process, especially if free text is involved, and it usually requires a human reader. The reader, whose qualifications may range from a trained "medical record analyst" or other health professional to an untrained research assistant, may be required to decipher illegible handwriting, translate obscure abbreviations and acronyms, and understand the clinical content sufficiently to extract the desired information. Registry personnel should develop formal chart abstraction guidelines, documentation, and coding forms for the analysts and reviewers to use. Generally, the guidelines include instructions to search for particular types of data that will go into

137

the registry (e.g., specific diagnoses or lab results). Often the analyst will be asked to code the data, using either standardized codes from a codebook (e.g., the ICD-9 code [International Classification of Diseases, 9th Revision]) corresponding to a text diagnosis in a chart, or codes that may be unique to the registry, (e.g., a severity scale of 1 to 5). All abstraction and coding instructions must be carefully documented and incorporated into a data dictionary for the registry. Because of the "noise" in unstructured, hard-copy documents (e.g., spurious marks or illegible writing) and the lack of precision in natural language, the clinical data abstracted by different abstracters from the same documents may differ. This is a potential source of error in a registry.

To reduce the potential for this source of error, registries should ensure proper training on the registry protocol and procedures, condition(s), data sources, data collection systems, and, most importantly, data definitions and their interpretation. While training should be provided for all registry personnel, it is particularly important for nonclinician data abstracters. Training time depends on the nature of the source (charts or CRFs), complexity of the data, and number of data items. A variety of training methods, from live meetings to online meetings to interactive multi-media recordings, have all been used with success.[247] Training often includes test abstractions using sample charts. For some purposes, it is best practice to train abstracters on using standardized test charts. Such standardized tests can be further used both to obtain data on the inter-rater reliability of the case report forms, definitions, and coding instructions and to determine whether individual abstracters can perform up to a defined minimum standard for the registry. Registries that rely on medical chart abstraction should consider reporting on the performance characteristics associated with abstraction, such as inter-rater reliability.[248] Some key considerations in standardizing medical chart abstractions are:

- Standardized materials (e.g., definitions, instructions).
- Standardized training.

- Testing with standardized charts.
- Reporting of inter-rater reliability.

Electronic medical record. The electronic medical record (EMR) will play an increasingly important role as a source of clinical data for registries. The medical community is currently in a transition period in which the primary repository of a patient's medical record is changing from the traditional hard-copy chart to the EMR. The main function of the EMR is to aggregate all clinical electronic data about a patient into one logical computer schema, in the same way that a hard-copy medical chart aggregates paper records from various personnel and departments responsible for the care of the patient. Depending on the extent of implementation, the EMR may include patient demographics, diagnoses, procedures, progress notes, orders, flow sheets, medications, and allergies. The primary sources of data for the EMR are the health care providers. Data may be entered into the EMR through keyboards or touch-screens in medical offices or at the bedside. In addition, the EMR system is usually interfaced to ancillary systems (see below), such as laboratory, pharmacy, radiology, and pathology. Ancillary systems, which usually have their own databases, export relevant patient data to the EMR system, which imports the data into its database.

Since EMRs include the majority of clinical data available about a patient, they can be a major source of patient information for a registry. What an EMR usually does not include is registry-specific (primary source) data that are collected separately from hard-copy or electronic forms. In the next several years, suitable EMR system interfaces may be able to present data needed by registries in accordance with registry-specified requirements either within the EMR (which then populates the registry) or in an electronic data capture system (which then populates the EMR). EMRs already serve as secondary data sources in some registries, and this practice will continue to grow as EMRs become more widely used. In these situations, data may be extracted from the EMR, transformed into registry format, and loaded into the registry, where they will reside in the registry database together

138

with registry-specific data imported from other sources. In a sense, this is similar to medical chart abstraction except that it is performed electronically. There are two key differences. First, the data are "abstracted" once for all records. In this context, abstraction refers to the mapping and other decisionmaking that needs to be made to bring the EMR data into the registry database. It does not eliminate the potential for interpretive errors, as described later in this chapter, but it centralizes that process, making the rules clear and easily reviewed. Second, the data are uploaded electronically, eliminating the extra data entry.

While EMRs offer interesting potential for registries, the reality is that only a minority of U.S. patients currently have their data stored in systems that are capable of retrieval at the level of a data element. Furthermore, only a small number of these systems currently store data in structured formats with standardized data definitions for those data elements that are common across different vendors. A significant amount of attention is currently focused on both interchange formats between clinical and research systems (e.g., from Health Level Seven [HL-7][249] to Clinical Data Interchange Standards Consortium[250] models) and the problems of data syntax. (See Chapter 4.)

Other data sources. Some of the clinical data used to populate registries may be derived from repositories other than EMRs. Examples of other data sources include billing systems, laboratory databases, and other registries. Chapter 5 discusses the potential uses of other data sources in more detail.

Data Entry Systems

Once the primary and any secondary data sources for a registry have been identified, the registry team can determine how data will be entered into the registry database. Many techniques and technologies exist for entering or moving data into the registry database, including paper CRFs, direct data entry, facsimile or scanning systems, and electronic CRFs. There are also different models for how quickly those data reach a central repository for cleaning, reviewing, monitoring, or reporting. Each

approach has advantages and limitations, and each registry must balance flexibility (the number of options available) with data availability (when the central repository is populated), data validity (whether all methods are equally able to produce clean data), and cost. Appropriate decisions depend on many factors, including the number of data elements, number of sites, location (local preferences that vary by country, language differences, and availability of different technologies), registry duration, followup frequency, and available resources.

Paper CRFs. With paper CRFs, the clinician enters clinician data on the paper form at the time of the clinical encounter or other data collectors abstract the data from medical records after the clinical encounter. CRFs may include a wide variety of clinical data on each patient gathered from different sources (e.g., medical chart, laboratory, pharmacy) and from multiple patient encounters. Before the data on formatted paper forms are entered into a computer, the forms should be reviewed for completeness, accuracy, and validity. Paper CRFs can be entered into the database by either direct data entry or computerized data entry via scanning systems.

With direct data entry, a computer keyboard is used to enter data into a database. Key entry has a variable error rate depending on personnel, so an assessment of error is usually desirable, particularly when a high volume of entry is performed. Double data entry is a method of increasing the accuracy of manually entered data by quantifying error rates as discrepancies between two different data entry personnel, and improving data accuracy by having up to two individuals enter the data and a third person review and manage discrepancies. With upfront data validation checks on electronic entry interfaces, the likelihood of data entry errors significantly decreases. Therefore, the choice of single versus double data entry should be driven by the ability of each method to achieve a specific error rate in key measures in the particular circumstance and by the requirements of the registry for a particular error rate. Double data entry, while a standard of practice for registrational trials, may

139

add significant cost. Its use should be guided by the need to reduce an error rate in key measures and the likelihood of accomplishing that by double data entry as opposed to other approaches. In some situations, assessing the data entry error rates by re-entering a sample of the data is sufficient for reporting purposes.

With hard-copy structured forms, entering data using a scanner and special software to extract the data from the scanned image is possible. If data are recorded on a form as marks in checkboxes, the scanning software enables the user to map the location of each checkbox to the value of a variable represented by the text item associated with the checkbox and determine whether the box is marked. The presence of a mark in a box is converted by the software to its corresponding value, which can then be transmitted to a database for storage. If the form contains hand-printed or typed text or numbers, optical character recognition (OCR) software is often effective in extracting the printed data from the scanned image. However, the print font must be of high quality to avoid translation errors, and spurious marks on the page can cause errors. Error checking is based on automated parameters specified by the operator of the system for exception handling. The comments on assessing error rates in the section above are applicable for scanning systems as well.

Electronic CRFs (eCRFs). An eCRF is defined as an auditable electronic record designed to record information required by the clinical trial protocol to be reported to the sponsor on each trial subject.[251] An eCRF allows clinician-reported data to be entered directly into the electronic system by the data collector (the clinician or other data collector). Site personnel in many registries still commonly complete an intermediate hard-copy worksheet representing the CRF and subsequently enter the data into the eCRF. While this approach increases work effort and error rates, it is not yet practical for all data entry to be performed at the bedside, during the clinical encounter, or in the midst of a busy clinical day.

An eCRF may originate from local computerized databases (including those on an individual computer, a local area network server, or a hand-held device) or directly from a central database server via an Internet-based connection or a private network. For registries that exist beyond a single site, the data from the local system must subsequently communicate with a central data system. An eCRF may be presented visually (e.g., computer screen) or aurally (e.g., telephonic data entry, such as interactive voice response systems). Specific circumstances will favor different presentations. For example, in one clozapine patient registry that is otherwise similar to Case Example 21, both pharmacists and physicians can obtain and enter data via a telephone-based interactive voice response system as well as a Web-based system.[252] The option is successful in this scenario because telephone access is ubiquitous in pharmacies, and the eCRF is very brief.

A common method of electronic data entry is to use Web-based data entry forms. Such forms may be used by patients, providers, and interviewers to enter data into a local repository. The forms reside on servers, which may be located at the site of the registry or co-located anywhere on the Internet. To access a data entry form, a user on a remote computer with an Internet connection opens a browser window and enters the address of the Web server. Typically, a login screen is displayed and the user enters a user identification and password, provided by personnel responsible for the Web site or repository. Once the server authenticates the user, the data entry form is displayed, and the user can begin entering data. As described in "Cleaning Data," many electronic systems can perform data validation checks or edits at the time of data entry. When data entry is complete, the user submits the form, which is sent over the Internet to the Web server.

Hand-held devices, such as personal digital assistants (PDAs) and cell phones, may also be used with Web-based or other forms to submit data to a server. Mobility has recently become an important attribute for clinical data collection. Software has been developed that enables wireless PDAs and cell phones to collect data and transmit them over the Internet to database servers in fixed locations. As wireless technology continues to evolve and data transmission rates increase, these will become more important data entry devices for patients and clinicians.

Advantages and Disadvantages of Data Collection Technologies

When the medical record or ancillary data are in electronic format, they may be abstracted to the CRF by a data collector or, in some cases, uploaded electronically to the registry database. The ease of extracting data from electronic systems for use in a registry depends on the design of the interfaces of ancillary and registry systems and the ability of the EMR or ancillary system software to serve up the requested data. However, as system vendors increasingly adopt standards for medical systems called HL-7 and interchange models between schema, transferring data from one system to another will likely become easier. The American Health Information Community[253] is actively working toward improved standards with organizations such as the National Institute of Standards and Technology (NIST).[254]

Electronic interfaces are necessary to move data from one computer to another. If clinical data are entered into a local repository from an eCRF form or entered into an EMR, the data must be extracted from the source data set in the local repository, transformed into the format required by the registry, and loaded into the registry database for permanent storage. This is called an "extract, transform, and load" (ETL) process. Unless the local repository is designed to be consistent with the registry database in terms of the names of variables and their values, data mapping and transformation can be a complex task. In some cases, manual transfer of the data may be more efficient and less time consuming than the effort to develop an electronic interface.

If an interface between a local electronic system and registry system is developed, it is still necessary to communicate to the ancillary system the criteria for

retrieval and transmission of a patient record. Typically, the ancillary data are maintained in a relational database, and the system needs to run an SQL (Structured Query Language) query against the database to retrieve the specified information. An SQL query may specify individual patients by an identifier (e.g., a medical record number) or by values or ranges of specific variables (e.g., all patients with hemoglobin A1C over 8 mg/dl). The results of the query are usually stored as a file (e.g., ASCII, CSV, CDISC ODM) that can be transferred to the registry system across the interface. A variety of interface protocols may be used to transfer the data.

Because data definitions and formats are not yet standardized nationally, transfer of data from an EMR or ancillary system to a registry database is prone to error. Careful evaluation of the transfer specifications for interpretive or mapping errors is a critical step that should be verified by the registry coordinating center. Furthermore, a series of test transfers and validation procedures should be performed and documented. Finally, error checking must be part of the transfer process because new formats or other errors not in the test databases may be introduced during actual practice, and these need to be identified and isolated from the registry itself. Even though each piece of data may be accurately transferred, the data may have different representations on the different systems (e.g., value discrepancies such as the meaning of "0" vs. "1," fixed vs. floating point numbers, date format, integer length, and missing values). In summary, any system used to extract EMR records into registry databases should be validated and include an interval sampling of transfers to ensure that uploading of this information is consistent over time.

The ancillary system must also notify the registry when an error correction occurs in a record already transferred to the registry. Registry software must be able to receive that notification, flag the erroneous value as invalid, and insert the new, corrected value into its database. Finally, it is important to recognize that the use of an electronic-to-electronic interchange requires not only testing but also validation of the integrity and quality of the data transferred. Few ancillary systems or electronic medical records systems are currently validated to a defined standard. For registries that intend to report data to the FDA or to other sponsors or data recipients with similar requirements— including electronic signatures, audit trails, and rigorous system validation—the ways in which the registry interacts with other systems must be carefully considered.

Cleaning Data

Data cleaning refers to the correction or amelioration of data problems, including missing values, incorrect or out-of-range values, or responses that are logically inconsistent with other responses in the database. While all registries strive for "clean data," in reality, this is a relative term. How and to what level the data will be cleaned should be addressed upfront in a data management manual that identifies the data elements that are intended to be cleaned, describes the data validation parameters or logical checks for out-of-range values, and explains how missing values and values that are logically inconsistent will be handled.

Data management manual. Data managers should develop formal data review guidelines for the reviewers and data entry personnel to use. The guidelines should include information on how to handle missing data; invalid entries (e.g., multiple selections in a single-choice field, alphabetic data in a numeric field); erroneous entries (e.g., patients of the wrong gender answering gender-based questions); and inconsistent data (e.g., an answer to one question contradicting the answer to another one). The guidelines should also include procedures to attempt to remediate these data problems. For example, with a data error on an interview form, it may be necessary to query the interviewer or the patient, or to refer to other data sources that may be able to resolve the problem. Documentation of any data review activity and remediation efforts, including dates, times, and results of the query, should be maintained.

Automated data cleaning. Ideally, automated data checks are preprogrammed into the database for presentation at the time of data entry. These data checks are particularly useful for cleaning data at the site level while the patient or medical record is readily accessible. Even relatively simple edit checks, such as range values for laboratories, can have a significant effect on improving the quality of data. Many systems allow for the implementation of more complex data edit checks, and these checks can substantially reduce the amount of subsequent manual data cleaning. A variation of this method is to use data cleaning rules to deactivate certain data fields so that erroneous entries cannot even be made. A combination of these approaches can also be used. For paper-based entry methods, automated data checks are not available at the time the paper CRF is being completed but can be incorporated when the data are later entered into the database.

Manual data cleaning. Data managers perform manual data checks or queries to review data for unexpected discrepancies. This is the standard approach to cleaning data that are not entered into the database at the site (e.g., for paper CRFs entered via data entry or scanning). By carefully reviewing the data using both data extracts analyzed by algorithms and hand review, data managers identify discrepancies and generate "queries" to send to the sites to resolve. Even eCRF-based data entry with data validation rules may not be fully adequate to ensure data cleaning for certain purposes. Anticipating all potential data discrepancies at the time that the data management manual and edit checks are developed is very difficult. Therefore, even with the use of automated data validation parameters, some manual cleaning is often still performed.

Query reports. The registry coordinating center should generate, on a periodic basis, query reports that relate to the quality of the data received based on the data management manual and, for some purposes, additional concurrent review by a data manager. The content of these reports will differ depending on what type of data cleaning is required for the registry purpose and how much automated data cleaning has already been performed. Query reports may include missing data, "out-of-range" data, or data that appear to be inconsistent (e.g., positive pregnancy test for a male patient). They may also identify abnormal trends in data, such as sudden increases or decreases in laboratory tests compared to patient historical averages or clinically established normal ranges. Qualified registry personnel should be responsible for reviewing the abnormal trends with designated site personnel. The most effective approach is for sites to provide one contact representative for purposes of queries or concerns by registry personnel. Depending on the availability of the records and resources at the site to review and respond to queries, resolving all queries can sometimes be a challenge. Creating systematic approaches to maximizing site responsiveness is recommended.

Data tracking. For most registry purposes, tracking of data received (paper CRFs), data entered, data cleaned, and other parameters are important components of active registry management. By comparing indicators, such as expected to observed rates of patient enrollment, CRF completion, and query rates, the registry coordinating center can identify problems and potentially take corrective action—either at individual sites or across the registry as a whole.

Coding data. As further described in Chapter 4, the use of standardized coding dictionaries is an increasingly important tool in the ability to aggregate registry data with other databases. As the health information community adopts standards, registries should routinely apply them unless there are specific reasons not to use such standard codes. While such codes should be implemented in the data dictionaries during registry planning, including all codes in the interface is not always possible. Some free text may be entered as a result. When free text data are entered into a registry, recoding these data using standardized dictionaries (e.g., MedDRA, WHODRUG, SNOMED®) may be worthwhile. There is cost associated with recoding, and in general, it should be limited to data elements that will be used in analysis or that need to be combined or reconciled with other datasets, such as when a

common safety database is maintained across multiple registries and studies.

Storing and securing data. When data on a form are entered into a computer for inclusion in a registry, the form itself, as well as a log of the data entered, should be maintained for the regulatory archival period. Data errors may be discovered long after the data have been stored in the registry. The error may have been made by the patient or interviewer on the original form or during the data entry process. Examination of the original form and the data entry log should reveal the source of the error. If the error is on the form, correcting it may require re-interviewing the patient. If the error occurred during data entry, the corrected data should be entered and the registry updated. By then, the erroneous registry data may have been used to generate reports or create cohorts for population studies. Therefore, instead of simply replacing erroneous data with corrected data, the registry system should have the ability to flag data as erroneous without deleting them and to insert the corrected data for subsequent use.

143

Once data are entered into the registry, the registry must be backed up on a regular basis. There are two basic types of backup, and both types should be considered for use as best practice by the registry coordinating center. The first type is real-time disk backup, which is done by the disk storage hardware used by the registry server. The second is a regular (e.g., daily) backup of the registry to removable media (e.g., tape, CD-ROM, DVD). In the first case, as data are stored on disk in the registry server, they are automatically replicated to two or more physical hard drives. In the simplest example, called "mirroring," registry data are stored on a primary disk and an exact replica is stored on the mirrored disk. If either disk fails, data continue to be stored on the mirrored disk until the failed disk is replaced. This failure can be completely transparent to the user, who may continue entering and retrieving data from the registry database during the failure. More complex disk backup configurations exist, in which arrays of disks are used to provide protection from single disk failures.

The second type of daily backup is needed for disaster recovery. Ideally, a backup copy of the registry database stored on removable media should be maintained off site. In case of failure of the registry server or disaster that closes the data center, the backup copy can be brought to a functioning server and the registry database restored, with the only loss of data being for the interval between the regularly scheduled backups. The lost data can usually be reloaded from local data repositories or re-entered from hard copy.

Managing Change

Like all other registry processes, the extent of change management will depend on the types of data being collected, the source(s) of the data, and the overall timeframe of the registry.

There are two major drivers behind the need for change during the conduct of a registry: internal-driven change to refine or improve the registry or the quality of data collected and external-driven change that comes as a result of changes in the environment in which the registry is being conducted.

Internal-driven change is generally focused on changes to data elements or data validation parameters that arise from site feedback, queries, and query trends that may point to a question, definition, or CRF field that was poorly designed or missing. If this is the case, the registry can use the information coming back from sites to add, delete, or modify the database requirements, CRFs, definitions, or data management manual as required. External-driven change generally arises in multiyear registries as new information about the disease and/or product under study becomes available or as new therapies or products are introduced into clinical practice. Change and turnover in registry personnel is another type of change, and one that can be highly disruptive if procedures are not standardized and documented.

Proper management of change is crucial to the maintenance of the registry. A consistent approach to change management, including decisionmaking, documentation, data mapping, and validation, is an important aspect of maintaining the quality of the registry and the validity of the data. While the specific change management processes might depend on the type and nature of the registry, change management in registries that are designed to evaluate patient outcomes requires, at the very least, the following structures and processes:

- *Detailed manual of procedures*: As described earlier, a detailed manual that is updated on a regular basis—containing all the registry policies, procedures, and protocols, as well as a complete data dictionary listing all the data elements and their definitions—is vital for the functioning of a registry. The manual is also a crucial component for managing and documenting change management in a registry.

- *Governing body*: As described in Chapter 2, registries require oversight and advisory bodies for a number of purposes. One of the most important is to manage change on a regular basis. Keeping the registry manual and data definitions up to date is one of the primary responsibilities of this governing body. Large prospective registries, such as the National Surgical Quality Improvement Program, have found it necessary to delegate the updating of data elements and definitions to a special Definitions Committee.

- *Infrastructure for ongoing training*: As mentioned above, change in personnel is a common issue for registries. Specific processes and an infrastructure for training should be available at all times to account for any unanticipated changes and turnover of registry personnel or providers who regularly enter data into the registry.

- *Method to communicate change*: Since registries frequently undergo change, there should be a standard approach and timeline for communicating to sites when changes will take place.

In addition to instituting these structures, registries should also plan for change from a budget perspective (Chapter 2) and from an analysis perspective (Chapter 10).

144

Special Case: Performance-Linked Access System (PLAS)

A performance-linked access system (PLAS), also known as a restricted access or limited distribution system, can be described as a special application of a registry. Unlike a disease and exposure registry, a PLAS is part of a detailed risk minimization action plan that sponsors develop as a commitment to enhance the risk-benefit balance of a product when approved for the market. The purpose of a PLAS is to mitigate a certain known drug-associated risk by ensuring that product access is linked to a specific performance measure. Examples include systems that monitor laboratory values, such as white blood cell counts during clozapine administration to prevent severe leukopenia or routine pregnancy testing during thalidomide administration to prevent in utero exposure to this known teratogenic compound. Additional information on PLAS can be found in *Guidance for Industry: Development and Use of Risk Minimization Action Plans*.[255] (See Case Example 21.)

Quality Assurance

Observational studies based on patient registries are being used today to support the results and assist in the planning of randomized controlled trials. Some are even substituting for clinical trials in the assessment of the comparative safety and effectiveness of specific pharmacologic interventions.[256] It is therefore imperative that patient registries be held to high standards of quality, particularly when they are intended to evaluate patient outcomes. Methods of quality assurance may vary depending on the intended purpose of the registry, and they generally fall under three main categories: quality assurance of data, quality assurance of registry procedures, and quality assurance of computerized systems. The level of quality assurance that can be obtained is always limited by budgetary constraints. A risk-based approach that focuses on the most important sources of error or procedural lapses from the perspective of the registry's purpose should be defined during

inception and design phases. For example, a registry describing the natural history of a disease and a registry determining the safety of a product may have very different quality assurance plans.

Assurance of Data Quality

Structures, processes, policies, and procedures need to be put in place to ascertain the quality of the data in the registry and to ensure against several types of errors, including:

* *Errors in interpretation or coding*: An example of this type of error would be two abstracters looking for the same data element in a patient's medical record but extracting different data from the same chart. Variations in coding of specific conditions or procedures also fall under the category of interpretive errors. Avoidance or detection of interpretive error includes adequate training on definitions, testing against standard charts, testing and reporting on inter-rater reliability, and re-abstraction.

* *Errors in data entry, transfer, or transformation accuracy*: These occur when data are entered into the registry inaccurately—for example, a laboratory value of 2.0 is entered as 20. Avoidance or detection of accuracy errors can be achieved through upfront data quality checks (such as ranges and data validation checks), re-entering samples of data to assess for accuracy, and rigorous attention to data cleaning.

* *Errors of intention*: Examples of intentional distortion of data (often referred to as "gaming") are inflated reporting of preoperative patient risk in registries that compare risk-adjusted outcomes of surgery or selecting only cases with good outcomes to report ("cherry-picking"). Avoidance or detection of intentional error can be challenging. Some approaches include checking for consistency of data between sites, assessing screening log information against other sources (e.g., billing data), or performing onsite audits (including monitoring source records) either at random or "for cause."

145

Case Example 21: Developing a Performance-Linked Access System	
Description	The Clozapine Patient Registry is one of several national patient registries for patients taking clozapine. The registry is a performance-linked access system (PLAS), mandated by the U.S. Food and Drug Administration, that collects patient lab data and contact information and investigates any adverse events that may be connected to clozapine.
Sponsor	IVAX Pharmaceuticals (a member of the Teva Group)
Year Started	1997
Year Ended	Ongoing
No. of Sites	40,000 registered health care providers (physicians and pharmacists)
No. of Patients	47,000

Challenge

Clozapine is indicated for patients with severe schizophrenia who fail standard therapy and for reducing the risk of recurrent suicidal behavior in schizophrenia or schizoaffective disorder. However, it has potentially serious side effects that require careful medical supervision. The primary goal of the registry is to prevent clozapine from being prescribed and dispensed to patients with a known history of clozapine-induced agranulocytosis and to detect leukopenic events (decrease in white blood cell counts).

Because of the potential serious side effects, the U.S. Food and Drug Administration (FDA) requires manufacturers of clozapine to maintain a patient monitoring system. Designed as a performance-linked access system, the registry needs to assure the eligibility of patients, pharmacies, and physicians; monitor white blood cell (WBC) and absolute neutrophil count (ANC) reports for low counts; assure compliance with lab report submission timelines; and respond to inquires and reports of adverse events.

Proposed Solution

The registry was developed to meet these goals. Patients must be enrolled in the registry prior to receiving clozapine, and they must be assigned to a dispensing pharmacy and treating physician. After the patient has initiated therapy, a current and acceptable WBC count and ANC value are required prior to dispensing clozapine. Once a patient is enrolled and eligibility is confirmed, a 1-, 2-, or 4-week supply of clozapine can be dispensed, depending on patient experience and the physician's prescription.

Health care professionals are required to submit lab reports to the registry based on the patients' monitoring frequency. Patients are monitored weekly for the first 6 months. If there are no low counts, the patient can be monitored every 2 weeks for an additional 6 months. Afterward, the patient may qualify for monitoring every 4 weeks (depending on the physician's prescription).

The registry provides reminders if lab data are not submitted according to the schedule. If a low count is identified, registry staff will inform the health care providers to make sure that they are aware of the event.

Results

By linking access to clozapine to a strict schedule of lab data submissions, the sponsor can ensure that only eligible patients are taking the drug, detect low counts, prevent inappropriate rechallenge (or re-exposure) in at-risk patients, and monitor the patient population for any adverse events. This system provides the sponsor with data on the frequency and severity of adverse events while ensuring that only the proper patient population receives the drug.

(continued)

Case Example 21: Developing a Performance-Linked Access System (continued)
Key Point
A PLAS can ensure that only appropriate patients receive a treatment. These systems can also help sponsors to monitor the patient population to learn more about adverse events and the frequency of these events.
For More Information
Reid WH. Access to care: clozapine in the public sector. Hosp Community Psychiatry 1990 Aug;40(8):870-3.

Steps for assuring data quality include:

- *Training*: Educate data collectors/abstracters in a structured manner.

- *Data completeness*: When possible, provide sites with immediate feedback on issues such as missing or out-of-range values and logical inconsistencies.

- *Data consistency*: Compare across sites and over time.

- *Onsite audits for a sample of sites*: Review screening logs and procedures and/or samples of data.

To further minimize or identify these errors and to ensure the overall quality of the data, the following should be considered.

A designated individual accountable for data quality at each site. Sites submitting data to a registry should have at least one person who is accountable for the quality of these data, irrespective of whether the person is collecting the data as well. The site coordinator should be fully knowledgeable of all protocols, policies, procedures, and definitions in a registry. The site coordinator should ensure that all site personnel involved in the registry are knowledgeable and that all data

transmitted to registry coordinating centers are valid and accurate.

Assessment of training and maintenance of competency of personnel. Thorough training and documentation of maintenance of competency for both site and registry personnel are imperative to the quality of the registry. A detailed and comprehensive operations manual, as described earlier, is crucial for the proper training of all personnel involved in the registry. Routine cognitive testing (surveys) of health care provider knowledge of patient registry requirements and appropriate product use should be performed to monitor maintenance of the knowledge base and compliance with patient registry requirements. Retraining programs should be initiated when survey results provide evidence of lack of knowledge maintenance. All registry training programs should provide means by which the knowledge of the data collectors about their registries and their competence in data collection can be assessed on a regular basis, particularly when changes in procedures or definitions are implemented.

Data quality audits. As described above, the level to which registry data will be cleaned is influenced by the objectives of the registry, the type of data being collected (e.g., clinical data vs. economic data), the sources of the data (e.g., primary vs. secondary), and the timeframe of the registry (e.g., 3-month followup vs. 10-year followup). These registry characteristics often affect the types and number of data queries that are generated both electronically and manually. In addition to identifying missing values, incorrect or out-of-range values, or responses that are logically inconsistent with other responses in the database, specifically trained registry personnel can review the data queries to identify possible error trends and to determine whether additional site training is required. For example, such personnel may identify a specific patient outcome question or eCRF field that is generating a larger than average proportion of queries, either from one site or across all registry

147

sites. Using this information, the registry personnel can conduct targeted followup with the sites to retrain them on the correct interpretation of the eCRF field in question, with the goal of reducing the future query rate on that particular question or field. These types of "training tips" can also be addressed in a registry newsletter as a way to maintain frequent, but unobtrusive, communication with the registry sites.

Should the registry purpose require a more stringent verification of the data being entered into the database by registry participants, registry planners may decide to conduct audits of the registry sites. Like queries discussed above, the audit plan for a specific registry will be influenced by the purpose of the registry, the type of data being collected, the source of the data, and the overall timeframe of the registry. In addition, registry developers must find the appropriate balance between the extensiveness of an audit and the impact on overall registry costs. Based on the objectives of the registry, a registry developer can define specific data fields (e.g., key effectiveness variables or adverse event data) on which the audit can be focused.

The term "audit" may describe examination or verification, may take place on site (sometimes called monitoring) or off site, and may be extensive or very limited. The audit can be conducted on a random sample of participating sites (e.g., 5-20 percent of registry sites); "for cause" (meaning only when there is an indication of a problem, such as one site being an outlier compared with most others); on a random sample of patients; or using sampling techniques based on geography, practice setting (academic center vs. community hospital), patient enrollment rate, or query rate. The approach to auditing the quality of the data should reflect the most significant sources of error with respect to the purpose of the registry. Finally, the timeframe of the registry may help determine the audit plan. A registry with a short followup period (e.g., 3 months) may require only one round of audits at the end of the study prior to database lock and data analysis. For registries with multiyear followup, registry personnel may conduct site audits every 1 or 2 years for the duration of the registry. In

addition to the site characteristics mentioned above, sites that have undergone significant staffing changes during a multiyear registry should be considered prime audit targets to help confirm adequate training of new personnel and to quickly address possible inter-rater variability. To minimize any impact on the observational nature of the registry, the audit plan should be documented in the registry manual.

Registries that are designed for the evaluation of patient outcomes and the generation of scientific information and that utilize medical chart abstracters should assess inter-rater reliability in data collection with sufficient scientific rigor for their intended purpose(s). For example, in one registry that uses abstractions extensively, a detailed system of assessing inter-rater reliability has been devised and published; in addition to requiring that abstracters achieve a certain level of proficiency, a proportion of charts are scheduled for re-abstraction on the basis of predefined criteria. Statistical measures of reliability from such re-abstractions are maintained and reported (e.g., kappa statistic).[257]

Subsequent to audits (onsite or remote), communication of findings with site personnel should be conducted in a face-to-face manner along with followup written communication of findings and opportunities for improvement. As appropriate to meet registry objectives, the sponsor may request corrective actions from the site. Site compliance may also be enhanced with routine communication of data generated from the patient registry system to the site for reconciliation.

Registry Procedures and Systems

External audits of registry procedures. If registry developers determine that external audits are necessary to assure the level of quality for the specific purpose(s) of the registry, they should be conducted in accordance with pre-established criteria. Pre-established criteria could include monitoring of sites with high patient enrollment or prior audit history with findings that require attention or monitoring based on level of site experience, rate of serious adverse event reporting, or identified problems. The registry coordinating center may perform monitoring of a sample of sites, which could be focused on one or several areas. This approach could range from review of procedures and interviewing site personnel, to checking screening logs, to monitoring individual case records.

The importance of having a complete and detailed registry manual that describes policies, structures, and procedures cannot be overemphasized in the context of quality assurance of registry procedures. Such a manual serves both as a basis for conducting the audits and as a means of documenting changes emanating from these audits. As was stated in relation to data quality audits, feedback of the findings of registry procedure audits should be communicated to all stakeholders and documented in the registry manual.

Assurance of system integrity and security. All aspects of data management processes should fall under a rigorous life-cycle approach to system development and quality management. Each process is clearly defined and documented. The concepts described below are consistent across many software industry standards and health care industry standards (e.g., 21 CFR Part 11, legal security standards), although some specifics may vary. The processes and procedures described should be regularly audited by an internal quality assurance function at t he registry coordinating center. When third parties other than the registry coordinating center perform activities that interact with the registry systems and data, they are typically assessed for risk and are subject to regular audits by the registry coordinating center.

System development and validation. All software systems used for patient registries should follow the standard principles of software development. The life-cycle model refers to a common model that is well described in the software industry.

In parallel, quality assurance of system development utilizes approved specifications to create a validation plan for each project. Test cases are created by trained personnel and systematically executed, with results recorded and reviewed. Depending on regulatory requirements, a final

validation report is often written and approved. Unresolved product and process issues are maintained and tracked in a "bug" tracking system. Processes are similarly documented and audited. The information from these audits is captured, summarized, and reviewed with the applicable group with the aim of ongoing process improvement and quality improvement.

Security

All registries maintain health information, and, therefore, security is an important issue. The HIPAA (Health Insurance Portability and Accountability Act of 1996) Security Rule lists the standards for security for electronic protected health information to be implemented by health plans, health care clearinghouses, and certain health care providers.[258] Although these standards are specific to electronic protected health information, the principles themselves are more broadly applicable.

Security is achieved not simply by technology but by clear processes and procedures. Overall responsibility for security is typically assigned. Security procedures are well documented and posted. The documentation is also used to train staff.

System security plan. A system security plan consists of documented policies and standard operating procedures defining the rules of systems, including administrative procedures, physical safeguards, technical security services, technical security mechanisms, electronic signatures, and audit trails, as applicable. The rules delineate roles and responsibilities. Included in the rules are the policies specifying individual accountability for actions, access rights based on the principle of least privilege, and the need for separation of duties. These principles and the accompanying security practices provide the foundation for the confidentiality and integrity of clinical trial data. The rules also detail the consequences associated with noncompliance.

Security assessment. Clinical data maintained in a registry can be assessed for the appropriate level of security. Standard criteria exist for such

149

assessments and are based on the type of data being collected. Part of the validation process is a security assessment of the systems and operating procedures. One of the goals of such an assessment is effective risk management, based on determining possible threats to the system or data and identifying potential vulnerabilities.

Education and training. All staff members of the registry coordinating center should be provided with periodic training on aspects of the overall systems, security requirements, and any special requirements of specific patient registries. Individuals should receive training relating to their specific job responsibilities and document that appropriate training has been received.

Access controls. Access to systems and data should be based on the principles of least privilege and separation of duties. No individual should be assigned access privileges that exceed job requirements, and no individual should be in a role that includes access rights that would allow circumvention of controls or the repudiation of actions within the system. In all cases, access should be limited to authorized individuals.

Electronic signatures. Logical access to systems and computerized data should require an electronic signature—either based on an encrypted digital certificate stored on a password-protected device or in the form of a unique user ID and password combination—that is assigned to the individual whose identity has been verified and whose job responsibilities require such access. Electronic signatures provide one of the foundations of individual accountability, helping to ensure an accurate change history when used in conjunction with secure, computer-generated, time-stamped audit trails.

Most systems utilize an electronic signature. For registries that report data to FDA, such signatures must meet criteria specified in 21 CFR Part 11 for general signature composition, use, and control (11.100, 11.200, and 11.300). However, even registries that do not have such requirements should view these as reasonable standards. Before an individual is assigned an electronic signature, it is

important to verify the person's identity and train the individual in the significance of the electronic signature. In cases where a signature consists of a user ID and a password, both management and technical means should be used to ensure uniqueness and compliance with password construction rules. Password length, character composition, uniqueness, and validity life cycle should be based on industry best practices and guidelines published by the NIST. Rules should be established for situations in which passwords are compromised. As passwords expire, new password information should be sent to the individual by a secure method. Electronic signatures provide the basis for authentication and logical access to critical systems and data. Since the authenticity, integrity, and auditability of data stored in electronic systems depend on accurate individual authentication, management of electronic signatures is an important topic.

Intrusion detection and firewalls should be employed on sites accessible to the Internet, with appropriate controls and rules in place to limit access to authorized users. Desktop systems should be equipped with antivirus software, and servers should run the most recent security patches. System security should be reviewed throughout the course of the registry to ensure that management, operational, personnel, and technical controls are functioning properly.

Validation. Systems that store electronic records (or depend on electronic or handwritten signatures of those records) that are required to be acceptable to FDA must be validated according to the requirements set forth in the 21 CFR Part 11 Final Rule,[259] dated March 20, 1997. The rule describes the requirements and controls for electronic systems that are used to fulfill records requirements set forth in agency regulations (often called "predicate rules") and for any electronic records submitted to the agency. FDA publishes nonbinding guidance documents from time to time that outline its current thinking regarding the scope and application of the regulation. The current guidance document is *Guidance for Industry, Part 11, Electronic Records;*

Electronic Signatures – Scope and Application,[260] dated August 2003. Other documents that are useful for determining validation requirements of electronic systems are *Guidance for Industry, Computerized Systems Used in Clinical Trials,*[261] dated April 1999, and *General Principles of Software Validation; Final Guidance for Industry and FDA Staff,*[262] dated January 11, 2002.

Resource Considerations

Costs for registries can be highly variable, depending on the overall goals. Costs are also associated with the total number of sites, the total number of patients, and the geographical reach of the registry program. Each of the elements described in this chapter has an associated cost.

Table 12 provides a list of some of the activities of the registry coordinating center as an example. Not all registries will require or can afford all of the functions, options, or quality assurance techniques described in this chapter. Registry planners must evaluate benefit vs. available resources to determine the most appropriate approach to achieve their goals.

151

Table 12: Data Activities Performed During Registry Coordination	
Data management	• Defines all in-process data quality control steps, procedures, and metrics • Defines the types of edit checks that are run against the data • Defines required file-format specifications for electronic files, as well as schedules and processes for transfers of data • Defines quality acceptance criteria for electronic data, as well as procedures for handling exceptions • Develops guidelines for data entry • Identifies areas of manual review where electronic checks are not effective • Develops and maintains process for reviewing, coding, and reporting adverse event data • Develops and maintains archiving process • Develops and documents the process for change management • Develops and maintains process for query tracking and creates standard reports to efficiently identify outstanding queries, query types per site, etc. • Relates queries to processes and activities (e.g., CRF design) requiring process improvements • Follows up on query responses and errors identified in data cleaning by performing accurate database updates • Defines registry-specific dictionaries and code lists • Performs database audits as applicable • Conducts user testing of systems and applications per written specifications • Establishes quality criteria and quality error rate acceptance limits • Evaluates data points that should be audited and identifies potential sources of data errors for audits • Identifies root cause of errors in order to recommend change in process/technology to assure the error does not occur again (continuous improvement) • Ensures that sampling audit techniques are valid and support decisions made about data • Outlines all other data flow, including external data sources
Documentation	• Documents the process, procedures, standards, and checklist(s) and provides training • Documents and maintains process and standards for identifying signals and trends in data • Documents database quality control actions performed
Reporting	• Generates standard reports of missing data from the patient database • Creates tools to track and inventory CRFs and reports anticipated vs. actual CRF receipts
Note: CRF = case report form.	

Chapter 9. Adverse Event Detection, Processing, and Reporting

The U.S. Food and Drug Administration (FDA) defines an adverse drug experience as any adverse event (AE) associated with the use of a drug in humans, whether or not considered drug related.[263] For clinical safety data from clinical and investigational studies, an International Conference on Harmonisation guideline defines an AE as an untoward medical occurrence in a patient administered a pharmaceutical product, whether or not related or considered to have a causal relationship with the treatment.[264] AEs are categorized for regulatory purposes according to the seriousness and expectedness of the event. For adverse events occurring during postmarketing studies and information concerning potential adverse experiences derived during planned contacts and active solicitation of information from patients, such as registries of an FDA-approved product,[265,266] the requirements for mandatory reporting include an additional categorization of "relatedness" that addresses whether or not there is a reasonable possibility that the drug caused the adverse experience.[267] For medical devices, reportable events include AEs and/or product problems. They are defined as events in which the device may have caused or contributed to a death or serious injury (AEs) or may have malfunctioned and would likely cause or contribute to death or serious injury if the malfunction were to recur (product problems).

Most registries have the opportunity to identify and capture information on AEs for biopharmaceutical products and/or medical devices. Although there are no regulations in the United States that specifically require registries to capture and process AE reports (aside from reporting requirements for registries that are sponsored by regulated industries), there is an implicit requirement from the perspective of promoting public health: any individual who believes a serious and previously unknown AE may have occurred because of exposure to a medical product should be encouraged to report that AE either to the product sponsor or directly to the FDA.

AE reporting depends, in part, on the ability to include an identifiable patient.[268] However, not all registries have direct contact with individual patients. AEs can be detected through retrospective analysis of a population database where direct patient contact does not occur, as well as through interaction with patients. Patient interactions could include clinical interactions or data collection by phone, Internet, or other means; perusal of electronic medical records or insurance claims data would not be considered direct patient interactions. Reporting is rarely required for individual AEs observed in aggregate population data, since there is no direct patient interaction where an association might be suggested or inferred. Nevertheless, if aggregate or epidemiologic analyses suggest an AE is associated with exposure to a drug or medical product, it is desirable that this information be forwarded to the manufacturer of that product, who will determine any need for and timing of reporting of study results to a regulatory authority.

Figure 2 provides a broad overview of the reporting requirements for AEs and shows how the reporting differs according to whether the registry has direct patient interaction and whether it receives sponsorship and/or financial support from a "regulated industry." These industries may include entities with products subject to FDA regulation, including products with FDA approval, an FDA-granted license, and unapproved marketed drug products, and others such as manufacturers, packers, and distributors.

This chapter addresses the identification, processing, and reporting of AEs that are detected in situations in which the registry has individual patient contact. This document is not a formal regulatory or legal document; therefore, any information or suggestions presented herein do not supersede, replace, or otherwise interpret Federal guidance documents that touch on these subjects. Registry sponsors are encouraged to discuss plans

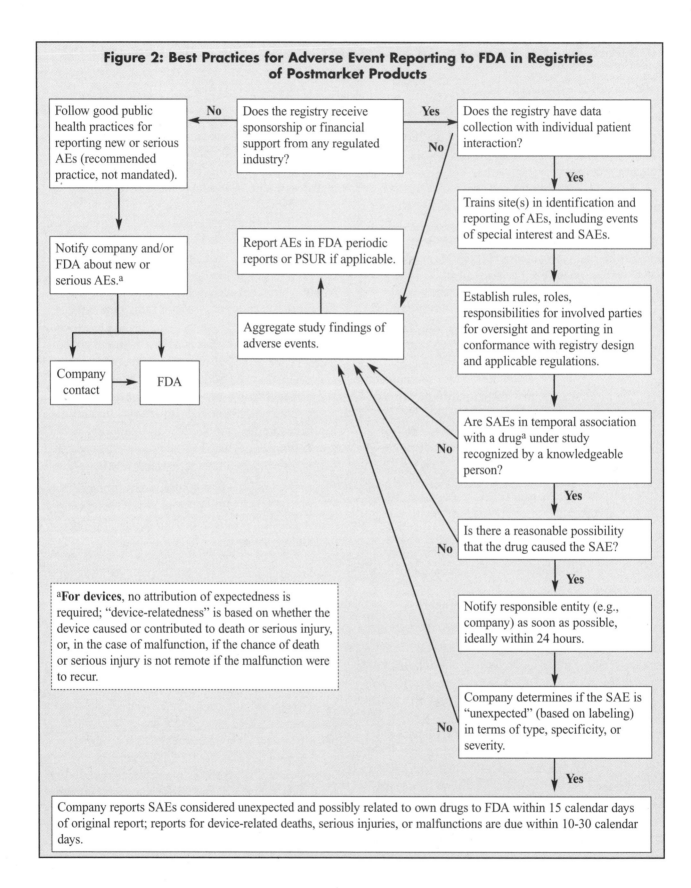

Figure 2: Best Practices for Adverse Event Reporting to FDA in Registries of Postmarket Products

154

for AE collection and processing with local health authorities when planning a registry.

Medical devices are significantly different from pharmaceuticals in the manner in which AEs and product problems present themselves, in the etiology of their occurrence, and in the regulation governing defining, and reporting of these occurrences, as well as postmarketing study requirements. This chapter is focused on AEs related to pharmaceutical products. Other sources provide more information about defining and reporting of device-related AEs and product problems and about postmarketing studies (including those involving registries).[269,270,271]

AE Detection and Recording by the Registry

All AE reporting begins with a suspicion by the site physician (or responsible person who obtains or receives information) that some adverse event has happened to the patient and that the event has a reasonable possibility of being causally related to the drug or device being used; this is referred to as the "becoming aware" principle. It is important to develop a plan for detecting, processing, and reporting AEs for any registry that has direct patient contact. If the registry receives sponsorship in whole or part from a regulated industry (for drugs or devices), then the sponsor has mandated reporting requirements, including stringent timelines. (See AE reporting requirements for registry sponsors later in this chapter.) The process for detecting and reporting AEs should be established in collaboration with the sponsor and any oversight committees. (See Chapter 2.) Once the plans have been developed, sites should be trained about how to identify AEs and to whom they should be reported.

AE reporting is based on categorization of the adverse event according to the seriousness of the event, expectedness of the event based on labeling, and presumed causality or possible association with use of the product, as follows:

- *Seriousness*: Serious drug-related AEs include those that result in death, are life threatening (an event in which the patient was at risk of death at the time of the event), require or prolong inpatient hospitalization, result in persistent or significant disability or incapacity, or result in a congenital anomaly. Important medical events may also be considered serious when, based on medical judgment, they may jeopardize the person exposed and may require medical or surgical intervention to prevent one of the outcomes listed above (e.g., death, prolonged hospitalization).

- *Expectedness*: All drug-related AEs that are previously unobserved or undocumented are referred to as "unexpected" in that the nature and severity are not consistent with information provided in the relevant product information (e.g., approved professional package insert or product label).

- *Relatedness*: "Relatedness" is intended to indicate that an evaluation has been made in which it was determined that the response that occurred in the individual had a reasonable possibility of being related to exposure to the product. This assessment of causality is based on factors such as biological plausibility, prior experience with the product, and temporal relationship between product exposure and onset of the event, as well as de-challenge (to determine if the adverse event resolves) and re-challenge (to determine if the adverse event reoccurs). Many terms and scales are used to describe the degree of causality, including terms such as "certainly," "definitely," "probably," "possibly," or "likely" related or not related, but there is no standard nomenclature.[272]

AE reports for a pharmaceutical or biological product should provide information about the four basic elements of an AE report: an identifiable patient, an identifiable reporter, a suspect drug or biological product, and an adverse event or fatal outcome. Typically, forms such as a questionnaire or an AE case report form may be used to collect information regarding an AE. When solicitation of specific AEs is not prespecified, it is good practice, although not required, to permit AE detection by asking general questions, such as "Have you had any problems since your last visit or since we last

155

spoke?" and then following up any such reports with probes as to what happened, diagnoses, and other documentation.

Collecting AE Data in a Registry

he collection of AE data by a registry generally is either intentionally solicited (meaning that the data are part of the uniform collection of information in the registry) or unsolicited (meaning that the AE information is volunteered or noted in an unsolicited manner and not as a required data element through a case report form). As described further below, it is good practice for a registry to specify when and how AE information, and any other events of special interest, should and should not be solicited from patients by physicians or other responsible parties (referred to as "sites" hereafter) and, if that information has been obtained, how and when the site should inform the appropriate persons. While an AE may be reported to the manufacturer, FDA (via MedWatch), or the registry (and then from the registry to the manufacturer), it is strongly encouraged that the protocol document the procedures that should be followed and that the sites be trained in these procedures, as well as general obligations and public health considerations.

Determining whether the registry should use the case report form to collect AEs should be based on the principles described in Chapter 4, which refer to the scientific importance of the information for evaluating the specified outcomes of interest. This may mean that all, some, or no adverse events are collected on the case report forms. However, if some AEs are collected in an intentional solicited manner (such as routine collection of a primary or secondary outcome via an AE case report form) and others come to attention in an unsolicited, "spontaneous" way (e.g., reporting an AE in the course of registry contact, such as a call to the sponsor or registry Help Desk), then from a practical perspective it is even more important to have a clear process so that sites are not confused and AEs that require reporting are identified. In this scenario, one best practice that has been introduced in electronic registry studies is to have a notification sent promptly to the sponsor's safety group when a case report form is submitted that has specific or

potential information that a serious AE has occurred. This process allows for rapid followup by the sponsor as needed.

AE Reporting by the Registry

Once suspicion has been aroused that an unexpected serious event has a reasonable possibility of being causally related to a drug, the AE should be reported to FDA through MedWatch, to the company that manufactures the product, or to the registry coordinating center. A system needs to be developed such that all appropriate events are captured and duplicate reporting is avoided to the extent possible. Generally, AE reports are submitted directly to the manufacturer, since they are often most efficient at evaluating, processing, and reporting for regulatory purposes within the required time periods. Alternatively, sites could report AEs directly to FDA; however, this often means companies are not notified of the AE and are not able to follow it up. In fact, companies are not necessarily notified by the FDA if an AE report comes directly to FDA, since only certain reports are shared with industry and reporters have an option to request that the information not be shared directly with the company.[273] When sites report AEs directly to FDA, this process can also risk inadvertent duplication of information for events recorded both by the registry and the company.

Ideally, the practice for handling AEs and serious adverse events (SAEs) should be applied to all treatments (including comparators) recorded in the registry, so that all subjects are treated similarly. Systematic collection of all AEs provides a unique resource of consistent and contemporaneously collected comparison information that can be used at a later date to conduct epidemiologic assessments of relatedness (or causality). In fact, a strong advantage of registries with systematic data collection and internal comparators is that they provide both numerators and denominators for safety events; thus reporting of known AE rates in the context of a safety evaluation provides useful information on real-world performance. Reporting AEs without this denominator information is less useful from a surveillance perspective.

For postmarketing registries that are not financially supported by pharmaceutical companies, health care providers at registry sites should be instructed that if they suspect or otherwise become aware of a serious and unexpected AE that has a reasonable possibility of being causally related to a drug or product, they should report the event directly to the product manufacturer (who must then report to FDA under regulation) or to FDA's MedWatch program (or local health authority if the study is conducted outside of the United States). Reporting can be facilitated by providing the MedWatch[274] template, as well as information regarding the process for submission and MedWatch contact information.

For registries that are sponsored or financially supported in full or part by a regulated industry and that study a single product, the most efficient monitoring system is one in which all physicians participating in the registry report all AEs directly to the sponsor (manufacturer) or centralized designated responsible personnel, who then reports to the regulatory authorities, in order to avoid duplicate reporting. However, when products other than those cxclusively manufactured by the sponsor are involved, sponsors will need to determine how to process AE reports that are received for comparator products. Sponsors are not generally obligated to report AEs for their competitors, but from a public health perspective, specifying how the site should address those AEs (e.g., report directly to the comparator product's manufacturer or to FDA) is good practice. Options for the sponsor include (1) recommending that the AEs of comparators be reported directly to the manufacturer or to FDA; (2) collecting all AEs and forwarding the AE report directly to the comparator's manufacturer (who would then, in turn, report to FDA); and (3) actually reporting the AE for the comparator product directly to FDA.

The MedWatch form[274] should be used for postmarketing reporting for drugs and therapeutic biologics; for vaccines, consult the Vaccine Adverse Event Reporting System (VAERS).[275] Foreign events may be submitted on a CIOMS form (the World Health Organization's Council for International Organizations of Medical Sciences),[276,277,278] or a letter can be generated that includes the relevant information in narrative format.

In most circumstances where a serious drug-associated AE is suspected, sites are encouraged to submit to sponsors supportive data, such as lab values, vital signs, and examinations, along with the SAE report form. The sponsor then transfers the information provided by sites to a format that is required for submission to the health authority.

Serious AEs that are unexpected and possibly related to drug exposure should be submitted to the sponsors as quickly as possible after becoming aware of the event so that the sponsor may, in turn, comply with 15-calendar-day reporting requirements. This submission can be accomplished by phone or fax, or by means of automated rules built into the vehicle used for data collection (such as automatic triggers that can be designed into electronic data capture programs).

Coding 157

Coding AEs into a standard nomenclature should be done by trained experts to assure accuracy and consistency. Reporters, patients, health care providers, and registry personnel should do their best to capture the primary data clearly, completely, and in as "natural" clinical language as possible. Since reporters may use different verbatim terms to describe the same particular AE, it is recommended that sponsors apply coding conventions to code the verbatim terms, e.g., MedDRA (International Conference on Harmonisation). Coding the different verbatim language to preferred terms allows similar events to be appropriately grouped. This also creates consistency among the terms for evaluation and maximizes the likelihood that safety signals will be detected.

Sponsors should review the accuracy of the coding of verbatim AEs into appropriate terms. Review of the coding process should focus on the use of terms that do not accurately communicate the severity or magnitude of the AE or possibly mischaracterize the AE. Review of the coded terms compared with reported verbatim terms should be performed in order to ensure consistency and accuracy of the AE reporting and to minimize variability of coding of similar adverse event terms. Attention to consistency is especially important, as many different individuals may code AEs over time and this contributes to variability in the coding process.

In addition to monitoring AEs individually for complete clinical evaluation of the safety data, sponsors should consider grouping and analyzing clinically relevant coded terms that could represent similar toxicities or syndromes. Combining terms may provide a method to detect less common and serious events that would otherwise be obscured. However, sponsors should be careful when combining related terms to avoid amplifying a weak signal or obscuring important overall findings.

In addition to monitoring individual AEs, sites and registry personnel should be attentive to toxicities that may cluster into syndromes.

AE Management

158

In some cases, such as a safety registry created as a condition of approval, a Data Safety Monitoring Board (DSMB) or Adjudication Committee may be established with the primary role of periodically reviewing the data as they are generated by the registry. Such activities are generally discussed directly with the health authorities, such as FDA. These authorities are typically involved in the design and critique of protocols for postmarketing drug studies. Ultimately, registry planning and the registry protocol should anticipate and clearly delineate the roles, responsibilities, process, forms, and lines of communication about AE reporting for sites; registry personnel; the DSMB or Adjudication Committee, if one exists; and the sponsoring organization. Definitions and approaches should be documented for determining what is considered unexpected and possibly related to drug or device exposure. Management of AE reporting should be clearly stated in the registry protocol, including the roles, responsibilities, processes, and methods for handling AE reports by the various parties conducting the registry and responsibilities to perform followup activities with the site to ensure that complete information is obtained.

Sponsors who are stakeholders in a registry should have a representative of their internal drug safety surveillance group participate in the design and review of the registry protocol and have a role in the data collection and reporting process (discussed in Chapter 2) to facilitate appropriate and timely reporting and communication.

For postmarketing studies financially sponsored by manufacturers, the overall company AE monitoring systems are usually operated by personnel experienced in drug safety surveillance (also known as pharmacovigilance, regulatory safety, and safety and risk management). If sites need to report or discuss an AE, they can call the contact number provided for the registry and are then prompted to press a number if reporting an AE. This number then transfers them to drug safety surveillance so they can interact directly with personnel in this division and bypass the registry coordinating group. These calls may or may not be tracked by the registry. Alternatively, the registry system can provide instructions to the site on how to report AEs directly to the sponsor's drug safety surveillance division. Through this method, the sponsor provides a separate contact number for AE reporting (independent of the registry Help Desk) that places the site in direct contact with drug safety surveillance personnel. This process minimizes the possibility of duplicate AE reports and the potentially complicated reconciliation of two different systems collecting AE information. Use of this process is critical when dealing with products that are available via a registry system as well as outside of a registry system and allows sites to have one designated drug safety surveillance representative for interaction.

Sponsors are strongly encouraged to hold discussions with the health authorities when considering the design of the AE monitoring system for a registry that is designed specifically for surveillance of drug or device safety. These discussions should be focused on the purpose of the registry, the "best fit" model for AE monitoring, and the timing of routine registry updates. With respect to internal operations chosen by the sponsor to support the requirements of an AE monitoring system, anecdotal feedback suggests that health authorities expect compliance with the agreed-upon requirements. Details regarding the implementation are the responsibility of the sponsor.

It should also be noted that FDA's proposed rule for Safety Reporting Requirements for Human Drug and Biologics Products suggests that one point of contact should be provided for all AE reporting, and preferably, this individual should be a licensed physician. Although this proposed rule is still not in effect, the sponsor should consider appointment of such an individual who can provide responses to health authorities, upon request, regarding AEs reported via the registry system.

AE Required Reporting for Registry Sponsors

Understanding the reporting requirements of the sponsor directly affects how registries collect and report AEs. Sponsors that are regulated industries are subject to the requirements shown in Table 13. ICH guidelines describe standards for expedited reporting[279,280] and provide recommendations for

periodic safety update reports[281] that are generally accepted globally.

Requirements for regulated industries that sponsor or financially support a registry include expedited reporting of serious and unexpected AEs made known to them via spontaneous reports. For studies such as registries, the 15-calendar-day notification applies if the regulated industry believes there is a reasonable possibility that the unexpected SAE was causally related to product exposure. Best practices for international reporting are that all "affiliates" of a sponsor report serious, unexpected, and possibly related events to the sponsor in a timely fashion, ideally within 5 calendar days; this allows the sponsor, in turn, to complete notification to the responsible regulatory authority within a total of 15 calendar days. Events that do not meet the requirements of expedited reporting (such as nonserious events or serious events considered expected or not related) may require submission through inclusion in an appropriate safety update, such as the New Drug Application (NDA) Annual Report, Periodic Report, or Periodic Safety Update Reports (PSUR), as applicable.[282] In many cases,

159

Table 13. Overview of Adverse Event Reporting Requirements for Marketed Products[a]		
Type of requirement	**Drugs**	**Devices**
U.S. postmarket regulations	21 CFR 310.305, 21 CFR 314.80, 21 CFR 314.98, 21 CFR 600.80	21 CFR 803
Required reporting source	Regulated industries	Manufacturer, importer, user facility
Required reports	Serious, unexpected, and with a reasonable possibility of being related to drug exposure	Death; serious injury; device malfunction
Alternative reports	Not applicable	Summary reports (periodic line-listing of reports of well-known events)
Timeframe for reporting	15 calendar days for required reports	10 to 30 calendar days, depending on source
Reporting form	MedWatch 3500A (for mandatory reporting required of a regulated industry) MedWatch 3500 (voluntary)	
Web sites	www.fda.gov/medwatch	www.fda.gov/cdrh/mdr
[a] International Conference on Harmonisation (ICH) guidances describe standards for expedited reporting[279,280] and provide recommendations for periodic safety update reports[281] that are generally accepted globally.		

sponsors are also required to provide registry safety updates to the health authority. Thus, sponsors may coordinate registry safety updates (i.e., determining the date for creating the data set [data cut off dates]) with the timing of the NDA Annual Report, Periodic Report, PSUR, or other agreed-upon periodic reporting format. Devices have different reporting requirements. (See www.fda.gov/cdrh/mdr.) In any event, sponsors should discuss safety reporting requirements for their specific registries with the applicable health authorities (such as FDA and European Medicines Agency [EMEA]) before finalizing their registry protocol.

In some cases, a registry sponsor may encourage the site to systematically report all potential SAEs to the sponsor. Given the potential for various interpretations by different sites in assessing the seriousness, expectedness, and relatedness of a particular AE—and therefore, inconsistency across sites in the evaluation of a particular adverse event—this method has certain advantages. However, this approach results in substantially greater demands on the sponsor to evaluate all reports. Further, U.S. and international regulations differ as to whether the site or industry prevails if there is a disagreement about presumed expectedness or relatedness. For these reasons, planning for good and consistent training in AE reporting requirements across sites is the preferred approach for a patient registry.

Regardless of who assesses presumed relatedness and expectedness, sponsors should be prepared to manage the increased volume of AE reports and sponsor registry staff should be trained to understand company policy and regulations on AE reporting in order to ensure compliance with local regulations. This training includes the ability to identify and evaluate the attributes of each adverse event and determine the reportability status to the health authority in keeping with local regulation. Sponsors are encouraged to appoint a health care practitioner to this role in order to ensure appropriate assessment of the seriousness or severity of an AE.

When biopharmaceutical or device companies are not sponsoring, financially supporting, or participating in a registry in any way, then AE reporting is dependent upon the "become aware" principle. If any agent or employee of the company receives information regarding an AE report, the agent or employee must document receipt and comply with internal company policy and regulatory requirements regarding AE reporting to assure compliance with applicable drug and device regulations.

Special Case: Performance-Linked Access System (PLAS)

A performance-linked access system (PLAS), also known as a restricted access or limited distribution system, can be described as a special application of a registry. Unlike the less structured disease or exposure registries discussed above, a PLAS is part of a detailed risk minimization action plan that sponsors develop as a commitment to enhance the risk-benefit balance of an approved product. The purpose of a PLAS is to mitigate a certain known drug-associated risk by ensuring that product access is tightly linked to some preventive and/or monitoring measure. Examples include systems that monitor laboratory values, such as white blood cell counts during clozapine administration to prevent severe leukopenia or routine pregnancy testing during thalidomide administration to prevent in utero exposure of this known teratogenic compound. Although different in the structured nature of their protocols, both PLAS and other registries collect a battery of information using standardized instruments in a prospective manner.

A PLAS may carry special AE reporting requirements. If such requirements exist, they should be made explicit in the registry protocol, with clear definitions of roles, responsibilities, and processes. Training of involved health care providers, such as physicians, nurses, and pharmacists, can be undertaken with written instructions or via telephone and/or face-to-face counseling. Training of these health care providers should also extend beyond AE reporting to the specific requirements of the PLAS in question. Such training may include the intended use and associated risk of the product, appropriate patient enrollment, and specific patient monitoring requirements, including guidelines for product discontinuation and management of AEs, as well as topics to cover during comprehensive counseling of patients. The objectives of the PLAS system should be clearly stated (e.g., prevention of in utero exposure during therapy via routine pregnancy testing) and registration forms that document the physician's and pharmacist's attestation of their commitment to requirements of the patient registry system that should be completed prior to prescribing or dispensing the product.

Chapter 10. Analysis and Interpretation of Registry Data To Evaluate Outcomes

Registries have the potential to produce databases that are an important source of information regarding health care patterns, decisionmaking, and delivery, and their association with patient outcomes. Registries, for example, can provide valuable insight into the safety and/or effectiveness of an intervention or the efficiency, timeliness, quality, and patient-centeredness of a health care system. The utility and applicability of registry data heavily rely on the quality of the data analysis plan and the ability to interpret the results.

Analysis and interpretation of registry data begin with a series of core questions:

- *Study purpose*: Were the objectives/hypotheses predefined or post hoc?

- *Patient population*: Who was studied?

- *Data quality*: How were the data collected, reviewed, and verified?

- *Data completeness*: How were missing data handled?

- *Data analysis*: How were the analyses chosen and performed?

While the scientific opportunities that may result from a well-designed registry are clear, there are inherent challenges to making appropriate inferences. A principal concern with registries is that of making inferences without regard to the quality of data, since quality standards have not been previously well established or consistently reported. In some registries, comparison groups may be less robustly defined than in more formal observational designs (e.g., cohort, case-control studies). Information provided about the external validity of a registry sample is often limited as well.

This chapter explains how analysis plans are constructed for registries, how they differ depending on their purpose, and how registry design and conduct can affect analysis and interpretation. The analytic techniques generally used for registry data

are presented, addressing how conclusions may be drawn from the data and what caveats are appropriate. The chapter also describes how timelines for data analysis can be built in at registry inception and how to determine when the registry data are complete enough to begin analysis.

Hypotheses and Purposes of the Registry

While it may be relatively straightforward to develop hypotheses for registries intended to evaluate safety and effectiveness, not all registries have elegantly testable or simple hypotheses, and the study methodology and presence or absence of a priori hypotheses or research questions may affect the interpretation of registry data. The many possible scenarios are well illustrated by examples at the theoretical extremes.

On one extreme, a study may evolve out of a clear and explicit prespecified research question and hypothesis. In such a study, there may have been preliminary scientific work that laid the conceptual foundation and plausibility of the proposed study. The investigators fully articulate the objectives and analytic plan before embarking on any analysis. The outcome is clearly defined and the statistical approach documented. Secondary analyses are identified and may be highlighted as hypothesis generating. The investigators have no prior knowledge of analyses in this database that would bias them in the formulation of their study objective. The study is conducted and published regardless of the result. The paper states clearly that the objective and hypothesis were prespecified. For registries that are intended to support national coverage determinations with data collection as a condition of coverage, the specific coverage decision question may be specified a priori as the research question, in lieu of a hypothesis.

On the other extreme, a study may evolve out of an unexpected observation in a database in the course of doing analyses for another purpose. A study could also evolve from a concerted effort to discover associations—for example, as part of a large effort to understand disease causation. In such a study, the foundation for the study is developed post hoc, or after making the observation. Because of the way in which the observation was found, the rationale for the study is developed retrospectively. The paper does not state clearly that the objective and hypothesis were not prespecified.

Of course, there are many examples that fall between these extremes. An investigator may suspect an association for many variables, but find the relationship for only one of them. The investigator decides to pursue only the positive finding and develop a rationale for a study or grant. The association was sought, but it was sought along with associations for many other variables and outcomes.

164

Thus, while there is substantial debate about the importance of prespecified hypotheses,[283,284] there is general agreement that it is informative to reveal how the study was developed. Transparency in the methods is needed so that readers may know whether these studies are the result of hypotheses developed independently of the study database, or whether the question and analyses evolved from experience with the database and multiple iterations of exploratory analyses. Both types of studies have value.

Patient Population

The purpose of a registry is to provide information about a specific patient population to which all study results are meant to apply. To determine how well the study results apply to the target population, four populations, each of which is a subset of the preceding population, need to be considered, along with how well each population represents the preceding population. These four populations are shown in Figure 3.

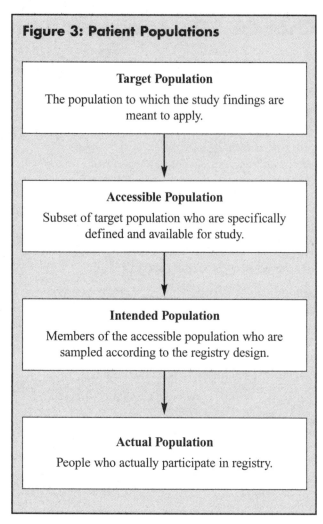

Figure 3: Patient Populations

Target Population
The population to which the study findings are meant to apply.

Accessible Population
Subset of target population who are specifically defined and available for study.

Intended Population
Members of the accessible population who are sampled according to the registry design.

Actual Population
People who actually participate in registry.

The *target population* is defined by the study's purpose. To assess the appropriateness of the target population, one must ask the question, Is this really the population that we need to know about? For example, the target population for a registry of oral contraceptive users would include women of childbearing age who could become pregnant and are seeking to prevent pregnancy. Studies often miss important segments of the population in an effort to make the study population more homogeneous. For example, it is less informative than desirable if a study to assess a medical device that is used to treat patients for cardiac arrhythmias defines only men as its target population, because the device is designed for use in both men and women.

The *accessible population* is defined using inclusion criteria and exclusion criteria. The inclusion criteria define the population that will be used for the study and generally include geographic (e.g., hospitals or clinics in the New England region), demographic, disease-specific, and temporal (e.g., specification of the included dates of hospital or clinic admission), as well as other criteria. Conversely, the exclusion criteria seek to eliminate specific patients from study and may be driven by an effort to assure an adequate-sized population of interest for analysis. The same goals may be said of inclusion criteria, since it is difficult to separate inclusion from exclusion criteria (e.g., inclusion of adults aged 18 and over vs. exclusion of children under age 18).

The accessible population may lose representativeness to the extent that convenience plays a part in its determination, because people who are easy to enroll in the registry may differ in some critical respects from the population at large. Similarly, to the extent that homogeneity plays a part in determining the accessible population, it is less likely to be representative of the entire population because certain population subgroups will be excluded.

Factors to be considered in assessing the accessible population's representativeness of the target population include all the factors mentioned above that are used as inclusion and exclusion criteria. One method of evaluating representativeness is to describe the demographics and other key descriptors of the registry study population and contrast its composition with patients with similar characteristics who are identified from an external database, such as might be obtained from health insurers, health maintenance organizations, and the Surveillance Epidemiology and End Results (SEER) cancer registries.

However, simple numerical/statistical representativeness is not the main issue. Rather, representativeness should be evaluated in the context of the purpose of the study. (See Case Example 22.) For example, suppose that the purpose of the study is to assess the effectiveness of a drug in U.S. residents with diabetes. If the accessible population includes no children, then the study results very well may not apply to children, since children often metabolize drugs very differently than adults.

On the other hand, consider the possibility that the accessible population is generally drawn from a geographically isolated region, whereas the target population may be the entire United States or the world. In that case, the accessible population is not geographically representative of the target population, but that would have little or no impact on the representativeness of the study findings to the target population if the action of the drug (or its delivery) does not vary geographically (which we would generally expect to be the case, unless pertinent racial/genetic or dietary factors were involved). Therefore, in this example, the lack of geographical representativeness would not affect interpretation of results.

The reason for using an *intended population*, rather than using the whole accessible population for the study, is simply a matter of convenience and practicality. The issues to consider in assessing how well the intended population represents the accessible population are similar to those for assessing how well the accessible population represents the target population. The main difference is that the intended population may be specified by a sampling scheme, which often tries to strike a balance among representativeness, convenience, and budget. If the intended population is a random sample of the accessible population, it may be reasonably assumed that it will represent the accessible population; however, for many if not most registries, a complete roster of the accessible population does not exist. More commonly, the intended population is compared with the accessible population in terms of pertinent variables.

On the other hand, to the extent that convenience or other design (e.g., stratified random sample) is used to choose the intended population, one must consider the extent to which the sampling of the accessible population—by means other than random sampling—has decreased the representativeness of the intended population. For example, suppose that, for the sake of convenience, only patients who attend clinic on Mondays are included in the study. If patients who attend clinic on Monday are similar

165

Case Example 22: Using Registry Data To Evaluate Outcomes by Practice

Description	The Epidemiologic Study of Cystic Fibrosis (ESCF) Registry was a multicenter, encounter-based, observational, post-marketing study designed to monitor product safety, define clinical practice patterns, explore risks for pulmonary function decline, and facilitate quality improvement for cystic fibrosis (CF) patients. The registry collected comprehensive data on pulmonary function, microbiology, growth, pulmonary exacerbations, CF-associated medical conditions, and chronic and acute treatments for children and adult CF patients at each visit to the clinical site.
Sponsor	Genentech, Inc.
Year Started	1993
Year Ended	Patient enrollment completed in 2005; followup ongoing
No. of Sites	215 sites over the life of the registry
No. of Records	32,414 patients and 832,705 encounters recorded

Challenge

Although guidelines for managing cystic fibrosis patients have been widely available for many years, little is known about variations in practice patterns among care sites and their associated outcomes. To determine whether differences in lung health existed between groups of patients attending different CF care sites and to determine whether these differences were associated with differences in monitoring and intervention, data on a large number of CF patients from a wide variety of CF sites were necessary.

As a large, observational, prospective registry, ESCF collected data on a large number of patients from a range of participating sites. At the time of the outcomes study, the registry was estimated to have data on over 80 percent of CF patients in the United States, and it collected data from more than 90 percent of the sites accredited by the U.S. Cystic Fibrosis Foundation. Because the registry contained a representative population of CF patients, the registry database offered strong potential for analyzing the association between practice patterns and outcomes.

Proposed Solution

In designing the study, the team decided to compare CF sites using lung function (i.e., FEV1 values), a common surrogate outcome for respiratory studies. Data from 18,411 patients followed in 194 care sites were reviewed, and 8,125 patients from 132 sites (minimum of 50 patients per site) were included. Only sites with at least 10 patients in a specified age group (6-12, 13-17, 18 and older) were included for evaluation of that age group. For each age group, sites were ranked in quartiles based on the median FEV1 value at each site. The frequency of patient monitoring and use of therapeutic interventions were compared between upper and lower quartile sites after stratification for disease severity.

Results

Substantial differences in lung health across different CF care sites were observed. Within-site rankings tended to be consistent across the three age groups. Patients who were cared for at higher ranking sites had more frequent monitoring of their clinical status, measurements of lung function, and cultures for respiratory pathogens. These patients also received more interventions, particularly intravenous antibiotics for pulmonary exacerbations. The study concluded that frequent monitoring and increased use of appropriate medications in the management of CF are associated with improved outcomes.

(continued)

<table>
<tr><td>

Case Example 22: Using Registry Data To Evaluate Outcomes by Practice (continued)

Key Point

Stratifying patients by quartile of lung function, age, and disease severity allowed comparison of practices among sites and revealed practice patterns that were associated with better clinical status. The large numbers of patients and sites allowed for sufficient information to create meaningful and informative stratification and resulted in sufficient information within those strata to reveal meaningful differences in site practices.

For More Information

Johnson C, Butler SM, Konstan MW et al. Factors influencing outcomes in cystic fibrosis: a center-based analysis. Chest 2003;123:20-27.

Padman R, McColley SA, Miller DP et al. Infant care patterns at Epidemiologic Study of Cystic Fibrosis sites that achieve superior childhood lung function. Pediatrics 2007;119:E531-537.

</td></tr>
</table>

in every relevant respect to other patients, that may not constitute a limitation. But if Monday patients are substantially different from patients who attend clinic on other days of the week (e.g., well-baby clinics are held on Mondays) and if those differences affect the outcome that is being studied (e.g., proportion of baby visits for "well babies"), then that sampling strategy would substantially alter the interpretations from the registry and would be considered a meaningful limitation.

Finally, the extent to which the *actual population* is not fully representative of the intended population is generally a matter of real-world issues that prevent the initial inclusion of study subjects or adequate followup. In assessing representativeness, one must consider the likely underlying factors that caused those subjects not to be included in the analysis of study results and how that might affect the interpretations from the registry. For example, consider a study of a newly introduced medication, such as an antiinflammatory drug that is thought to

be as effective as other products with fewer side effects but is more costly. Inclusion in the actual population may be influenced by prescribing practices governed by a health insurer (such as the new drug being approved for reimbursement only for patients who have "failed" treatment with other antiinflammatory products, resulting in an actual population that is systematically different from the target population of potential antiinflammatory drug users). The actual population may be refractory to treatment or have more comorbidities (e.g., gastrointestinal problems) and be specifically selected for treatment beyond the intention of the study-specified inclusion criteria. In fact, registries of newly introduced drugs and devices may often include patients who are different from the ultimate target population.

A related issue is that of "early adopters," in which practitioners who are quick to use a novel health care intervention or therapy differ from those who use it only once it is well established. For example, a registry of the use of a new surgical technique may initially enroll largely academic physicians and only much later enroll community-based surgeons. If the outcomes of the technique differ between the academic surgeons (early adopters) and community-based surgeons (later adopters), then the initial results of the registry may not reflect the true effectiveness of the technique in widespread use.

Selective information about followup can also affect the representativeness of the actual population. For example, in the extreme scenario, subjects who die during the course of a study may be erroneously characterized as lost to followup and not accurately identified as deceased, and subsequently not identified for inclusion in the study results. In this scenario, the worst effects of the exposure may easily be missed.[a]

---

[a]This type of selection bias is particularly difficult to assess through comparison with external data sources, such as health insurance databases, since deaths are generally not "billable" or coded events, and it is difficult to distinguish whether an insurance plan member has changed plans, discontinued enrollment, or died.

Data Quality Issues

In addition to a full understanding of study design and methodology, analysis of registry events and outcomes requires an assessment of data quality. One must consider whether most (or all) important covariates were collected, whether the data were complete, and whether missing data were handled correctly.

Collection of All Important Covariates

Registry information is often collected for one purpose (e.g., provider performance feedback) but then used for another (e.g., addressing a specific clinical research question). While using an available database for multiple purposes is a reasonable goal, one needs to be sure that all the information necessary to address a specific research question was collected in a manner that is sufficient to answer the question.

For example, suppose the research question addresses the comparative effectiveness of two treatments for a given disease using an existing registry. To be meaningful, the registry should have accurate, well-defined, and complete information, including potential confounding factors, on the population (those with disease X); on other potential confounding factors; on the exposure (whether patients received treatment A or B); and on the patient outcome(s) of interest. Confounding factors are variables that influence both the exposure (treatment selection) and the outcome in the analyses. These factors can include patient factors (age, gender, race, socioeconomic factors, disease severity, or comorbid illness); provider factors (experience, skills); and system factors (type of care setting, quality of care, or regional effects). While it is not possible to identify all confounding factors in planning a registry, it is desirable to give serious thought to what will be important and how the necessary data can be collected. Analysis of registries requires information about such variables so that the confounding covariates can be accounted for using one of several analytic techniques covered

in upcoming sections of this chapter. In addition, as described in Chapter 3, eligibility for entry into the registry may be restricted to individuals within a certain range of values for potential confounding factors to reduce their effects. Such restrictions may also affect the generalizability of the registry.

Data Completeness

Assuming a registry has the necessary data elements, the next step is to be assured that the data are complete. Missing data can be a challenge for any registry-based analysis. Missing data include situations where a variable is directly reported as missing or unavailable, where a variable is "nonreported" (i.e., the observation is blank), where the reported data may not be interpretable (e.g., the subjects provide responses that may be subject to recall bias), or where the value must be imputed to be missing because of data inconsistency or out-of-range results. Before analyzing a registry database, the database should be "cleaned" (discussed in Chapter 8), and attempts should be made to obtain as much missing data as realistically possible from source documents. Inconsistent data (e.g., answer yes to a question at one point and no to the same question at another) and out-of-range data (a 500-year-old patient) should be corrected. Finally, the degree of data completeness should be summarized for the researcher and eventual consumer of analyses from the registry.

Handling Missing Data

The intent of any analysis is to make valid inferences from the data. Missing data can threaten this goal by both reducing the information yield of the study and, in many cases, introducing bias. The first step in knowing how to handle missing data is to understand why the data are missing. Missing data fall into three classic categories:[286]

- *Missing completely at random (MCAR)*: Instances where there are no differences between subjects with missing data and those with complete data. In such random instances, missing data only reduce study power without introducing bias.

168

- *Missing at random (MAR)*: Instances where missing data depend on known or observed values but not unmeasured data. In such cases, accounting for these known factors in the analysis will produce unbiased results.
- *Missing not at random (MNAR)*: Here, missing data depend on events or factors not measured by the researcher and thus potentially introduce bias.

To gain insight into which of the three categories of missing data are in play, one can compare the distribution of observed variables for patients with specific missing data to the distribution of those variables for patients for whom those same data are present. Alternatively, one can attempt to "predict a missing variable" using logistic regression analysis where the dependent variable is a dummy variable representing the missing data.

There are several means of managing missing data within an analysis. For example, a "complete case" strategy limits the analysis to patients with complete information for all variables. This is the default strategy used in many standard analytic packages (e.g., SAS, Cary, NC). A simple deletion of all incomplete observations, however, is not appropriate or efficient in all circumstances, and it may introduce significant bias if the deleted cases are substantively different from the retained, complete cases (i.e., not MCAR). In observational studies with prospective, structured data collection, missing data are not uncommon, and the "complete case" strategy is inefficient and not generally used. For example, patients with diabetes who were hospitalized because of inadequate glucose control might not return for a scheduled followup visit at which HbA1c was to be measured. Those missing values for HbA1c, then, would probably differ from the measured values because of the reason for which they were missing, and they would be categorized as MNAR. In an example of MAR, the availability of the results of certain tests or measurements may depend on what is covered by patients' health insurance (a known value) since registries typically do not pay for testing. Patients without this particular measurement may still contribute meaningfully to the analysis. In order to not exclude

patients with missing data, one of several imputation techniques may be used to estimate the missing data.

Imputation is a common strategy in which average values are substituted for missing data, using strategies such as unconditional and conditional mean, multiple hot-deck, and expectation maximum, among others.[287,288] For data that are captured at multiple time points, investigators often "carry forward" a last observation. However, such a technique can be problematic if early dropouts occur and a response variable is expected to change over time. "Worst-case" imputation is another means of substitution in which investigators test the sensitivity of a finding by substituting a "worst case" value for all missing results. While this is conservative, it offers a "lower bounds" on an association rather than an accurate assessment. One particular imputation method that has received significant attention in recent analyses has been termed "multiple imputations." Rubin first proposed the idea to impute more than one value for a missing variable as a means of reflecting the uncertainty around this value.[289] The general strategy is to replace a missing value with multiple values from an approximate distribution for missing values. This produces multiple "complete data sets" for analysis from which a single summary finding is estimated.

A recent review provides insight, using cancer registry data, into the issues of how prognostic models for decisionmaking can be influenced by data completeness and missing data.[290] Burton and Altman reviewed 100 published multivariable cancer prognostic models published in seven leading cancer journals in 2002. They found that the proportion of complete cases was reported in only 39 studies, while the percentage missing for important prognostic variables was reported in 52 studies. Comparison of complete cases with incomplete cases was provided in 10 studies, and the methods used to handle missing data were summarized in 32 studies. The most common techniques used for handling missing data were complete case analysis (12), dropping variables with high numbers of missing cases from model consideration (6), and some simple author imputation rule (6). One article

169

used multiple imputation techniques. The reviewers concluded there was room for improvement in the reporting and handling of missing data within registry studies.[291]

Readers interested in learning more about methods for handling missing data and the potential for bias are directed to two other useful reviews, one by Greenland and Finkle[292] and the other by Hernan and colleagues.[293]

It is important to keep in mind that the impact of data completeness will differ, depending on the extent of missing data and the intended use of the registry; it is less likely to influence descriptive research than research that is intended to support decisionmaking. For all registries, it is important to have a strategy on how to handle missing data and how to explicitly report on data completeness to facilitate interpretation of study results.

Data Analysis

170

This section provides an overview of practical considerations regarding data analysis of a registry. As the name suggests, a descriptive study focuses on describing frequency and patterns of various elements of a patient population, whereas an analytical study focuses on examining associations between patients or treatment characteristics and health outcomes of interest (e.g., comparative effectiveness).

Statistical methods commonly used for descriptive purposes include those that summarize information from continuous variables (e.g., mean, median) or from categorical variables (e.g., proportions, rates). Registries may use incidence (the proportion of the population that develops the condition over a specified time interval) and prevalence (the proportion of the population that has the condition at a specific point in time) to describe the population. Another summary estimate that is often used is an incidence rate. The incidence rate (also known as absolute risk) takes into account both the number of people in a population who develop the outcome of interest and the person-time at risk, or the length of time contributed by all people during the period when they were in the population and the events were counted.

For studies that include patient followup, an important part of the description of study conduct is characterization of how many patients are "lost" or drop out during the course of conducting a registry and at what point they are "lost." Figure 4 illustrates key points of information that provide a useful description of losses to followup and study dropouts.

For analytical studies, the association between a risk factor and outcome may be expressed as attributable risk, relative risk, odds ratio, or hazard ratio, depending on the nature of data collected, the duration of the study, and the frequency of the outcome. Attributable risk, a concept developed in the field of public health and preventive medicine, is defined as the proportion of disease incidence that can be attributed to a specific exposure, and it may be used to indicate the impact of a particular exposure at a population level. The vast amount of information and large sample sizes often found in registries also support use of various modeling techniques, such as using propensity scores to create strata of patients with similar risk sets or to create propensity scores to use in multivariate risk modeling.[294,295,296,297] The standard textbooks cited here have detailed discussions regarding epidemiologic and statistical methods commonly used for the various analyses supported by registries.[298,299,300,301,302]

For economic analyses, the analytic approaches often encountered are cost-effectiveness analyses and cost-utility studies. To examine cost effectiveness, costs are compared with clinical outcomes measured in units such as life expectancy or years of disease avoided.[303] Cost-utility analysis, a closely related technique, compares costs with outcomes adjusted for quality of life (utility) using measures known as quality-adjusted life years (QALYs). Since most new interventions are more effective but also more expensive, another analytic approach examines the incremental cost-effectiveness ratio (ICER) and contrasts that to the willingness to pay. (Willingness-to-pay analyses are generally conducted on a country-by-country basis,

Figure 4: The Flow of Participants Into an Analysis

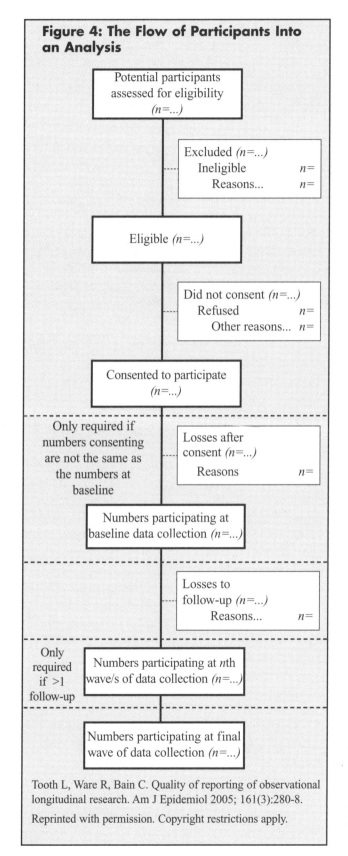

Tooth L, Ware R, Bain C. Quality of reporting of observational longitudinal research. Am J Epidemiol 2005; 161(3):280-8.

Reprinted with permission. Copyright restrictions apply.

since various factors relating to national health insurance practices and cultural issues affect willingness to pay.) The use of registries for cost-effectiveness evaluations is a fairly recent development, and consequently, the methods are evolving rapidly. More information about economic analyses can be found in standard textbooks.[304,305,306,307,308,309]

It is important to emphasize that cost-effectiveness analyses, much like safety and clinical-effectiveness analyses, require prospective collection of specific data elements suited to the purpose. Although cost-effectiveness-type analyses are becoming more important and registries can play a key role in such analyses, traditionally registries have not collected much information on quality of life or resource use that can be linked to cost data.[310] To be used for cost-effectiveness analysis, registries must be developed with that purpose in mind.

Developing a Statistical Analysis Plan

Need for a statistical analysis plan. It is important to develop a statistical analysis plan (SAP) that describes the analytical principles and statistical techniques to be employed to address the primary and secondary objectives, as specified in the study protocol or plan. Generally, the SAP for a registry study that is intended to support decisionmaking, such as a safety registry, is likely to be more detailed than the SAP for a descriptive study or health economics study. A registry may require a primary "master SAP," as well as subsequent, supplemental SAPs. Supplemental SAPs might be triggered by new research questions emerging after the initial "master SAP" was developed or because the registry evolved over time (e.g., additional data collected, data elements revised). Although the evolving nature of data collection practices in some registries poses challenges for data analysis and interpretation, it is important to keep in mind that the ability to answer questions emerging during the course of the study is one of the advantages (as well as challenges) of a registry. In the specific case of long-term rare disease registries, many of the relevant research questions of interest cannot be

171

defined a priori but arise over time as disease knowledge and treatment experience are accrued. Supplemental SAPs can be developed only when enough data become available to analyze for a particular research question. At times, the method of statistical analysis may have to be modified to accommodate the amount and quality of data available. Such supplemental analysis should be considered as prospectively defined analysis rather than exploratory analyses (sometimes referred to as "fishing expeditions"), in that the research question and SAP are formulated *before* the data analyses are conducted, and results are used to answer specific questions or hypotheses. The key to success is to provide sufficient details in the SAP that, together with the study protocol and the case report form(s), dictate the overall process of the data analysis and reporting.

Preliminary analysis to assist SAP development. During SAP development, one particular aspect of a registry that is somewhat different from a randomized controlled study is the necessity to understand the "shape" of the data collected in the study. This may be crucial for a number of reasons.

Given the broad inclusion criteria that most registries tend to propose, there might be a wide distribution of patients, treatment, and/or outcome characteristics. The distribution of age, for example, may help to determine if more detailed analyses should be conducted in the "oldest old" age group (80 years and over) to help understand health outcomes in this subgroup that might be different from outcomes for their younger counterparts.

Unless a registry is designed to limit data collection to a fixed number of regimens, in theory, the study population could experience many "regimens," considering the combination of various dose levels, drug names, and even more importantly, frequency and timing of medication use (e.g., acute, chronic, intermittent). The scope and complexity of these variations constitute one of the most challenging aspects of analyzing a registry, since treatment is given at each individual physician's discretion. Grouping of treatment into "regimens" should be carefully conducted, guided by clinical experts in that therapeutic area. The full picture of treatment

patterns may become clear only after a sizable number of the patients have been enrolled. Consequently, the treatment definition in a SAP may be refined during the course of the study. Furthermore, there may be occasions where a particular therapeutic regimen is used in a much smaller number of patients than anticipated, so specific study objectives focusing on this group of patients might become unfeasible. Also, the registry might have enrolled many patients who would normally be excluded from a clinical trial because of significant contraindications related to comorbidity or concomitant medication use; in this case, the SAP may need to define how these patients will be analyzed (either as a separate group or as part of the overall study population) and how these different approaches might affect the interpretation of the study results.

There is a need to evaluate the presence of potential sources of bias and, to the extent feasible, utilize appropriate statistical measures to address such biases. For example, the bias known as "confounding by indication"[311] results from the fact that physicians do not prescribe medicine at random: the reason a patient is put on a particular regimen is often associated with his/her underlying disease severity and may, in turn, affect treatment outcome. To detect such a bias, the distribution of various prognostic factors at baseline is compared for patients who receive a treatment of interest and those who do not. Another example is "channeling bias," where drugs with similar therapeutic indications are prescribed to groups of patients with prognostic differences.[312] To detect such a bias, registry developers and users must document the characteristics of the exposed and nonexposed participants and either demonstrate their comparability or use statistical techniques to adjust for differences. (Additional information about biases often found in registries is detailed in Chapter 3.) In addition to such biases, analyses need to account for factors that are interrelated, also known as interaction terms.[313] The presence of interaction terms may also be identified after the data are collected. All of these issues should be taken into account in an SAP based on understanding of the patient population in the registry.

Timing of Analyses During the Study

Unlike a typical clinical trial, registries, especially those that take several years to complete, may conduct "intermediate" analyses before all patients have been enrolled and/or all data collection has been completed. Such midcourse analyses may be undertaken for several reasons. First, many of these registries focus on safety outcomes, which may be catastrophic. For such safety studies, it is important for all parties involved to actively monitor the frequency of such events at regular predefined intervals so that further risk assessment or risk management can be considered. The timing of such analyses may be influenced by regulatory requirements. Second, it may be of interest to examine treatment practices or health outcomes during the study to capture any emerging trends. Finally, it may also be important to provide intermediate analysis to document progress, often as a requirement for continued funding.

While it is useful to conduct such intermediate analysis, careful planning should be given to the process and timing. The first questions are whether a sufficient number of patients have been enrolled and whether a sufficient number of events have occurred. Both can be estimated based on the speed of enrollment and rate of patient retention, as well as the expected incidence rate of the event of interest. The second issue is whether sufficient time has elapsed after the initial treatment with a product that, biologically speaking, it is plausible for events to have occurred. (For example, some events can be observed after a relatively short duration, such as site reactions to injections, compared with cancers, which may have a long induction or latency.) If there are too few patients or insufficient time has elapsed, premature analyses may lead to the inappropriate conclusion that there is no occurrence of a particular event. Similarly, uncommon events occurring by random chance in a limited sample may be incorrectly construed as a safety signal. On the other hand, it is inappropriate to delay analysis so long that an opportunity might be missed to observe emerging (safety) outcomes. Investigators should use sound clinical and epidemiological judgment when planning intermediate analysis and,

whenever possible, use data from previous studies to help to determine the feasibility and utility of such an analysis.

When planning the timing of the analysis, it may be helpful to consider substudies if emerging questions require data that were not collected originally. Substudies often involve data collection based on biological specimens or specific laboratory procedures. They may, for example, take the form of nested case-control studies. In other situations, a research question may be applicable only to a subset of patients, such as patients who become pregnant while in the study. It may also be desirable to conduct substudies among patients in a selected site or patient group to confirm the validity of study measurement. In such instances, a supplemental SAP should be developed that describes the statistical principles and methods.

Factors To Be Considered in the Analysis

Registry results are most meaningful when they are specific to well-defined endpoints or outcomes in a specific patient population with a specific treatment status. Registry analyses may be more meaningful if variations of study results across patient groups, treatment methods, or subgroups of endpoints are reported. In other words, analysis of a registry should explicitly provide the following information:

- *Patient*: What are the characteristics of the patient population in terms of demographics, such as age, gender, race/ethnicity, insurance status, and clinical and treatment characteristics (e.g., past history of significant medical conditions, disease status at baseline, and prior treatment history)?

- *Exposure (or treatment)*: Exposure could be therapeutic treatment such as medication or surgery, a diagnostic or screening tool, behavioral factors such as alcohol or smoking habits, or other factors such as genetic predisposition. What are the distributions of the exposure in the population? Is the study objective specific to any one form of treatment?

173

- *Endpoints (or outcomes)*: Effectiveness (and comparative-effectiveness) outcomes include survival, disease recurrence, symptom severity, quality of life, and cost effectiveness. Safety outcomes include infection, cancer, organ rejection, and mortality, for example. Are the study data on all-cause mortality or cause-specific mortality? Is information available on pathogen-specific infection (bacterial vs. viral, for example)? Was followup obtained equally across comparison groups? (See Case Example 23.)

- *Time*: Results should be described in a "time-appropriate" fashion. For example, is the risk consistent over time (in relation to initiation of treatment) in a long-term study? If not, what time-related risk measures should be reported in addition to (or instead of) cumulative risk? When exposure status changes frequently, what is the method of capturing the population at risk? Many observational studies of intermittent exposures (e.g., use of nonsteroidal antiinflammatory drugs or pain medications) use time windows of analysis, such as looking at events following first use of a drug after a prescribed interval (e.g., 2 weeks) without drug use. Other factors that are important for registry analyses include consideration of comparators to assist in determining whether an observed effect is, in fact, different from what would be expected otherwise in similar patients and consideration of how to address different lengths of observation for people who enroll in a registry at different time periods.

- *Potential for bias*: Successful analysis of observational studies depends to a large extent on the ability to measure and analytically address the potential for bias. Refer to Chapter 3 for a description of potential sources of bias.

Choice of comparator. An example of a troublesome source of bias is the choice of comparator. When participants of a cohort are classified into two or more groups of individuals according to certain study characteristics (such as treatment status, with the "standard of care" group as the comparator), the registry is said to have an internal, or concurrent, comparator. The theoretical advantage to such an internal comparator design is that patients are likely to be more similar to than different from each other (in contrast to comparisons between registry subjects and external groups of subjects) except for their treatment status. In addition, consistency in data collection methods may also make the comparison more valid. Internal comparators are particularly useful for treatment practices that change over time.

Unfortunately, it is not always possible to have or sustain a valid internal comparator. For example, there may be significant medical differences between patients who receive a particularly effective therapy and those who do not (e.g., underlying disease severity or contraindications), or it may not be feasible to maintain a long-term cohort of patients who are not treated with such a medication. It is known that external information about treatment practices (such as scientific publications or presentations) can result in physicians changing their practice of medicine such that they no longer prescribe the previously accepted standard of care. There may be a systematic difference between physicians who are early adopters and those who start using the drug or device after its effectiveness has been more widely accepted. Early adopters may also share other practices that differentiate them from their later adopting colleagues.

In the absence of a good internal comparator, one may have to leverage external comparators to provide critical context to help interpret data revealed by a registry. An external or historical comparison occurs when members of another study or another database that have similar disease or treatment characteristics are compared with registry subjects. Such data may be viewed as a context for anticipating the rate of an event. One widely used comparator is the SEER cancer registry data, because SEER provides detailed annual incidence rates of cancer stratified by cancer site, age group, gender, and tumor staging at diagnosis. A procedure for formalizing comparisons with external data is known as standardized incidence rate or ratio;[314] when used appropriately, it can be interpreted as a proxy measure of risk or relative risk.

Case Example 23: Using Registry Data To Study Patterns of Use and Outcomes

Description	The Palivizumab Outcomes Registry was designed to characterize the population of infants receiving prophylaxis for respiratory syncytial virus (RSV) disease, to describe the patterns and scope of the use of palivizumab, and to gather data on hospitalization outcomes.
Sponsor	MedImmune, Inc.
Year Started	2000
Year Ended	2004
No. of Sites	256
No. of Patients	19,548 infants

Challenge

RSV is a significant cause of hospitalization, sometimes resulting in death for premature infants during their first 2 years of life. In 1998, the U.S. Food and Drug Administration (FDA) approved palivizumab as a prophylaxis for RSV in pediatric patients at high risk for RSV disease, after clinical trials demonstrated the efficacy of the product in preventing RSV hospitalizations. Two large retrospective surveys conducted after FDA approval studied the effectiveness of palivizumab in infants, again showing that it reduces the rate of RSV hospitalizations. Despite the consistency of findings between the clinical trials and retrospective studies, questions remained about the target population and treatment patterns. The manufacturer wanted to create a prospective study that would identify infants receiving palivizumab to better understand the population receiving the prophylaxis for RSV disease and to study the patterns of use and the hospitalization outcomes.

Proposed Solution

The manufacturer decided to create a multicenter registry study to collect data on infants receiving palivizumab injections. The registry was initiated during the 2000-01 RSV season. Over 4 consecutive years, 256 sites across the United States enrolled infants who had received palivizumab for RSV under their care, provided that the infant's parent or legally authorized representative gave informed consent for participation in the registry. Infants were enrolled at the time of their first injection, and data were obtained on palivizumab injections, demographics, and risk factors, as well as on medical and family history.

Followup forms were used to collect data on subsequent palivizumab injections, including dates and doses, during the RSV season. These data were then used to determine compliance with the prescribed injection schedule by comparing the number of injections actually received with the number of expected doses. Data were also collected for all enrolled infants hospitalized for RSV at the time of hospitalization. Adverse events were not collected and analyzed separately for purposes of this registry.

Results

From September 2000 through May 2004, the registry collected data on 19,548 infants. The analysis presented injection rates and hospitalization rates for all infants by month of injection and by site of first dose (pediatrician's office or hospital). The observed number of injections per infant was compared with the expected number of doses based on the month the first injection was given. Over 4 years of data collection, less than 2 percent (1.3 percent) of all infants were hospitalized for RSV. Infants who had greater adherence to the recommended injection schedule had lower RSV hospitalization rates. This analysis demonstrates the effectiveness of a palivizumab prophylaxis for RSV in a large cohort of high-risk infants from a geographically diverse group of practices and clinics. The registry data also showed that the use of palivizumab was mostly consistent with the guidelines of the American Academy of Pediatrics.

175

(continued)

Case Example 23: Using Registry Data To Study Patterns of Use and Outcomes (continued)

The registry succeeded in collecting nearly complete demographic information and more than 99 percent of followup information on all enrolled infants, a level of completeness much higher than had been achieved in the retrospective studies.

Key Point

A simple stratified analysis was used to describe the characteristics of infants receiving injections for RSV. Infants in the registry had a low hospitalization rate, and these data support the effectiveness of this treatment outside of a controlled clinical study. Risk factors for RSV hospitalizations were described and quantified by presenting the number of infants with RSV hospitalization as a percentage of all enrolled infants who were hospitalized. These data supported an analysis of postlicensure effectiveness, in addition to describing the patient population and treatment patterns.

For More Information

The Palivizumab Outcomes Study Group. Palivizumab prophylaxis of respiratory syncytial virus in 2000-2001— results from the Palivizumab Outcomes Registry. Pediatr Pulmonol 2003;35:484-9.

The IMpact-RSV Study Group. Palivizumab, a humanized respiratory virus monoclonal antibody, reduces hospitalization from respiratory syncytial virus infection in high-risk infants. Pediatrics 1998;102:531-7.

176

Use of an external comparator, however, may present significant challenges. For example, SEER and a given registry population may differ from each other for a number of reasons. The SEER data cover the general population, and have no exclusion criteria pertaining to history of smoking or cancer screening, for example. On the other hand, a given registry may consist of patients who have an inherently different risk of cancer than the general population, resulting from the registry having excluded smokers and others known to be at high risk of developing a particular cancer. Therefore, the SEER population would be expected to overestimate the expected incidence rate in the absence of a treatment of interest.

Regardless of the choice of comparator, similarity between the groups under comparison should not be assumed without careful examination of the study patients. Different comparator groups may potentially result in very different inferences for safety and effectiveness evaluations; therefore, analysis of registry findings using different comparator groups may be used in sensitivity analyses to determine the robustness of a registry's findings. Sensitivity analysis refers to a procedure used to determine the sensitivity of the study result to alterations of a parameter. If a small parameter alteration leads to a relatively large change in the results, the results are said to be sensitive to that parameter. This procedure may be used to determine how the final study results might change when taking into account those lost to followup. A simple hypothetical example is presented in Table 14.

Table 14 illustrates the extent of change in the incidence rate of a hypothetical outcome assuming varying degrees of loss to followup, and differences in incidence between those for whom there is information and those for whom there is no information due to loss to followup. In the first example, where 10 percent of the patients are lost to followup, the estimated incidence rate of 111/1,000 people is reasonably stable; it does not change too much when the (unknown) incidence in those lost to followup changed from 0.5 times the observed to 5 times the observed, with the corresponding incidence rate that would have been observed

Table 14: A Hypothetical Simple Sensitivity Analysis

[Impact of loss to followup on incidence rates per 1,000 in a study of 1,000 patients]

Various assumptions of the observed incidence rate	Assuming a 10-percent loss to followup	Assuming a 30-percent loss to followup
Incidence rates based on patients who stayed in the study	111 (100/900)	110 (77/700)
Assuming the incidence of patients lost to followup is X times the rate of incidence estimated in those who stayed in the study:		
X=0.5	106	94
X=1	111	110
X=2	122	143
X=5	156	242

ranging from 106 to 156 per 1,000). On the other hand, when the loss to followup increases to 30 percent, the corresponding incidence rates that would have been observed range from 94 to 242. This procedure could be extended to a study where there is more than one cohort of patients, with one being exposed and the other being nonexposed. In that case, the impact of loss to followup on the relative risk could be estimated by using sensitivity analysis.

Patient censoring. At the time of a registry analysis, events may not have occurred for all patients. For these patients, the data (e.g., survival) are said to be "censored," indicating that the observation period of the registry was stopped before all events occurred. In these situations, it is unclear when the event will occur, if at all. In addition, a registry may enroll patients until a set stop date, and patients entered into the registry earlier will have a greater probability of having an event than those entered more recently because of the longer followup. An important assumption (and one that needs to be assessed in a registry) is that patients entered into the registry late have the same prognosis as those entered early. This may be a particularly problematic assumption in registries that assess innovative (and changing) therapies. Patients and outcomes observed initially in the registry may differ from patients and outcomes observed later in the registry timeframe (or not at all). Patients with censored data, however, contribute important

information to the registry analysis and should not be excluded from the SAP. One method of analyzing censored data is to use the Kaplan-Meier method[315] to estimate the conditional probability of the event occurring. In this method, for each time period, the probability is calculated that those who have not experienced an event before the beginning of the period will still not have experienced it by the end of the period. The probability of an event occurring at any given time is then calculated from the product of the conditional probabilities of each time interval.

In summary, the development of a good SAP requires careful considerations of study design features and the nature of the data collected. Most typical cohort study analytical methods can be applied, and there is no one-size-fits-all approach. Efforts should be made to carefully evaluate the presence of biases and to control for identified potential biases during data analysis. This requires close collaboration among clinicians, epidemiologists, statisticians, study coordinators, and others involved in the design, conduct, and interpretation of the registry.

Interpretation of Registry Data

Interpretation of registry data is needed so that the lessons from the registry can be applied to the target population and used to change future health care and patient outcomes. Proper interpretation of

177

registry data allows users not only to evaluate the hypotheses tested in the current registry but also to generate new hypotheses to be tested by future registries or randomized controlled trials. If the purpose of the registry is explicit, the actual population studied is reasonably representative of the target population, the data quality monitored, and the analyses performed so as to reduce potential biases, then the interpretation of the registry data should allow a realistic picture of the safety, effectiveness, or value of a clinical evaluation, the quality of medical care, or the natural history of the disease process studied. Each of these topics needs to be discussed in the interpretation of the registry data, and potential shortcomings should be explored. Assumptions or biases that could have influenced the outcomes of the analyses should be highlighted and separated from those that do not affect the interpretation of the registry results. The use of a comparator that is of the highest reasonably possible quality is integral to the proper interpretation of the analysis.

178

Once analyzed, registries provide important feedback to several groups. One group is the registry developers. Analysis and interpretation of the registry will demonstrate strengths and limitations of the original registry design and allow the developers to make needed design changes for

future versions of the registry. Another group comprises the study sponsors and related oversight/governance groups, such as the Scientific Committee and Data Monitoring Committee. (Refer to Chapter 2 for more information on registry governance and oversight.) Interpretation of the analyses allows the oversight committees to offer recommendations concerning continued use and/or adaptation of the registry and to evaluate patient safety. The final group is the end users of the registry output, such as patients or other health care consumers, health services researchers, health care providers, and policymakers. These are the people for whom the data were collected and who may use the results to choose a treatment or intervention to provide or undergo, to determine the need for additional research programs to change clinical practice, to develop clinical practice guidelines, or to determine policy. All three user groups work toward the ultimate goal of each registry—improving patient outcomes.

Section III.
Evaluating Registries

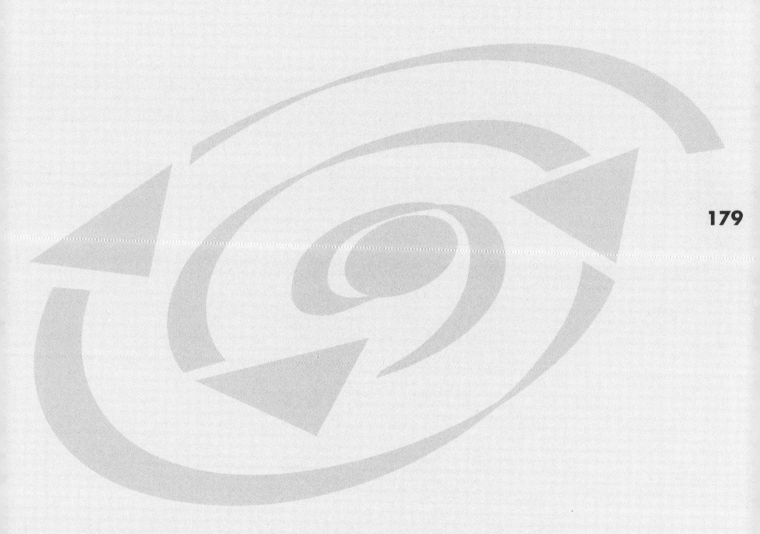

Chapter 11. Assessing Quality

Registries are undertaken for many purposes, ranging from descriptive studies intended to contribute to scientific understanding of patient outcomes to studies used to inform policy decisions. Some are undertaken with great urgency, whereas others proceed with more deliberation. Budgetary support ranges from spartan to adequate. Most importantly, registries often serve multiple purposes and change over time to accommodate these various purposes—in fact, these are hallmarks of registries. Although all registries can provide useful information, there are levels of rigor that enhance validity and make the information from some registries more useful for guiding decisions than others.

To date, no standards have been developed by which to guide evaluation of registries, and the research into quality aspects of registries has been sparse.[316] Previous chapters of this handbook have described various attributes and characteristics that constitute good registries and "good registry practice." This chapter provides an overview of key components of the design, execution, and analysis of a registry that promote reliability and validity of data on patient outcomes.

The aim of this chapter is to provide a simple and user-friendly system that allows registries to be described and evaluated in the context of the purpose for which they are conducted. Information is presented to help distinguish between:

- Basic good registry practices that are desirable to meet certain purposes.

- Future directions for practices that could enhance scientific rigor but may not be achievable because of practical constraints.

The items listed as "basic elements of good practice" are applicable to all patient registries. While it may not be practical or feasible to achieve all of the basic elements of good practice, it is useful to consider these characteristics in planning and evaluating registries. The information described in this handbook, and particularly in this chapter, is also designed to be used in reporting registry study results, much as CONSORT guidelines have been used to improve reporting of clinical trials.[317]

Defining Quality

This chapter has adapted a definition of "quality" that was developed for randomized controlled trials;[318] the term is used to refer to the confidence that the design, conduct, and analysis of the trial or registry can be shown to protect against bias (systematic error) and errors in inference—that is, erroneous conclusions drawn from a study.[319] As used here, quality refers both to the data and to the conclusions drawn from analyses of these data. For more information about the types of biases that can affect observational studies, as well as strategies for addressing and even avoiding these biases to the extent feasible, see Chapters 3 and 10. For more information about bias, validity, and inference, readers are encouraged to consult epidemiologic textbooks.[320,321,322]

Measuring Quality

There are two major difficulties with assessing quality in registries:

- It can often be difficult to differentiate between the quality of the design, the study conduct, and the information available.

- There is a lack of empirical evidence for evaluating parameters purported to indicate quality and impact on the evidence produced from registries.

In addition, registries vary widely in methodology, scope, and objectives, and therefore attributes that are important in one scenario may be less important in another. Furthermore, registries may be very useful vehicles for providing clinically relevant real-world information, even when they meet relatively few of the basic elements of good practice (typically because of budgetary limitations). In many cases, some data are better than no data, and even registries that fall short of including all the basic elements of good registry practice may still provide valuable insights about real-world medical and consumer practices and disease etiology. Evaluations of the quality of any registry must therefore be done with respect to the context-specific purpose of the registry, must take into account both the internal and external validity of the data, and should be tempered by considerations of cost and feasibility.

The most commonly used method to assess quality of studies is a quality scale; there are numerous quality scales of varying length and complexity in existence, with strong views being expressed both for and against their use.[318,323,324] Different scales emphasize distinctive dimensions of quality and therefore can produce disparate results when applied to a given study. In most situations, a summary score is derived by adding individual item scores, with or without weighting. This method, however, ignores whether the various items may lead to a bias toward the null (suggesting the erroneous interpretation that there is no effect) or tend to exaggerate the appearance of an effect when none really exists, and the final score produced does not reflect individual components.[325]

Rather than develop a checklist, the approach suggested here is to undertake a quality component analysis, an investigation of the components that may affect the results obtained.[325] In the quality component analysis, a differentiation is made between two domains: *research* quality, which pertains to the scientific process (in this instance, the design and operational aspects of the registry), and *evidence* quality, which relates to the data/findings emanating from the research process.[326,327,328] According to Lohr,[329] "The level of confidence one might have in evidence turns on the underlying robustness of the research and the analysis done to synthesize that research."

To select the quality components for analysis, several key elements identified in previous research studies, among many consulted, were Guidelines for Good Pharmacoepidemiology Practice,[330] the ICH (International Conference on Harmonisation of Technical Requirements for Registration of Pharmaceuticals for Human Use) Guideline on Good Clinical Practice,[331] the Council for International Organizations of Medical Sciences (CIOMS) International Guidelines for Ethical Review of Epidemiological Studies,[332] the Evidence Report/Technology Assessment of Systems to Rate the Strength of Scientific Evidence by West and colleagues,[324] the guidance document prepared by Klaucke and colleagues from the Centers for Disease Control and Prevention with regard to assessing the overall quality of a surveillance system,[333] and Goldberg's review of registry evaluation methods.[334]

The results of the quality component analysis must be considered in conjunction with context-specific substantive components that relate to the disease area, the type of registry, and the purpose of the registry. (See Table 15.) For example, a disease-specific registry that has been designed to look at natural history should not be deemed low quality simply because it is not large enough to detect rare treatment effects.

Quality Domains

The quality domains shown here are the domains described earlier in this handbook. For *research*, the quality domains are planning; design; data elements and data sources; and ethics, privacy, and governance. For *evidence*, the quality domains are described separately for registry participants; data elements and data sources; data quality assurance; analysis; and reporting.

Table 16 shows the basic elements of good registry practice for research, and Table 17 shows additional practices that have the potential to enhance scientific rigor, and thus the validity and reliability of information resulting from registries. Similarly, Table 18 shows the basic elements of good registry practice for evidence, and Table 19 shows additional practices that may enhance the evidence quality. It is important to weigh efforts taken to promote the accuracy and completeness of evidence in balance

182

with the public health urgency of a problem, the types of interventions that are available, and the risks to public health from coming to a wrong conclusion. These lists of components are most likely incomplete, but the level of detail provided should be useful for high-level quality distinctions.

Most importantly, the basic elements of good practice, as well as the potential enhancements to good practice, depend to a great extent on the resources and budget available to support registry-based research.

Table 15: Overview of Registry Purposes

- Determining clinical effectiveness, cost effectiveness, or comparative effectiveness of a test or treatment, including evaluating the acceptability of drugs, devices, or procedures for reimbursement.

- Measuring or monitoring safety and harm of specific products and treatments, including comparative evaluation of safety and effectiveness.

- Measuring or improving quality of care, including conducting programs to measure and/or improve the practice of medicine and/or public health.

- Assessing natural history, including estimating the magnitude of a problem; determining the underlying incidence or prevalence rate; examining trends of disease over time, conducting surveillance; assessing service delivery and identifying groups at high risk; documenting the types of patients served by a health provider; and describing and estimating survival.

183

Table 16: Research Quality for Registries—Basic Elements of Good Practice
Planning
• Sufficient thought has been given to identifying and capturing all the necessary aspects that are feasible to collect from the outset.
• A written registry plan documents the goals; design; target population; methods for data collection, including patient recruitment; data elements and data sources; a high-level data management plan; plans for protecting human subjects and for data review for quality; and a high-level analysis plan that contains sufficient detail to explain the main focus and proposed methods of analysis.
• The process for identifying serious events is described and a plan is created for reporting, as appropriate and consistent with regulatory requirements.
• A plan for communication of study results is addressed.
• Appropriate personnel and facilities are available, including facilities for secure storage of data.
• A process is established for documenting subsequent modifications to the registry plan.
Design
• The literature has been reviewed to guide appropriate data collection.
• The target population is described, including plans to recruit study subjects.
• Specific eligibility, inclusion, and exclusion criteria are specified.
• The size required to detect an effect, should one exist, or achieve a desired level of precision is specified, whether or not the sample size requirement is met.
• The followup time required to detect events of interest is specified, whether or not it is feasible to achieve; however, the followup time planned is adequate to address the main objective.
• Plans are made for how the analysis will be conducted, including what comparative information, if any, will be used to support study hypotheses or objectives.
Data elements and data sources
• Outcomes are clinically meaningful and relevant in that the information is useful to the medical community for decisionmaking .
• Operational definitions of outcomes are clearly defined.
• Important exposures, risk factors, and mitigating (or protective) factors are identified and collected to the extent feasible.
• The individual(s) responsible for the integrity of the data, computerized and hard copy, are identified; it is determined that they have the training and experience to perform the assigned tasks.
• Data collectors are trained using standard techniques.
• A data and coding dictionary is maintained to provide explicit definitions and describe coding used.
• A quality assurance plan has been created and addresses data editing and verification, as appropriate.
Ethics, privacy, and governance
• The issues of protection of human subjects—including privacy, informed consent, data security, and study ethics—have been carefully considered and addressed in accordance with local, national, and international regulations.
• The registry has received review by any required oversight committees (e.g., ethics committee, privacy committee, or institutional review board, as applicable).

Table 17: Research Quality for Registries—Potential Enhancements to Good Practice

Planning

- A formal protocol covers all the topics listed as basic elements of a study plan, covering some elements in depth. The protocol also includes objectives or hypotheses; governance, privacy, and ethics; plans for data entry; and reporting of study results. It may be helpful for stakeholders to have input in reviewing the protocol before it is finalized to assure clinical relevance and feasibility.

- The protocol includes a plan for training registry and site personnel about how to identify and report serious events that occur during the observation period and that could be causally related to the product or process under study, as appropriate.

- An advisory board has been established.

- A feasibility study or pilot test may be useful in certain situations, such as when studying hard-to-reach populations, when sensitive data are sought, and when critical registry methods are new or have not otherwise been tested. Feasibility assessment may include evaluation of factors such as means and likelihood of recruiting appropriate patients, as well as establishing and fine-tuning what data will be collected and the methods for data collection.

- A plan for quality assurance is described in the protocol. The sampling process is part of a risk-based strategy that focuses on detecting and quantifying the most likely causes of error and the types of error that are most likely to impact the registry purpose. For example, a registry might compare a random sample of patient data (e.g. 5 percent to 20 percent of patients and specific data variables) with patient charts or with a sample of registry sites based on "for-cause" reasons, or a combination of these approaches.

- The plan for generating and/or reviewing publications and presentations is defined. It includes review by knowledgeable parties.

- Plans for timely dissemination of information and a process for others to access the data are considered.

Design

- Use of concurrent comparators may offer an advantage over historical or external comparison groups in situations where treatments are evolving rapidly.

- The methods of data collection do not limit site participation such that the representativeness of site selection is compromised. While single methods of data collection to a centralized database (e.g., via Web) are most efficient, a single method may not suit all registries. Multiple methods of data collection may be required for some purposes (e.g., where access to computers or Internet is limited).

- Formal statistical calculations may be used to specify the size of the registry (number of patients or patient-years of observation) needed to measure an effect with a certain level of precision or to meet a specified statistical power to detect an effect, should one exist, whether or not the desired size is achievable within the practical study constraints. Precision and power considerations must be balanced against budgetary and feasibility constraints, and should not be used as a reason to avoid conducting research in areas where little exists.

(continued)

Table 17: Research Quality for Registries—Potential Enhancements to Good Practice (continued)

Data elements and data sources

- Whenever possible, coding used is consistent with nationally approved coding systems to promote comparability of information among studies. Standardized data dictionaries, such as the ICD-9 (International Classification of Diseases, 9th Revision), are used where applicable.
- It is preferable to use scales and tests that have been validated when such tools exist for the purpose needed.
- Rigor can be enhanced by external validation for a sample of data and/or data review by an adjudication committee for complex conditions or endpoints for which established procedures and/or coding are not used.
- To reduce losses to followup, safety studies can be enhanced by collecting enough information on individual identifiers to permit linkage with external databases such as the National Death Index where such databases exist, as appropriate. However, the desire for long-term followup should be balanced by considerations relating to the challenges posed by collecting individually identifiable data (as opposed to "de-identified data"), especially with regard to institutional review policies.
- Levels of quality assurance activities may be adapted based on observed performance. For example, they would be increased for sites that appear to be having difficulty in study conduct or data entry.

Ethics, privacy, and governance

- Potential conflicts of interest are considered and managed appropriately.
- Plans for timely review and dissemination of results are established at the outset.
- Publication policies are specified in advance of collecting data.
- Publishing results in the peer-reviewed literature is a desirable means of introducing information into the public domain.

Table 18: Evidence Quality for Registries—Basic Elements of Good Practice
Registry participants <ul><li>Registry participants are similar to the target population, and attention has been paid to minimizing selection bias to the extent feasible.</li><li>Eligibility (in terms of inclusion and exclusion criteria) is confirmed upon patient enrollment.</li><li>For safety studies, personnel are appropriately trained to ask about complaints or adverse events in a manner that is clear and specific (e.g., solicited vs. unsolicited) and to know how information should be reported to manufacturers and health authorities.</li><li>Completeness of information on eligible patients has been evaluated and described.</li></ul>
Data elements and data sources <ul><li>Information has been collected for relevant key exposures, risk factors, and mitigating or protective factors.</li><li>Patient outcomes are clinically relevant (in terms of information that will assist medical professionals with decisionmaking) and clearly defined. Definitions are provided, especially for complex conditions or outcomes that may not have uniformly established criteria (e.g., specify how an "injection site reaction" is operationally defined).</li><li>The followup period is reasonably sufficient to capture the main outcomes of interest.</li></ul>
Data quality assurance <ul><li>Data are reasonably complete.</li><li>Reasonable efforts have been expended to assure that appropriate patients have been systematically enrolled and followed in as unbiased a manner as possible.</li><li>Reasonable efforts have been devoted to minimize losses to followup.</li><li>Data checks are employed using range and consistency checks.</li></ul>
Analysis <ul><li>Accepted analytic techniques are used; these may be augmented by new or novel approaches.</li><li>The role and impact of missing data and potential confounding factors have been explored.</li></ul>
Reporting <ul><li>A report describes the methods, including target population and selection of study subjects, compliance with applicable regulatory rules and regulations, data collection methods, any transformation of variables and/or construction of composite endpoints, statistical methods used for data analysis, and a description of any circumstances that may have affected the quality or integrity of the data.</li><li>Results are reported for all the main objectives.</li><li>Followup time is described so that readers can assess the impact of the observation period on the conclusions drawn.</li><li>The report includes a clear statement of any conclusions drawn from the analysis of the registry's primary and secondary objectives and any implications of study results, as appropriate.</li><li>All authors who are acknowledged have had a meaningful role in the design, conduct, analysis, or interpretation of results.</li></ul>

187

Table 19: Evidence Quality for Registries—Potential Enhancements to Good Practice
Registry participants   • Selection bias is evaluated.   • The external validity is described (i.e., registry subjects are shown typical of the target population). It may also be informative to describe how the actual population was selected.   • For studies of comparative effectiveness and safety, contemporaneous data are collected for a comparison group to the extent that this is ethical and feasible, and that other clinically relevant, robust comparative data are not available.   • For registries where practice characteristics may impact outcome, diverse clinical practices are represented.
Data elements and data sources   • The exposure data used to support the main hypothesis are as specific as possible. For example, data identify a specific product, including manufacturer, if available.   • Results that can be confirmed by an unbiased observer—such as death, test results, and scores from validated measures for patient-reported results or clinical rating scales—enhance accuracy and reliability.   • The followup period is sufficient to capture outcomes of interest.
Data quality assurance   • Reproducibility of coding is evaluated.   • Potential sources of errors relating to accuracy and falsification are rigorously evaluated and quantified (e.g., through database and site reviews).   • For studies of safety, effectiveness, and comparative effectiveness, a sample of data are compared with patient records.   • Followup is reasonably complete for the registry purpose.   • Validated analytic tools are used for the main analysis (e.g., commercially available analytic packages are used).
Analysis   • Loss to followup is characterized at key stages during the conduct of the study.   • For safety studies, the risks and/or benefits of products, devices, or processes under study are quantitatively evaluated beyond simply evaluating statistical significance (e.g., rates, proportions, and/or relative risks are reported).   • Sensitivity analyses are useful to examine the effect of varying the study population inclusion/exclusion criteria, the assumptions regarding exposure, and the definitions of potential confounders and outcomes on the association between the a priori exposure of interest and the outcome(s).   • If models are used, the specific data elements that are included are described.
Reporting   • Consistency of results is compared and contrasted with other relevant research.   • Inferences about causal effects are based on a variety of factors, including the strength of the association, biases, and temporal relations. The practice of making inferences about causation largely on the outcome of tests of statistical significance is discouraged.

References

1. Available at: Webster's English Dictionary. http://www.m-w.com. Accessed January 17, 2007.

2. Brooke EM. The current and future use of registers in health information systems. Publication No. 8. Geneva: World Health Organization, 1974.

3. Available at: Frequently Asked Questions about Medical and Public Health Registries. The National Committee on Vital and Health Statistics. http://ncvhs.hhs.gov/9701138b.htm. Accessed January 17, 2007.

4. Labresh KA, Gliklich R, Liljestrand J et al. Using "Get With The Guidelines" improve cardiovascular secondary prevention. Jt Comm J Qual Patient Safety 2003 Oct;29(10): 539-50.

5. Kennedy L, Craig AM. Global registries for measuring pharmacoeconomic and quality-of-life outcomes: focus on design and data collection, analysis and interpretation. Pharmacoeconomics 2004;22(9):551-68.

6. U.S. Food and Drug Administration. FDA Guidance for Industry. Good pharmacovigilance and pharmacoepidemiologic assessment, March 2005.

7. Concato J, Shah N, Horwitz RI. Randomized, controlled trials, observational studies and the hierarchy of research designs. N Engl J Med 2000;342:1887-92.

8. Guyatt GH, Sackett DL, Sinclair JC et al. For the Evidence-Based Medicine Working Group: User's guides to the medical literature. 1X. A method for grading health care recommendations. Evidence-Based medicine working group. JAMA 1995;274:1800-4.

9. Concato J, Shah N, Horwitz RI. Randomized, controlled trials, observational studies, and the hierarchy of research designs. N Engl J Med 2000 Jun 22;342(25):1887-92.

10. Atkins D, Eccles M, Flottorp S et al. Systems for grading the quality of evidence and the strength of recommendations I: Critical appraisal of existing approaches The GRADE Working Group. BMC Health Services Research 2004;4:38.

11. The GRADE Working Group. Grading quality of evidence and strength of recommendations. BMJ 2004;(328):1-8.

12. Clancy CM, Eisenberg JM. Outcomes research: measure the end results of health care. Science 1998;282:245-6.

13. Lipscomb J, Snyder CF. The outcomes of cancer outcomes research. Med Care 2002;40[supplement]:III-3-III-10.

14. Available at: National Cancer Institute. Defining the Emerging Field of Outcomes Research. http://outcomes.cancer.gov/aboutresearch/index.html. Accessed July 6, 2006.

15. Lipsomb DJ, Hiatt RA. Cancer outcomes research and the arenas of application. J Natl Cancer Inst Monogr No. 33, 2004:1-7.

16. Hurtado MP, Swift EK, Corrigan JM. Crossing the quality chasm: a new health system for the 21st Century. Washington DC: National Academy Press, Institute of Medicine; 2001.

17. Schwamm LH, LaBresh KA, Pan W et al. Get With The Guidelines – Stroke produces sustainable improvements in hospital-based acute stroke care. Stroke 2006.

18. Schwamm LH, LaBresh KA, Pan W et al. Get With The Guidelines – Stroke improves the rate of "defect-free" acute stroke care. Stroke 2006.

19. Barranger J, O'Rourke E. Lessons learned from the development of enzyme therapy for Gaucher disease. J Inherit Metab Dis 2001 Apr 16;24(0):89-96.

20. Wennberg DE, Lucas FL, Birkmeyer JD et al. Variation in carotid endarterectomy mortality in the Medicare population. JAMA 1998;279:1278-81.

21. MacIntyre K, Capewell S, Stewart S et al. Evidence of improving prognosis in heart failure: trends in case-fatality in 66 547 patients hospitalized between 1986 and 1995. Circulation 2000;102:1126–31.

22. Konstam M. Progress in heart failure management? Lessons from the real world. Circulation 2000;102:1076.

23. Hutchins LF, Unger JM, Crowley JJ et al. Underrepresentation of patients 65 years of age or older in cancer-treatment trials. N Engl J Med 1999;341:2061-7.

24. Eichler HG, Kong SX, Gerth WC et al. Use of cost-effectiveness analysis in health-care resource allocation decision-making: how are cost-effectiveness thresholds expected to emerge? Value in Health 2004;7:518-28.

25. Palmer AJ. Health economics—what the nephrologist should know. Nephrol Dial Transplant 2005;20:1038-41.

26. Hodgson DC, Fuchs LS, Ayanian JZ. The impact of patient and provider characteristics on the treatment and outcomes of colorectal cancer. JNCI 2001;93(7):501-15.

27. Available at: https://www.cms.hhs.gov/regsguidance.asp. Accessed March 30, 2007.

References

28. Guidance for the Public, Industry, and CMS Staff: National Coverage Determinations with Data Collection as a Condition of Coverage: Coverage with Evidence Development. Document issued July 12 , 2006.

29. Connock M, Burls A, Frew E et al. The clinical effectiveness and cost-effectiveness of enzyme replacement therapy for Gaucher's disease: a systematic review. Health Technol Assessment 2006 Jul;10(24):1-152.

30. Devlin N, Parkin D. Does NICE have a cost-effectiveness threshold and what other factors influence its decisions? A binary choice analysis. Health Econ 2004; 13:437-52.

31. Connock M, Juarez-Garcia A, Frew E et al. Systematic review of the clinical effectiveness and cost-effectiveness of enzyme replacement therapies for Fabry's disease and mucopolysaccharidosis type 1. Health Technol Assess 2006 Jun;10(20):iii-iv, ix-113.

32. Matchar DB, Oddone EZ. McCrory DC et al. Influence of projected complication rates on estimated appropriate use rates for carotid endarterectomy. Appropriateness Project Investigators. Academic Medical Center Consortium. Health Serv Res 1997 Aug; 32(3):325-42.

33. Epstein M. Guidelines for good pharmacoepidemiology practice. ISPE commentary. Pharmacoepidemiol Drug Saf 2005;14:589-95.

34. Updated guidelines for evaluating public health surveillance systems. MMWR Recommendations and Reports 2001 July 27;50(RR13):1-5.

35. Solomon DJ, Henry RC, Hogan JG et al. Evaluation and implementation of public health registries. Public Health Rep 1991;106(2):142-50.

36. Glaser SL, Clarke CA, Gomez SL. Cancer surveillance research: a vital subdiscipline of cancer epidemiology. Cancer Causes Control 2005 Nov 16;(9):1009-19.

37. Kennedy L , Craig A. Global registries for measuring pharmacoeconomic and quality-of-life outcomes: focus on design and data collection, analysis, and interpretation. Pharmacoeconomics 2004;22(9):551-68.

38. Bookman MA. Using tumor registry resources in analyzing concordance with guidelines and outcomes. Oncology 2000 Nov;14(11A):104-7.

39. Alter DA, Venkatesh V, Chong A. Evaluating the performance of the Global Registry of Acute Coronary Events risk-adjustment index across socioeconomic strata among patients discharged from the hospital after acute myocardial infarction. Am Heart J 2006 Feb;151(2):323-31.

40. Hernan MA, Hernandez-Dias S, Werler MM et al. Causal knowledge as a prerequisite for confounding evaluation: an application to birth defects epidemiology. Am J Epidemiol 2002;155(2):176-84.

41. Woodward M. Epidemiology. New York: Chapman & Hall, 2005. Chapter 8, Sample size determination.

42. Mangano DT, Tudor IC, Dietzel C. For the Multicenter Study of Perioperative Ischemia Research Group and the Ischemia Research and Education Foundation. The risk association with aprotinin in cardiac surgery. N Engl J Med 2006;354:353-65.

43. Newton J, Garner S. Disease registers in England. Institute of Health Sciences. University of Oxford. Report commissioned by the Department of Health Policy Research Programme, February 2002.

44. Retchin SM, Wenzel RP. Electronic medical record systems at academic health centers: advantages and implementation issues. Acad Med 1999 May;74(5):493-8.

45. Tunis SR. A clinical research strategy to support shared decision making. Health Aff (Millwood) 2005 Jan-Feb;24(1):180-84.

46. Ray WA, Stein CM. Reform of drug regulation – beyond an independent drug-safety board. N Engl J Med 2006;354(2):194-201.

47. Strom BL. How the US drug safety system should be changed. JAMA 2006;295:2072-5.

48. Okie S. Safety in numbers – monitoring risks of approved drugs. N Engl J Med 2005;352(12):1173-6.

49. Editorial. Sponsorship, authorship and accountability. Ann Intern Med 2001;125(6):463-6.

50. Available at: International Committee of Medical Journal Editors. Uniform requirements for manuscripts submitted to biomedical journals: writing and editing for biomedical publication. www.icmje.org. Updated February, 2006.

51. Strom BL. Pharmacoepidemiology. 3rd ed. Chichester, England: John Wiley, 2000.

52. Chow SC, Chang M, Pong A. Statistical consideration of adaptive methods in clinical development. J Biopharm Stat 2005;15(4):575-91.

53. Travis LB, Rabkin CS, Brown LM et al. Cancer survivorship—genetic susceptibility and second primary cancers: research strategies and recommendations. J Natl Cancer Inst 2006 Jan 4;98(1):15-25.

54. Sackett DL, Haynes RB, Tugwell P. Clinical epidemiology. Boston: Little, Brown and Company, 1985. p. 228.

55. Hennekens CH, Buring JE. Epidemiology in medicine. 1st ed. Boston: Little, Brown and Company, 1987.

56. Schoebel FC, Gradaus F, Ivens K et al. Restenosis after elective coronary balloon angioplasty in patients with end stage renal disease: a case-control study using quantitative coronary angiography. Heart 1997;78:337-42.

57. Oral contraceptive use and the risk of endometrial cancer. The Centers for Disease Control Cancer and Steroid Hormone Study. JAMA 1983 Mar 25;249(12):1600-4.

58. Oral contraceptive use and the risk of ovarian cancer. The Centers for Disease Control Cancer and Steroid Hormone Study. JAMA 1983 Mar 25;249(12):1596-9.

59. Long-term oral contraceptive use and the risk of breast cancer. The Centers for Disease Control Cancer and Steroid Hormone Study. JAMA 1983 Mar 25;249(12):1591-5.

60. Speck CE, Kukull WA, Brenner DE et al. History of depression as a risk factor for Alzheimer's disease. Epidemiology 1995 Jul;6(4):366-9.

61. Rothman K, Greenland S. Modern epidemiology. Philadelphia: Lippincott Williams & Wilkins,1998. p. 108.

62. Vigneswaran R, Aitchison SJ, McDonald HM et al. Cerebral palsy and placental infection: a case-cohort study. BMC Pregnancy Childbirth 2004;4:1.

63. Ong AT, Daemen J, van Hout BA et al. Cost-effectiveness of the unrestricted use of sirolimus-eluting stents vs. bare metal stents at 1 and 2-year follow-up: results from the RESEARCH Registry. Eur Heart J 2006;27:2996-3003.

64. Hulley SB, Cumming SR. Designing clinical research. Baltimore: Williams & Wilkins, 1988.

65. Hunter D. First, gather the data. N Engl J Med 2006;354:329-31.

66. Mangano DT, Tudor IC, Dietzel C. The risk association with aprotinin in cardiac surgery. Multicenter study of Perioperative Ischemia Research Group and the Ischemia Research and Education Foundation. N Engl J Med 2006;354:353-65.

67. Wacholder S, McLaughlin JK, Silverman DT et al. Selection of controls in case-control studies. I. Principles. Am J Epidemiol 1992;135:1019-28.

68. Wacholder S, Silverman DT, McLaughlin JK et al. Selection of controls in case-control studies. II. Types of controls. Am J Epidemiol 1992;135:1029-41.

69. Wacholder S, Silverman DT, McLaughlin JK et al. Selection of controls in case-control studies. III. Design options. Am J Epidemiol 1992;135:1042-50.

70. Available at: National Cancer Institute. Surveillance Epidemiology and End Results. http://seer.cancer.gov. Accessed January 17, 2007.

71. Rothman K, Greenland S. Modern epidemiology. Philadelphia: Lippincott Williams & Wilkins, 1998. p. 116.

72. Concato J. Shah, N, Horowitz R. Randomized, controlled trials, observational studies, and the hierarchy of research designs. N Engl J Med 2000;342:1887-92.

73. Benson K, Hartz AJ. A comparison of observational studies and randomized, controlled trials. N Engl J Med 2000;342:1878-86.

74. Black N. Why we need observational studies to evaluate the effectiveness of health care. BMJ 1996 May 11;212(7040):1215-8.

75. Rothman K. Modern epidemiology. Boston: Little Brown, 1986. p. 83.

76. Petri H, Urquhart J. Channeling bias in the interpretation of drug effects. Stat Med 1991 Apr;10(4):577-81.

77. Johnston SC. Identifying confounding by indication through blinded prospective review. Am J Epidemiol 2001;154:276-84.

78. Ray WA. Evaluating medication effects outside of clinical trials: new-user designs. Am J Epidemiol 2003 Nov 1;158(9).915-20.

79. Wattigney WA, Croft JB, Mensah GA et al. Establishing data elements for the Paul Coverdell National Acute Stroke Registry: Part 1: Proceedings of an expert panel. Stroke 2003 Jan;34(1):151-6.

80. Good PI. A manager's guide to the design and conduct of clinical trials. New York: John Wiley & Sons, Inc., 2002.

81. Cannon CP, Battler A, Brindis RG et al. American College of Cardiology key data elements and definitions for measuring the clinical management and outcomes of patients with acute coronary syndromes. A report of the American College of Cardiology Task Force on Clinical Data Standards (Acute Coronary Syndromes Writing Committee). J Am Coll Cardiol 2001 Nov 7;38:2114-30.

82. McNamara RL, Brass LM, Drozda JP Jr. et al. ACC/AHA key data elements and definitions for measuring the clinical management and outcomes of patients with atrial fibrillation: a report of the American College of Cardiology/American Heart Association Task Force on Clinical Data Standards (Writing Committee to Develop Data Standards on Atrial Fibrillation). Circulation 2004 Jun 29;109(25):3223-43.

191

83. Radford MJ, Arnold JM, Bennett SJ et al. ACC/AHA key data elements and definitions for measuring the clinical management and outcomes of patients with chronic heart failure: a report of the American College of Cardiology/American Heart Association Task Force on Clinical Data Standards (Writing Committee to Develop Heart Failure Clinical Data Standards): developed in collaboration with the American College of Chest Physicians and the International Society for Heart and Lung Transplantation: endorsed by the Heart Failure Society of America. Circulation 2005 Sept 20;112:1888-916.

84. Available at: Clinical Data Interchange Standards Consortium. E-Newsletter. http://www.cdisc.org/newsletter/article.asp?issue=200507&n=7. Accessed January 15, 2007.

85. Available at: Biomedical Informatics, LTD. HL7 and CDISC mark first anniversary of renewed associate charter agreement, joint projects result from important healthcare-clinical research industry collaboration. http://news.biohealthmatics.com/PressReleases/2005/10/12/000000003206.aspx. Accessed January 16, 2007.

86. Kim K. Clinical data standards in health care: five case studies. iHealthReports. California HealthCare Foundation. http://www.chcf.org/topics/view.cfm?itemID=112795. Accessed January 15, 2007.

87. Institute of Medicine. Crossing the quality chasm: a new health system for the twenty-first century. Washington: National Academy Press, 2001.

88. Guyatt GH, Feeny DH, Patrick DL. Measuring health-related quality of life. Ann Intern Med 1993 April 15;118(8):622-9.

89. Torrance GW. Measurement of health state utilities for economic appraisal: a review. J Health Econ 1986 Mar;5(1):1-30.

90. Torrance GW. Utility approach to measuring health-related quality of life. J Chronic Dis 1987;40(6):593-603.

91. Feeny D, Furlong W, Boyle M et al. Multi-attribute health status classification systems: health utilities index. Pharmacoeconomics 1995 Jun;7(6):490-502.

92. Torrance GW, Furlong W, Feeny D et al. Multi-attribute preference functions: health utilities index. Pharmacoeconomics 1995 Jun;7(6):503-520.

93. Guyatt GH, Feeny DH, Patrick DL. Measuring health-related quality of life. Ann Intern Med 1993 Apr 15;118(8):622-9.

94. Green CP, Porter CB, Bresnahan DR et al. Development and evaluation of the Kansas City Cardiomyopathy Questionnaire: a new health status measure for heart failure. J Am Coll Cardiol 2000;35:1245-55.

95. Spertus JA, Peterson ED, Conard MW et al. Monitoring clinical changes in patients with heart failure: a comparison of methods. Am Heart J 2005;150:707-15.

96. Spertus JA, Winder JA, Dewhurst TA et al. Monitoring the quality of life in patients with coronary artery disease. Am J Cardiol 1994;74:1240-4.

97. Patrick DL, Deyo RA. Generic and disease-specific measures in assessing health status and quality of life. Med Care 1989 Mar;27:S217-32.

98. Assessing health status and quality-of-life instruments: attributes and review criteria. Qual Life Res 2002 May; 1(3):193-205.

99. Iezzoni LI. Risk adjustment for measuring healthcare outcomes, second edition. Chicago: Health Administration Press, 1997.

100. Goldberg J, Gelfand HM, Levy PS. Registry evaluation methods: a review and case study. Epidemiol Rev 1980;2:210-20.

101. Sorensen HT, Sabroe S, Olsen J. A framework for evaluation of secondary data sources for epidemiological research. Int J Epidemiol 1996;25(2):435-42.

102. Bland JM, Altman DG . Statistical methods for assessing agreement between two methods of clinical measurement. Lancet 1986;I:307-10.

103. Available at: Research Data Assistance Center. http://www.resdac.umn.edu. Accessed January 16, 2007.

104. Available at: National Center for Health Statistics. http://www.cdc.gov/nchs/ndi.htm. Accessed January 16, 2007.

105. Available at: National Technical Information Service. Social Security Administration's Death Master File. http://www.ntis.gov/products/pages/ssa-death-master.asp. Accessed January 16, 2007.

106. Doody MM, Hayes HM, Bilgrad R. Comparability of National Death Index Plus and standard procedures for determining causes of death in epidemiologic studies. Ann Epidemiol 2001;11(1):46-50.

107. Sathiakumar N, Delzell E, Abdalla O. Using the National Death Index to obtain underlying cause of death codes. J Occup Environ Med 1998;40(9):808-13.

108. Available at: U.S. Census Bureau. www.census.gov. Accessed January 16, 2007.

109. Available at: National Marrow Donor Program. http://www.marrow.org. Accessed January 16, 2007.

110. Available at: United States Renal Database. http://www.usrds.org. Accessed January 16, 2007.

111. 45 CFR 160.103: definition of health information; 45 CFR 46.102(f): definition of human subject.

112. 45 CFR Part 46.

113. Part C of Title XI of the Social Security Act, 42 USC §§ 1320d to 1320d-8 (2000), and section 264 of the Health Insurance Portability and Accountability Act of 1996, 42 USC § 1320d-2 note (2000); 45 CFR Parts 160 and 164.

114. National Commission for the Protection of Human Subjects of Biomedical and Behavioral Research, April 18, 1979. Available at: http://www.hhs.gov/ohrp/humansubjects/guidance/belmont.htm. Accessed May 5, 2006.

115. Public Law 93-348 (1974), Title II.

116. Council for International Organizations of Medical Sciences: 1991 International Guidelines for Ethical Review of Epidemiological Studies (hereinafter CIOMS Guidelines). Available at: http://www.cioms.ch/frame_1991_texts_of_guidelines.htm. Accessed May 5, 2006 and noted to be under revision. See especially sections entitled General Ethical Principles and Informed Consent.

117. Grant RW, Sugarman J. Ethics in human subjects research: do incentives matter? J Med Philos 2004 29(6):717-38.

118. CIOMS Guidelines, supra note 2, at paragraphs 11 and 12.

119. Department of Heath and Human Services, Office of the Inspector General: Recruiting human subjects: sample guidelines for practice. OEI-01-97-00196, June 2000. p. 5.

120. Department of Heath and Human Services, Office of the Inspector General: Recruiting human subjects: sample guidelines for practice. OEI-01-97-00196, June 2000. Appendix A.

121. CIOMS Guidelines, supra note 2, at paragraphs 18-21.

122. CIOMS Guidelines, supra note 2, at paragraph 26.

123. CIOMS Guidelines, supra note 2, at paragraph 40.

124. See generally CIOMS Guidelines, supra note 2, at paragraph 43.

125. See, for example, U.S. Department of Health and Human Services (HHS) regulations at 45 CFR Part 46; 21 CFR Parts 50 and 56 for research conducted in support of products regulated by the Food and Drug Administration (FDA).

126. Regulations identical to 45 CFR 46 Subpart A apply to research funded or conducted by a total of 17 Federal agencies, some of which may also require additional legal protections for human subjects.

127. The terms of the model Federal-wide assurance are available from the Office for Human Research Protection in the U.S. Department of Health and Human Services at: http://www.hhs.gov/ohrp/humansubjects/assurance/filasurt.htm. Accessed May 5, 2006.

128. Office for Human Research Protection. Guidance on Research Involving Coded Private Information or Biological Specimens, August 10, 2004. p. 3.

129. 45 CFR Part 46, Subpart A.

130. See, for example, International Society for Pharmacoepidemiology (ISPE). Guidelines for Good Pharmacoepidemiology Practices (GPP), August 2004. Pharmacoepidemiol Drug Safety 2005;14:589-95 on the essential elements of a protocol.

131. Part C of Title XI of the Social Security Act, 42 USC §§ 1320d to 1320d-8 (2000), and section 264 of the Health Insurance Portability and Accountability Act of 1996, 42 USC § 1320d-2 note (2000); 45 CFR Parts 160 and 164.

132. 45 CFR 160.102, Applicability, and 160.103, definitions of covered entity, health care provider, health plan, health care clearinghouse, and transaction.

133. 45 CFR 160.203.

134. 45 CFR 160.103 defines both "disclosure" and "use" for the purposes of the Privacy Rule.

135. 45 CFR 164.501.

136. 67 Fed Reg 53231, August 14, 2002.

137. 45 CFR 46.102(d).

138. U.S. Department of Health and Human Services, National Institutes of Health. Health services research and the HIPAA Privacy Rule. NIH Publication Number 05-5308, May 2005. See also U.S. Department of health and Human Services, National Institutes of Health. Research repositories, databases, and the HIPAA Privacy Rule. NIH Publication Number 04-5489, January 2004.

139. 45 CFR 164.512(b).

140. 45 CFR 164.501.

141. Centers for Disease Control and Prevention. HIPAA Privacy Rule and Public Health: Guidance from CDC and the U.S. Department of Health and Human Services. MMWR 2003;52 (early release).

142. 45 CFR 164.512(a).

143. 45 CFR 164.508(a).

144. 45 CFR 164.514(e).

145. 45 CFR 164.514(a)-(c).

146. 45 CFR 164.528.

193

References

147. 45 CFR 164.512(i)(1)(i).

148. 21 CFR 65.111(a)(7).

149. Available at: Centers for Disease Control and Prevention. Guidelines for Defining Public Health Research and Public Health Non-Research, revised October 4, 1999. http://www.cdc.gov/od/ads/opspoll1.htm. Accessed June 30, 2006. Gostin LO. Public health law: power, duty, restraint. Berkeley and Los Angeles, CA: University of California Press; New York: The Milbank Memorial Fund; 2000. p. 126-127 (hereinafter Public Health Law). See also CIOMS Guidelines, supra note 2, Introduction, noting that epidemiological practice and research may overlap.

150. Bellin E, Dubler NN. The quality improvement-research divide and the need for external oversight. Am J Public Health 2001; 91(9):1512-1517 (hereinafter Quality Improvement-Research Divide). Lindenauer PK, Benjamin EM et al. The Role of the institutional review board in quality improvement: a survey of quality officers, institutional review board chairs, and journal editors. Am J Med 2002;113(7): 575-9. Lo B, Groman M. Oversight of quality improvement: focusing on benefits and risks. Arch Intern Med 2003;163(12):1481-6.

151. Available at: Office for Human Research Protections. http://www.hhs.gov/ohrp. Accessed January 17, 2007.

152. National Institutes of Health. Health services research and the HIPAA Privacy Rule. Publication Number 05-5308, p. 2-3. See also 45 CFR 164.501 for the definition of health care operations.

153. A copy of the HHS version of the "Common Rule," 45 CFR Part 46, subpart A, and additional subparts B, C, and D regarding vulnerable populations may be obtained on the Web site of the Office for Human Research Protection (OHRP) in the U.S. Department of Health and Human Services. Available at: http://www.hhs.gov/ohrp/humansubjects/guidance/45cfr46.htm. Accessed May 8, 2006.

154. A copy of the "Privacy Rule," 45 CFR Parts 160 and 164, may be obtained on the Web site of the Office for Civil Rights (OCR) in the U.S. Department of Health and Human Services. Available at: http://www.hhs.gov/ocr/hipaa/finalreg.html. Accessed May 8, 2006.

155. The Common Rule as adopted by HHS contains special protections for certain defined "vulnerable" populations, i.e., women, human fetuses, neonates, prisoners, and children. See 45 CFR Part 46, Subparts B, C, D.

156. Available at: American College of Epidemiology: Policy Statement on Sharing Data from Epidemiologic Studies, May 2002. http://www.acepidemiology2.org/policystmts/DataSharing.pdf. Accessed May 8, 2006.

157. 45 CFR 46.102(d).

158. Available at: Centers for Disease Control and Prevention. National Program of Cancer Registries (NPCR). Description of SEER program. http://www.cdc.gov/cancer/npcr/css.htm section IV. Accessed July 9, 2006.

159. 45 CFR 164.512(b).

160. Lillienfeld DE, Stolley PD. Foundations of epidemiology (revised). Oxford University Press, 1994, at 104. See also Public Health Law, supra note 34, at 114, Table 5.

161. 45 CFR 164.512(d).

162. 45 CFR 164.512(d)(1).

163. 45 CFR 164.512(b)(1)(iii).

164. 45 CFR 46.102(d) and 45 CFR 164.501, respectively.

165. 45 CFR 46.102(d).

166. 45 CFR 164.501.

167. Available at: National Institutes of Health, U.S. Department of Health and Human Services. Health services research and the HIPAA Privacy Rule. NIH Publication No. 04-5489, Jan. 2004. p. 2-3. http://privacyruleandresearch.nih.gov/healthservicesprivacy.asp. Accessed May 19, 2006.

168. 45 CFR 164.501.

169. Available at: Centers for Disease Control and Prevention. Guidelines for Defining Public Health Research and Public Health Non-Research, revised October 4, 1999. http://www.cdc.gov/od/ads/opspoll1.htm. Accessed June 30, 2006. Public Health Law, supra note 3, p. 126-127. See also CIOMS Guidelines, supra note 6, Introduction, noting that epidemiological practice and research may overlap and Quality Improvement-Research Divide, supra note 39.

170. Quality Improvement-Research Divide, supra note 39, 1512-1517. Lindenauer PK, Benjamin EM et al. The role of the institutional review board in quality improvement: a survey of quality officers, institutional review board chairs, and journal editors. Am J Med 2002; 113(7):575-9. Lo B, Groman M. Oversight of quality improvement: focusing on benefits and risks. Arch Intern Med 2003;163(12):1481-6.

171. See 45 CFR 160.103 for the definition of individually identifiable health information and 45 CFR 164.514(a)-(c) and (e) on the de-identification of health information and limited data sets, respectively.

172. 45 CFR 46.102(f).

173. 45 CFR 46.111(a)(7).

174. 45 CFR 46.116(a)(5).

175. See 45 CFR 164.514(a)-(c) and (e) on the de-identification of health information and limited data sets, respectively.

176. 45 CFR 164.514(e)(2).

177. 45 CFR 164.514(b).

178. 45 CFR 164.514(b)(1).

179. 45 CFR 164.514(c).

180. 45 CFR 164.514(c).

181. 45 CFR 46.102(f).

182. 45 CFR 164.514(e)(2).

183. 45 CFR 164.514(e)(4).

184. 45 CFR 164.514(e)(4)(ii)(A).

185. 67 Fed Reg 53181, 53236, August 14, 2002.

186. 45 CFR 164.504(e).

187. 45 CFR 164.504(e).

188. 45 CFR 164.514(e)(2).

189. 45 CFR 164.514(e)(4)(ii)(C)(5).

190. 45 CFR 46.101(b)(4).

191. 45 CFR 164.508.

192. 45 CFR 164.508(c).

193. 45 CFR 164.502(a)(1).

194. 45 CFR 164.501.

195. 45 CFR 46.102(f).

196. 45 CFR 46.116.

197. 45 CFR 164.508(b)(3).

198. 45 CFR 46.116.

199. 45 CFR 164.512(i)(1)(i)(B).

200. 45 CFR 164.508(c)(1)(iv).

201. 45 CFR 46.116.

202. 67 Fed Reg 53181, 53226, August 14, 2002.

203. Available at: Department of Health and Human Services: Institutional review boards and the HIPAA Privacy Rule, August 2003. NIH Publication Number 03-5428. p. 15-16. http://privacyruleandresearch.nih.gov/pdf/IRB_Factsheet.pdf. Accessed May 9, 2006.

204. 45 CFR 164.508(c)(2)(iii).

205. Family Educational Rights and Privacy Act (FERPA), 20 USC 1232g, 34 CFR Part 99.

206. Public Health Services Act Section 301(d), 42 USC 241(d) as amended. See also 42 CFR Part 2a about research activities on mental health, including the use and effect of alcohol and other psychoactive drugs.

207. Available at: Office for Human Research Protection in the Department of Health and Human Services: Guidance on Certificates of Confidentiality, Feb. 25, 2003, Background. http://www.hhs.gov/ohrp/humansubjects/guidance/certconf.htm. Accessed May 9, 2006.

208. Available at: National Institutes of Health: Notice NOT-OD-02-037, released on March 15, 2002. http://grants1.nih.gov/grants/guide/notice-files/NOT-OD-02-037.html. Accessed May 9, 2006.

209. Information about obtaining a certificate of confidentiality is available at the "CoC Kiosk" on the NIH Web site. Available at: http://grants.nih.gov/grants/policy/coc/index.htm. Accessed May 9, 2006.

210. Available at: National Institutes of Health, Office of Extramural Research: Certificates of Confidentiality: Background Information, Web posting Feb. 14, 2006. http://grants.nih.gov/grants/policy/coc/background.htm. Accessed May 9, 2006.

211. Information about certificates of confidentiality is available at the "CoC Kiosk" on the NIH Web site. Available at: http://grants.nih.gov/grants/policy/coc/index.htm. Accessed May 9, 2006.

212. 42 USCS 290dd-2 and 290ee-3; 42 CFR Part 2.

213. 42 CFR 2.52(a).

214. 42 CFR 2.52(a).

215. Louisiana statute re protection of tobacco data from subpoena.

216. See, for example, Wis. Stat. 146.38.

217. See 45 CFR 164.512(i) and 46.116(d), respectively.

218. 45 CFR 164.512(i)(2)(ii).

219. 45 CFR 164.512(i)(1)(i).

220. 45 CFR 164.512(i)(2).

221. 45 CFR 164.512(i)(2)(iii) and (iv).

195

References

222. 45 CFR 46.116(d).

223. 21 CFR 50.20 and 50.23.

224. 45 CFR 164.528(a)(1).

225. 45 CFR 164.528(b).

226. 45 CFR 164.528(a)(1).

227. 45 CFR 164.528(b)(3) and (4).

228. 45 CFR 46.117(c)(1).

229. 45 CFR 46.117(c)(2).

230. 45 CFR 46.117(c).

231. 45 CFR 46.116(d)(4).

232. Available at: The Center for International Blood and Marrow Transplant Research. http://www.cibmtr.org/index.html. Accessed May 12, 2006.

233. 67 F.R. 53213, August 14, 2002.

234. 67 F.R. 53213, August 14, 2002.

235. Joyce C, Patry W, Leaffer M et al. Copyright law, 3rd Edition. New York and San Francisco: Matthew Bender & Co., Inc, 1994, reprinted 1997. "The Landscape of Copyright," p. 1-41.

236. American Medical Association House of Delegates, Connecticut Delegation: Guiding Principles, Collection and Warehousing of Electronic Medical Record Information. Resolution #802, received Sept. 16, 2005. Available at: http://www.ama-assn.org/meetings/public/interim05/802i05.pdf. Accessed May 20, 2006. Bailey S. Your data for sale? Boston Globe, Mar. 24, 2006. Available at: http://www.boston.com/business/globe/articles/2006/03/24/your_data_for_sale?mode=P. Accessed April 3, 2006.

237. Washington University v. Catalona, Case No. 4:03CV1065SNL (E.D. Mo., filed Mar. 31, 2006).

238. American College of Epidemiology. Policy Statement on Sharing Data from Epidemiologic Studies, May 2002. Available at: http://www.acepidemiology2.org/policystmts/DataSharing.pdf. Accessed May 19, 2006. National Institutes of Health, U.S. Department of Health and Human Services. Final NIH Statement on Sharing Research Data, Notice NOT-OD-03-032, Feb. 26, 2003. Available at: http://grants.nih.gov/grants/guide/notice-files/NOT-OD-03-032.html. Accessed May 20, 2006.

239. 17 USC § 101.

240. Feist Publications, Inc. v. Rural Telephone Service, Co., Inc., 499 U.S. 340, 345, 348 (1991).

241. Id., 340 et seq.; Harris RK, Rosenfield SS. Copyright Protection for Genetic Databases, 2005; Jurimetrics J. 45: 225-250 (hereinafter Genetic Databases).

242. Available at: Scios. Press release. http://www.sciosinc.com/scios/pr_1046368542. Accessed January 16, 2007.

243. Available at: Ameican Heart Association. Get With The Guidelines. http://www.americanheart.org/presenter.jhtml?identifier=1165. Accessed June 16, 2006.

244. Available at: Clinical Data Interchange Standards Consortium. www.cdisc.org. Accessed June 16, 2006.

245. Available at: National Institutes of Health Stroke Scale. http://www.ninds.nih.gov/doctors/NIH_Stroke_Scale.pdf. Accessed June 16, 2006.

246. Luck J, Peabody JW, Dresselhaus TR et al. How well does chart abstraction measure quality? A prospective comparison of standardized patients with the medical record. Am J Med 2000 Jun 1;108(8):642-9.

247. Reisch LM, Fosse JS, Beverly K et al. Training, quality assurance, and assessment of medical record abstraction in a multisite study. Am J Epidemiol 2003; 157:546-51.

248. Neale R, Rokkas P, McClure RJ. Inter-rater reliability of injury coding in the Queensland Trauma Registry. Emerg Med (Fremantle) 2003 Feb;15(1):38-41.

249. Available at: Health-Level Seven. www.hl7.org. Accessed June 16, 2006.

250. Available at: Clinical Data Interchange Standards Consortium. www.cdisc.org. Accessed June 16, 2006.

251. Available at: U.S. Food and Drug Administration. www.fda.gov/oral/compliance_ref/bimo/ffinalcct.pdf. Accessed June 16, 2006.

252. Gliklich R. Personal communication.

253. Available at: U.S. Department of Health and Human Services. http://www.hhs.gov/healthit/ahiccharter.pdf. Accessed June 16, 2006.

254. Available at: National Institute of Standards and Technology. http://www.nist.gov/. Accessed June 16, 2006.

255. Available at: U.S. Food and Drug Administration. Guidance for Industry: Development and Use of Risk Minimization Action Plans. http://www.fda.gov/cder/Guidance/6358fnl.htm. Accessed August 19, 2006.

256. Mangano DT, Tudor IC, Dietzel C. The risk associated with aprotinin in cardiac surgery. N Engl J Med 2006 Jan 26;354(4):353-65.

257. Fink AS, Campbell DA, Mentzer RM et al. The National Surgical Quality Improvement Program in non-Veterans Administration hospitals: initial demonstration of feasibility. Ann Surg 2002 Sept; 236(3): 344-54.

196

258. The HIPAA Security Rule: Health Insurance Reform: Security Standards, February 20, 2003. 68 FR 8334.

259. Available at: U.S. Food and Drug Administration. http://www.fda.gov/ora/compliance_ref/part11/FRs/background/pt11finr.pdf. Accessed June 19, 2006.

260. Available at: U.S. Food and Drug Administration. http://www.fda.gov/Cder/guidance/5667fnl.pdf. Accessed June 19, 2006.

261. Available at: U.S. Food and Drug Administration. http://www.fda.gov/ora/compliance_ref/bimo/ffinalcct.pdf. Accessed June 19, 2006.

262. Available at: U.S. Food and Drug Administration. http://www.fda.gov/cdrh/comp/guidance/938.pdf. Accessed June 19, 2006.

263. 21 CFR 314.80.

264. ICH E2A: Clinical safety data management: definitions and standards for expedited reporting, and 21CFR 310.305: Records and reports concerning adverse drug experiences on marketed products.

265. Guidance for Industry: Establishing Pregnancy Exposure Registries. Available at: http://www.fda.gov/cder/guidance/3626fnl.pdf. Accessed April 4, 2007.

266. Postmarketing Adverse Experience Reporting for Human Drug and Licensed Biological Products: Clarification of What to Report. Available at: http://www.fda.gov/cder/guidance/1830fn1.pdf. Accessed April 4, 2007.

267. 21 CFR 314.80.

268. Guidance for Industry Postmarketing Adverse Experience Reporting for Human Drug and Licensed Biological Products: Clarification of What to Report. USDHHS, FDA, CDER, and CBER. CLIN4 August 1997.

269. Baim DS, Mehran R, Kereiakes DJ et al. Postmarket surveillance for drug-eluting coronary stents: a comprehensive approach. Circulation 2006;113:891-7.

270. Available at: U.S. Food and Drug Administration. http://www.fda.gov/cdrh/mdr. Accessed March 22, 2007.

271. Gross TP, Witten CM, Uldriks C et al. A view from the US Food and Drug Administration. In: Johnson FE, Goldstone J, Virgo KS, Eds. The bionic patient: health promotion for people with implanted prosthetic devices. New Jersey: Humana Press, Inc., 2005. p, 61-87.

272. FDA Pharmacovigilance Guidance. Available at: www.fda.gov/cdrh/osb/guidance/316.pdf. Accessed April 4, 2007.

273. Available at: U.S. Food and Drug Administration. http://www.fda.gov/medwatch/report/mmp.htm. Accessed March 22, 2007.

274. Available at: U.S. Food and Drug Administration. www.fda.gov/medwatch. Accessed March 22, 2007.

275. Available at: Vaccine Adverse Event Reporting System. http://vaers.hhs.gov. Accessed March 22, 2007.

276. Available at: Council for International Organizations of Medical Sciences. http://www.cioms.ch. Accessed March 22, 2007.

277. 21 CFR 312.32.

278. 21 CFR 314.80(f)(1).

279. ICH Topic E 2 A. Clinical Safety Data Management: Definitions and Standards for Expedited Reporting. European Medicines Agency. CPMP/ICH/377/95. June 1995.

280. ICH Topic E 2 D. Post Approval Safety Data Management. European Medicines Agency. CPMP/ICH/3945/03. May 2004.

281. ICH E2C R1: Clinical Safety Data Management: Periodic Updated Safety Reports for Marketed Drugs. European Medicines Agency. CPMP/ICH/288/95. June 1997.

282. See 21CFR 314.80.

283. Cole P. The hypothesis generating machine. Epidemiology 1993;4(3):271-3.

284. Yusuf S, Wittes J, Probstfield J et al. Analysis and interpretation of treatment effects in subgroups of patients in randomized clinical trials. JAMA 1991;266(1):93-8.

285. Hulley SB, Cumming SR, Eds. Designing clinical research. Williams & Wilkins: Baltimore, MD, 1988.

286. Little RJA, Rubin DB. Statisticalanalysis with missing data. New York: John Wiley & Sons, 1987.

287. Barzi F, Woodward M. Imputation of missing values in practice: results from imputations of serum cholesterol in 28 cohort studies. Am J Epidemiol 2004;160:34-45.

288. Little RJA, Rubin DB. Statistical analysis with missing data. New York: John Wiley & Sons, 1987.

289. Rubin DB. Multiple imputations in sample surveys - a phenomenological Bayesian approach to nonresponse. Imputation and editing of faulty or missing survey data. U.S. Department of Commerce, 1978:1-23.

290. Burton A, Altman DG. Missing covariate data within cancer prognostic studies: a review of current reporting and proposed guidelines. Br J Cancer 2004;91:4-8.

291. Burton A Altman DG, Missing covariate data within cancer prognostic studies: a review of current reporting and proposed guidelines. British J of Cancer 2004;91:4-8.

197

292. Greenland S and Finkle WD. A critical look at methods for handling missing coverages in epidemiologic regression analyses. Amer J Epidemiol 1995;142(12):1255-1264.

293. Hernan MA, Hernandez-Dias S, Werler MM, Mitchell AA. Causal knowledge as a prerequisite for confounding evaluation: an application to birth defects epidemiology. Amer J Epidemiol 2002;155(2):176-84.

294. Mangano DT, Tudor IC, Dietzel C for the Multicenter Study of Perioperative Ischemia Research Group and the Ischemia Research and Education Foundation. The risk associated with aprotinin in cardiac surgery. N Engl J Med 2006;354:353-6.

295. Cepeda MS, Boston R, Farrar JT et al. Comparison of logistic regression versus propensity score when the number of events is low and there are multiple confounders. Am J Epidemiol 2003;158:280-7.

296. Sturmer T, Joshi M, Glynn RJ, et al. A review of the application of propensity score methods yielded increasing use, advantages in specific settings, but not substantially different estimates compared with conventional multivariable methods. J Clin Epidemiol 2006;59(5):437-47.

297. Glynn RJ, Schneeweiss S, Sturmer T. Indications for propensity scores and review of their use in pharmacoepidemiology. Basic Clin Pharmacol Toxicol 2006;98(3):253-9.

298. Rothman KJ, Greenland S, Eds. Modern epidemiology. Lippincott Williams & Williams, 1998.

299. Hennekens CH, Buring JE, Mayrent SL. Epidemiology in medicine. Little Brown & Co., 1987.

300. Kleinbaum DG, Kupper LL, Miller KE et al. Applied regression analysis and other multivariable methods. Duxbury Press, 1998.

301. Aschengrau A, Seage G. Essentials of epidemiology in public health. Jones & Bartlett, 2003.

302. Rosner B. Fundamentals of biostatistics, 5th edition. Duxbury Press, 2000.

303. Palmer AJ. Health economics – what the nephrologists should know. Nephrol Dial Transplant 2005;20:1038-41.

304. Neumann PJ. Using cost-effectiveness analysis to improve health care. Opportunities and barriers. Oxford University Press, 2004.

305. Tan-Torres Edejer T, Baltussen R, Adam T, et al. Making choices in health: WHO Guide to Cost-Effectiveness Analysis. World Health Organization: Geneva, 2004.

306. Drummond M, Stoddart G, Torrance G. Methods for the economic evaluation of health care programmes, 3rd edition. Oxford: Oxford University Press, 2005.

307. Muennig P. Designing and conducting cost-effectiveness analyses in medicine and health care. San Francisco: John Wiley & Sons, Inc., 2002.

308. Haddix AC, Teutsch SM, Corso PS. Prevention effectiveness: a guide to decision analysis and economic evaluation. Oxford University Press, 2003.

309. Gold MR, Siegel JE, Russell LB et al. Cost-effectiveness in health and medicine: The Report of the Panel on Cost-Effectiveness in Health and Medicine. New York: Oxford University Press, 1996.

310. Raffery J, Roderick P, Stevens A. Potential use of routine databases in health technology assessment. Health Technol Assess 2005;9(20):1-106.

311. Salas M, Hofman A, Stricker BH. Confounding by indication: an example of variation in the use of epidemiologic terminology. Am J Epidemiol 1999;149(11):981-3.

312. Petri H, Urquhart J: Channeling bias in the interpretation of drug effects. Stat Med 1991 Apr;10(4):577-81.

313. Rothman KJ. Causes (Commentary). Am J Epidemiol 1976;104(6):587-92.

314. Rothman KJ, Greenland S, Eds. Modern epidemiology. Lippincott Williams & Williams, 1998.

315. Bland JM, Altman DG. Statistical notes: Survival probabilities (the Kaplan-Meier method). BMJ 1998;317:1572-80.

316. Samsa GP, Matchar DV. Issues in the design and implementation of registries. White paper prepared for the Agency for Healthcare Research and Quality. August 22, 2005.

317. Moher D, Schulz KF, Altman D for the CONSORT group. The CONSORT Statement: revised recommendations for improving the quality of reports of parallel group randomized trials. JAMA 2001;285:1987-91.

318. Moher D, Jadad AR, Nichol G et al. Assessing the quality of randomized controlled trials: an annotated bibliography of scales and checklists. Control Clin Trials 1995;16:62-73.

319. Rothman KJ, Ed. Causal inference. Chestnut Hill, MA, 1988.

320. Rothman KJ, Greenland S. Modern epidemiology. Philadelphia: Lippincott Williams & Wilkins, 1998.

321. Weiss NS. Clinical epidemiology. The study of the outcome of illness. Oxford University Press, 2006.

322. Fletcher RH, Fletcher SW, Fletcher EH. Clinical epidemiology: the essentials. Williams & Wilkins, 1996.

323. Rothman KJ, Greenland S. Modern epidemiology, Philadelphia: Lippincott Williams & Wilkins, 1998. p. 135-61.

324. West S, King V, Carey TS et al. Systems to rate the strength of scientific evidence. Evidence Report/Technology Assessment No. 47. Rockville, MD: Agency for Healthcare Research and Quality. AHRQ Publication No. 02-E016, April 2002.

325. Greenland S. A critical look at some popular meta-analytic methods. Am J Epidemiol 1994; 140(3):290-6.

326. Available at: National Center for the Dissemination of Disability Research. http://www.ncddr.org. Accessed January 17, 2007.

327. Mosteller F, Boruch R, Eds. Evidence matters: randomized trials in education research. Washington, DC: The Brookings Institute, 2002.

328. Shavelson RJ, Towne L, Eds. Scientific research in education. Washington, DC: National Research Council, National Academy Press, 2002.

329. Lohr KN. Rating the strength of scientific evidence: relevance for quality improvement programs. Int J Qual Health Care 2004;16(1):9-18.

330. Guidelines for Good Pharmacoepidemiologic Practice. Pharmacoepidemiology and Drug Safety 2005;14:589-95. See www.pharmacoepi.org for latest updates to this policy.

331. Available at: ICH Guideline on Good Clinical Practice. http://www.emea.eu.int/pdfs/human/ich/013595en.pdf. Accessed January 17, 2007.

332. Available at: Council for International Organizations of Medical Sciences. http://www.cioms.ch/frame_1991_texts_of_guidelines.htm. Accessed January 17, 2007.

333. Klaucke D, Buehler J, Thacker S et al. Guidelines for evaluating surveillance systems. MMMR 1988;37(S5): 1-18.

334. Goldberg J, Gelfand HM, Levy PS. Registry evaluation methods: a review and case study. Epidemiol Rev 1980;2:210-20.

335. Harris RK, Rosenfield SS. Copyright protection for genetic databases. Jurimetrics J 2005;45:225-50.

336. 17 USC §106.

337. Available at: United States Copyright Office. http://www.copyright.gov. Accessed January 17, 2007.

338. 17 USC §201(a).

339. 17 USC §102(b). Feist Publications, Inc. v. Rural Telephone Service, Co., Inc., 499 U.S. 340 (1991).

340. 17 USC §201(b).

341. 17 USC §201(a).

342. 17 UCSC §107.

343. Genetic Databases, supra note 114 at 243.

199

Contributors

Chapter 1. Patient Registries

*Richard E. Gliklich, M.D.
President
Outcome Sciences, Inc. d/b/a Outcome
Principal Investigator, Outcome DEcIDE Center
Associate Professor, Harvard Medical School
Cambridge, MA

David Matchar, M.D.
Professor of Medicine
Director, Center for Clinical Health Policy Research
Duke University Medical Center
Durham, NC

Chapter 2. Planning a Registry

Thomas Gross, M.D., M.P.H.
Director, Division of Postmarket Surveillance
Center for Devices and Radiological Health
Food and Drug Administration
Rockville, MD

*Joel M. Kremer, M.D.
Pfaff Family Professor and Chair in Medicine,
  Albany Medical College
Director of Research, The Center for Rheumatology
President, The Consortium of Rheumatology
  Researchers of North America (CORRONA)
Albany, NY

C. Geoffrey McDonough, M.D.
Vice President, Global Medical Affairs
Genzyme Therapeutics
Cambridge, MA

Chapter 3. Registry Design

*Nancy A. Dreyer, M.P.H., Ph.D.
Chief of Scientific Affairs
Outcome Sciences, Inc. d/b/a Outcome
Cambridge, MA

Hesha J. Duggirala, Ph.D., M.P.H.
Epidemiologist, Division of Postmarket Surveillance
Center for Devices and Radiological Health
Food and Drug Administration
Rockville, MD

* **Indicates chapter coordinator.**

Gregory Samsa, Ph.D.
Associate Professor, Department of Biostatistics
  and Bioinformatics
Duke University School of Medicine
Durham, NC

Paul Stang, Ph.D.
Institute for Primary Care Research
Associate Professor, West Chester University, and
  Galt Associates
Blue Bell, PA

Chapter 4. Data Elements for Registries

Marc L. Berger, M.D.
Vice President, USHH Outcomes Research and
  Management
Merck & Co. Inc
West Point, PA

*Michelle A. Bertagna
Project Manager
Outcome Sciences, Inc. d/b/a Outcome
Cambridge, MA

Irene Katzan, M.D., M.S.
Director, Northeastern Ohio Stroke Outcomes
  Research Program
Cleveland Clinic Foundation
Center for Health Care Research & Policy,
  MetroHealth Medical Center
Cleveland, OH

John Spertus, M.D., M.P.H.
Professor of Medicine, University of Missouri –
  Kansas City
Director CV Education and Outcomes Research,
  Saint Luke's Mid America Heart Institute
Kansas City, MO

Chapter 5. Data Sources for Registries

Paul Eggers, Ph.D.
Program Director for Kidney and Urology
  Epidemiology
National Institute of Diabetes and Digestive and
  Kidney Diseases
Bethesda, MD

David J. Malenka, M.D.
Professor of Medicine
Dartmouth Medical School
Hanover, NH
Section of Cardiology
Dartmouth-Hitchcock Medical Center
Lebanon, NH

Joseph Selby, M.D., M.P.H.
Director of the Division of Research
Kaiser Permanente, Northern California
Oakland, CA

*Lisa G. Vincent, M.A., Ph.D.
Senior Director, Clinical Research and Development
Corporate Quality, Regulatory, and Clinical Affairs
Medtronic, Inc.
Minneapolis, MN

Chapter 6. Principles of Registry Ethics, Data Ownership, and Privacy

*Susan M. Adams, J.D.
Independent Consultant
Orford, NH

Holly L. Howe, Ph.D.
Executive Director
North American Association of Central Cancer Registries, Inc.
Springfield, IL

David W. Kaufman, Sc.D.
Assoc. Director, Slone Epidemiology Center
Professor of Epidemiology
Boston University School of Public Health
Boston, MA

Stuart Kim, J.D., M.S.
Regulatory Counsel
Cephalon, Inc.
Frazer, PA

Debra R. Lappin, J.D.
Senior Vice President
B&D Consulting LLC – Health and Life Sciences Practice
Washington, DC

Marianne Ulcickas Yood, D.Sc., M.P.H.
Principal Epidemiologist, EpiSource
Hamden, CT
Associate Research Scientist
Epidemiology and Public Health
Yale University School of Medicine
New Haven, CT

Chapter 7. Patient and Provider Recruitment and Management

*Fred Anderson, Ph.D.
Research Professor of Surgery
Director, Center for Outcomes Research
University of Massachusetts Medical School
Worcester, MA

Ralph Brindis, M.D., M.P.H.
Regional Senior Advisor for Cardiovascular Disease, Northern California Kaiser Permanente
Oakland, CA
Clinical Professor of Medicine, UCSF
Chief Medical Officer & Chairman
NCDR Management Board, American College of Cardiology,
Washington, DC

Jeanette M. Broering, R.N., M.S., M.P.H.
Director, Data Procurement & Quality Assurance
GU-Cancer Epidemiology & Population Science
Department of Urology
University of California, San Francisco
San Francisco, CA

Richard E. Gliklich, M.D.
President
Outcome Sciences, Inc. d/b/a Outcome
Principal Investigator, Outcome DEcIDE Center
Associate Professor, Harvard Medical School
Cambridge, MA

Robert E. Harbaugh, M.D.
Professor and Chairman, Department of Neurosurgery
Professor, Department of Engineering Science and Mechanics
Penn State University - Milton S. Hershey Medical Center
Hershey, PA

* Indicates chapter coordinator.

Chapter 8. Data Collection and Quality Assurance

Richard E. Gliklich, M.D.
President
Outcome Sciences, Inc. d/b/a Outcome
Principal Investigator, Outcome DEcIDE Center
Associate Professor, Harvard Medical School
Cambridge, MA

*Shukri F. Khuri, M.D.
Professor of Surgery, Harvard Medical School
Co-Founder, National Surgical Quality Improvement
  Program
VA Boston Healthcare System
West Roxbury, MA

Neal Mantick, M.S.
Formerly Director, Global Registry Programs,
  Genzyme Therapeutics
Currently Director of Registries, Abt Associates,
  Inc.
Lexington, MA

Barry Mirrer, M.S., C.Q.M.
Director of Quality
Outcome Sciences, Inc. d/b/a Outcome
Cambridge, MA

Neha Sheth, Pharm.D.
Senior Director, Risk Management Strategy
Pfizer Global Research and Development
Ann Arbor, MI

Joseph Terdiman, M.D., Ph.D.
Director of Information Technology
Division of Research
Kaiser Permanente
Oakland, CA

Chapter 9. Adverse Event Detection, Processing, and Reporting

Nancy A. Dreyer, M.P.H., Ph.D.
Chief of Scientific Affairs
Outcome Sciences, Inc. d/b/a Outcome
Cambridge, MA

Richard E. Gliklich, M.D.
President
Outcome Sciences, Inc. d/b/a Outcome
Principal Investigator, Outcome DEcIDE Center
Associate Professor, Harvard Medical School
Cambridge, MA

*Neha Sheth, Pharm.D.
Senior Director, Risk Management Strategy
Pfizer Global Research and Development
Ann Arbor, MI

Anne Trontell, M.D., M.P.H.
Senior Advisor on Pharmaceutical Outcomes
Center for Outcomes and Evidence
Agency for Healthcare Research and Quality
Rockville, MD

Chapter 10. Analysis and Interpretation of Registry Data To Evaluate Outcomes

Nancy A. Dreyer, M.P.H., Ph.D.
Chief of Scientific Affairs
Outcome Sciences, Inc. d/b/a Outcome
Cambridge, MA

Wei Dong, M.D., Ph.D.
Associate Director, Epidemiology
Genentech, Inc.
South San Francisco, CA

Harlan M. Krumholz, M.D., S.M.
Director of the Yale-New Haven Hospital Center for
  Outcomes Research & Evaluation
Harold H. Hines, Jr. Professor of Medicine and
  Epidemiology and Public Health
Yale University School of Medicine
New Haven, CT

Eric Peterson, M.D., M.P.H.
Physician Investigator
Duke Clinical Research Institute
Durham, NC

*Gillian D. Sanders, Ph.D.
Co-Director, Center for the Prevention of Sudden
  Cardiac Death
Associate Professor of Medicine
Duke Clinical Research Institute
Durham, NC

203

* **Indicates chapter coordinator.**

Dale R. Tavris, M.D., M.P.H.
Epidemiologist
Center for Devices and Radiological Health
Food and Drug Administration
Rockville, MD

Chapter 11. Evaluating Registries

*Nancy A. Dreyer, M.P.H., Ph.D.
Chief of Scientific Affairs
Outcome Sciences, Inc. d/b/a Outcome
Cambridge, MA

Sarah E. Garner, BPharm, Ph.D., MRPharm.S.
Technical Adviser
National Institute for Health and Clinical Excellence
  (NICE)
London, UK

*Indicates chapter coordinator.

Reviewers

Chapter 1. Patient Registries

Michael A. Carome, M.D.
Captain, U.S. Public Health Service
Associate Director for Regulatory Affairs
Office for Human Research Protections
Rockville, MD

Janet Hiller, M.P.H., Ph.D.
Professor of Public Health
Director, Adelaide Health Technology Assessment
  (AHTA)
University of Adelaide
Adelaide, Australia

Chapter 2. Planning a Registry

Michael A. Carome, M.D.
Captain, U.S. Public Health Service
Associate Director for Regulatory Affairs
Office for Human Research Protections
Rockville, MD

Patrice Desvigne-Nickens, M.D.
Leader, Cardiovascular Medicine Scientific
  Research Group
Clinical and Molecular Medicine Program
Division of Heart and Vascular Diseases
National Heart, Lung, and Blood Institute
Bethesda, MD

Gregg Fonarow, M.D.
Professor of Medicine
Director, Ahmanson-UCLA Cardiomyopathy Center
Director, UCLA Cardiology Fellowship Training
  Program
Co-Director, UCLA Preventative Cardiology
  Program
The Eliot Corday Chair in Cardiovascular Medicine
  and Science
David Geffen School of Medicine at UCLA
Los Angeles, CA

Peter I. Juhn, M.D., M.P.H.
Executive Director, Health Policy and Evidence-
  based Medicine
Johnson & Johnson – Corporate Office
New Brunswick, NJ

Catherine Koepper
Senior Project Manager, Global Registries
Genzyme Corporation
Cambridge, MA

Hugh Tilson, M.D., Dr.P.H.
Clinical Professor of Public Health Leadership
Adjunct Professor of Epidemiology and Health
  Policy
University of North Carolina School of Public
  Health
Chapel Hill, NC

Chapter 3. Registry Design

Michael A. Carome, M.D.
Captain, U.S. Public Health Service
Associate Director for Regulatory Affairs
Office for Human Research Protections
Rockville, MD

Sarah E. Garner, BPharm, Ph.D., MRPharm.S.
Technical Adviser
National Institute for Health and Clinical Excellence
  (NICE)
London, UK

Newell McElwee, Pharm.D., M.S.P.H.
Vice President, U.S. Outcomes Research
U.S. Medical Group
Pfizer, Inc.
New York, NY

Steven Pearson, M.D.
Associate Professor of Ambulatory Care and
  Prevention
Harvard Medical School
Boston, MA

Kenneth J. Rothman, Dr.P.H.
Vice President, Epidemiology
RTI Health Solutions
Research Triangle Park, NC

Chapter 4. Data Elements for Registries

Steven J. Atlas, M.D., M.P.H.
Assistant Professor of Medicine
Harvard Medical School
Associate Physician
General Medicine Division
Massachusetts General Hospital
Boston, MA

Michael A. Carome, M.D.
Captain, U.S. Public Health Service
Associate Director for Regulatory Affairs
Office for Human Research Protections
Rockville, MD

Gregg Fonarow, M.D.
Professor of Medicine
Director, Ahmanson-UCLA Cardiomyopathy Center
Director, UCLA Cardiology Fellowship Training
  Program
Co-Director, UCLA Preventative Cardiology
  Program
The Eliot Corday Chair in Cardiovascular Medicine
  and Science
David Geffen School of Medicine at UCLA
Los Angeles, CA

Janet Hiller, M.P.H., Ph.D.
Professor of Public Health
Director, Adelaide Health Technology Assessment
  (AHTA)
University of Adelaide
Adelaide, Australia

Robert Reynolds, Sc.D.
Senior Director, Global Head, Epidemiology Safety
  and Risk Management
Pfizer, Inc.
New York, NY

Chapter 5. Data Sources for Registries

Michael A. Carome, M.D.
Captain, U.S. Public Health Service
Associate Director for Regulatory Affairs
Office for Human Research Protections
Rockville, MD

Marie R. Griffin, M.D., M.P.H.
Professor of Preventive Medicine
Professor of Medicine
Vanderbilt University School of Medicine
Nashville, TN

William B. Saunders, Ph.D., M.P.H.
Director, Analytics & Research
Pharmaceutical Research Services
Premier, Inc.
Charlotte, NC

Marcus Wilson, Pharm.D.
President
HealthCore, Inc.
Wilmington, DE

Chapter 6. Principles of Registry Ethics, Data Ownership, and Privacy

Stephen W. Bernstein, J.D.
McDermott Will & Emery LLP
Boston, MA

Michael A. Carome, M.D.
Captain, U.S. Public Health Service
Associate Director for Regulatory Affairs
Office for Human Research Protections
Rockville, MD

John P. Fanning, LL.B.
Retired
Washington, DC

Sally Flanzer, Ph.D., C.I.P.
Human Protections Administrator
Office of Extramural Research, Education and
  Priority Populations
Agency for Healthcare Research and Quality
U.S. Department of Health and Human Services
Rockville, MD

206

Christina Heide
Senior Health Information Privacy Policy Specialist
Office for Civil Rights
U.S. Department of Health and Human Services
Washington, DC

Susan McAndrew, J.D.
Deputy Director for Health Information Privacy
Office for Civil Rights
U.S. Department of Health and Human Services
Washington, DC

Sara Rosenbaum, J.D.
Hirsh Professor and Chair Department of Health
  Policy
The George Washington University Medical Center
School of Public Health and Health Services
Washington, DC

**Chapter 7. Patient and Provider Recruitment
and Management**

Gregg Fonarow, M.D.
Professor of Medicine
Director, Ahmanson-UCLA Cardiomyopathy Center
Director, UCLA Cardiology Fellowship Training
  Program
Co-Director, UCLA Preventative Cardiology
  Program
The Eliot Corday Chair in Cardiovascular Medicine
  and Science
David Geffen School of Medicine at UCLA
Los Angeles, CA

Grannum R. Sant, M.D.
Vice President and Head of Urology
U.S. Medical Affairs
Sanofi-Aventis
Bridgewater, NJ

Jack V. Tu, M.D., Ph.D.
Senior Scientist
Institute for Clinical Evaluative Sciences
Ontario, Canada

**Chapter 8. Data Collection and Quality
Assurance**

Michael A. Carome, M.D.
Captain, U.S. Public Health Service
Associate Director for Regulatory Affairs
Office for Human Research Protections
Rockville, MD

Brenda K. Edwards, Ph.D.
Associate Director, Surveillance Research Program
Division of Cancer Control and Population Sciences
National Cancer Institute
Bethesda, MD

Stephen C. Hammill, M.D.
Professor of Medicine, Mayo Clinic College of
  Medicine
Director, Electrocardiography Laboratory
Rochester, MN

Robert Reynolds, Sc.D.
Senior Director, Global Head, Epidemiology Safety
  and Risk Management
Pfizer, Inc.
New York, NY

**Chapter 9. Adverse Event Detection, Processing,
and Reporting**

Thomas Gross, M.D., M.P.H.
Director, Division of Postmarket Surveillance
Center for Devices and Radiological Health
Food and Drug Administration
Rockville, MD

Susan T. Sacks, Ph.D.
Global Head, Epidemiology
Roche Drug Safety Risk Management
Nutley, NJ

**Chapter 10. Analysis and Interpretation of
Registry Data To Evaluate Outcomes**

Joseph A. Ladapo
Harvard Medical School
Boston, MA
Harvard University
Cambridge, MA

207

Newell McElwee, Pharm.D., M.S.P.H.
Vice President, U.S. Outcomes Research
U.S. Medical Group
Pfizer, Inc.
New York, NY

Gareth Parry, Ph.D.
Director, Quality Measurement & Analysis
Department of Medicine
Children's Hospital, Boston
Boston, MA

Walter L. Straus, M.D., M.P.H.
Executive Director
Policy, Public Health, & Medical Affairs
Merck & Co., Inc.
North Wales, PA

Chapter 11. Evaluating Registries

Shamiram Feinglass, M.D., M.P.H.
Senior Medical Officer
Coverage and Analysis Group, Office of Clinical
   Standards and Quality
Centers for Medicare & Medicaid Services
U.S. Public Health Service
Baltimore, MD

Peter Littlejohns, M.D.
Clinical and Public Health Director
National Institute for Health and Clinical Excellence
   (NICE)
London, UK

J. Michael McGinnis, M.D., M.P.P.
Senior Scholar
Institute of Medicine
National Academy of Sciences
Washington, DC

Suzanne L. West, M.P.H, Ph.D.
Research Associate Professor
Department of Epidemiology
School of Public Health
University of North Carolina at Chapel Hill
Chapel Hill, NC

Case Example Contributors

Case Example 1: Developing a Registry To Determine Policy

Michelle A. Bertagna
Project Manager
Outcome Sciences, Inc. d/b/a Outcome
Cambridge, MA

Stephen C. Hammill, M.D.
Professor of Medicine, Mayo Clinic College of
  Medicine
Director, Electrocardiography Laboratory
Rochester, MN

Case Example 2: Using Registries To Understand Rare Diseases

Betsy Bogard, M.S.
Project Manager, Global Registry Programs
Genzyme Corporation
Cambridge, MA

John Yee, M.D., M.P.H.
Senior Director, Global Medical Programs
Genzyme Corporation
Cambridge, MA

Case Example 3: Creating a Registry To Fulfill Multiple Purposes and Using a Publications Committee To Review Data Requests

Michelle A. Bertagna
Project Manager
Outcome Sciences, Inc. d/b/a Outcome
Cambridge, MA

Edna J. Stoehr
NRMI Clinical Trial Manager
Genentech, Inc.
South San Francisco, CA

Case Example 4: Assessing the Safety of Products Used During Pregnancy

Michelle A. Bertagna
Project Manager
Outcome Sciences, Inc. d/b/a Outcome
Cambridge, MA

Deborah Covington, Dr.P.H.
Director, Registries & Epidemiology
Kendle International Inc.
Wilmington, NC

Case Example 5: Designing a Registry To Study Outcomes

Michelle A. Bertagna
Project Manager
Outcome Sciences, Inc. d/b/a Outcome
Cambridge, MA

Sidney A. Cohen, M.D., Ph.D.
Group Director, Clinical Research
Cordis Corporation
Warren, NJ

Case Example 6: Analyzing Clinical Effectiveness and Comparative Effectiveness in an Observational Study

Michelle A. Bertagna
Project Manager
Outcome Sciences, Inc. d/b/a Outcome
Cambridge, MA

Barbara Lippe, M.D.
Principal Medical Director
Genentech, Inc.
South San Francisco, CA

Case Example 7: Using a Registry To Recruit Patients for Clinical Trials

Michelle A. Bertagna
Project Manager
Outcome Sciences, Inc. d/b/a Outcome
Cambridge, MA

Robert A. Sandhaus, M.D., Ph.D.
Medical Director and Executive V.P.
AlphaNet and Alpha-1 Foundation
Professor of Medicine
National Jewish Medical and Research Center
Denver, CO

Case Example 8: Selecting Data Elements for a Registry

Michelle A. Bertagna
Project Manager
Outcome Sciences, Inc. d/b/a Outcome
Cambridge, MA

Scott McKenzie, M.D.
Regional Director Outcomes Research
Ortho Biotech Clinical Affairs LLC
Dallas, TX

Case Example 9: Using Performance Measures To Develop a Data Set

Michelle A. Bertagna
Project Manager
Outcome Sciences, Inc. d/b/a Outcome
Cambridge, MA

Kenneth A. LaBresh, M.D.
SVP, Chief Medical Officer
MassPRO
Waltham, MA

Lee H. Schwamm, M.D.
Associate Professor of Neurology, Harvard Medical
  School
Associate Program Director, MIT – Clinical
  Research Center
Director, TeleStroke & Acute Stroke Services,
  Massachusetts General Hospital,
Boston, MA

Kathleen Turner, M.B.A.
Sr. Manager
Quality Improvement Initiatives
American Heart Association
Dallas, TX

Case Example 10: Developing and Validating a Patient-Administered Questionnaire

Michelle A. Bertagna
Project Manager
Outcome Sciences, Inc. d/b/a Outcome
Cambridge, MA

Grannum R. Sant, M.D.
Vice President and Head of Urology
U.S. Medical Affairs
Sanofi-Aventis
Bridgewater, NJ

Case Example 11: Understanding the Needs and Goals of the Registry Participants

Michelle A. Bertagna
Project Manager
Outcome Sciences, Inc. d/b/a Outcome
Cambridge, MA

John Spertus, M.D., M.P.H.
Professor of Medicine, University of Missouri –
  Kansas City
Director CV Education and Outcomes Research,
  Saint Luke's Mid America Heart Institute
Kansas City, MO

Case Example 12: Integrating Data From Multiple Sources With Patient ID Matching

Noam H. Arzt, Ph.D.
President
HLN Consulting, LLC
San Diego, CA

Michelle A. Bertagna
Project Manager
Outcome Sciences, Inc. d/b/a Outcome
Cambridge, MA

Case Example 13: Incorporating Data From Multiple Sources

Michelle A. Bertagna
Project Manager
Outcome Sciences, Inc. d/b/a Outcome
Cambridge, MA

Stephen Steinberg, M.D.
Medical Director
Liver Research Institute
Denver, CO

Case Example 14: Considering the Institutional Review Board Process During Registry Design

Brian P. Carey, J.D.
Partner
Foley Hoag LLP
Boston, MA

Barry A. Siegel, M.D.
Professor of Radiology and Medicine
Director, Division of Nuclear Medicine
Mallinckrodt Institute of Radiology
Washington University School of Medicine
St. Louis, MO

Case Example 15: Using Registries for Public Health Activities

Michelle A. Bertagna
Project Manager
Outcome Sciences, Inc. d/b/a Outcome
Cambridge, MA

Anne Cordon, M.P.H., C.H.E.S.
San Diego Regional Immunization Registry
  Manager
County of San Diego Health and Human Services
  Agency's Immunization Program
San Diego, CA

Therese Hoyle
Michigan Care Improvement Registry Coordinator
Michigan Department of Community Health
Lansing MI

Sandra Schulthies, M.S.
Data Operations Manager
Utah Statewide Immunization Information System
Salt Lake City, UT

Case Example 16: Issues With Obtaining Informed Consent

Janice A. Richards, R.N., B.A.
Project Manager
Registry of the Canadian Stroke Network
Toronto, Ontario, Canada

Jack V. Tu, M.D., Ph.D.
Senior Scientist
Institute for Clinical Evaluative Sciences
Ontario, Canada

Case Example 17: Building Value as a Means To Recruit Hospitals

Michelle A. Bertagna
Project Manager
Outcome Sciences, Inc. d/b/a Outcome
Cambridge, MA

Kathleen Turner, M.B.A.
Sr. Manager
Quality Improvement Initiatives
American Heart Association
Dallas, TX

Case Example 18: Using Registry Tools To Recruit Sites

Michelle A. Bertagna
Project Manager
Outcome Sciences, Inc. d/b/a Outcome
Cambridge, MA

Case Example 19: Using Proactive Awareness Activities To Recruit Patients for a Pregnancy-Exposure Registry

211

Michelle A. Bertagna
Project Manager
Outcome Sciences, Inc. d/b/a Outcome
Cambridge, MA

Susan Sinclair Roberts, Ph.D.
Associate Director, Registries and Epidemiology
Kendle International Inc.
Wilmington, NC

Case Example 20: Developing Data Collection Tools and Systems for Patient-Reported Data

Michelle A. Bertagna
Project Manager
Outcome Sciences, Inc. d/b/a Outcome
Cambridge, MA

Deborah S. Main, Ph.D.
Professor, Department of Family Medicine
University of Colorado at Denver and Health
  Sciences Center
Denver, CO

Case Example 21: Developing a Performance-Linked Access System

Michelle A. Bertagna
Project Manager
Outcome Sciences, Inc. d/b/a Outcome
Cambridge, MA

Michael Karukin, P.A., Ph.D.
Associate Director, Medical Affairs
IVAX Pharmaceuticals
Miami, FL

Case Example 22: Using Registry Data To Evaluate Outcomes by Practice

Michelle A. Bertagna
Project Manager
Outcome Sciences, Inc. d/b/a Outcome
Cambridge, MA

Jeffrey Wagener, M.D.
Medical Director
Genentech, Inc.
South San Francisco, CA

Case Example 23: Using Registry Data To Study Patterns of Use and Outcomes

Michelle A. Bertagna
Project Manager
Outcome Sciences, Inc. d/b/a Outcome
Cambridge, MA

Marnie L. Boron, Pharm.D.
Associate Director, Medical Affairs
MedImmune, Inc.
Gaithersburg, MD

Appendix A. An Illustration of Sample Size Calculations

For concreteness, assume that the outcome of interest is a dichotomous variable measured on each patient, such as the presence/absence of a complication associated with carotid endarterectomy (CE). (Typically, this literature considers complications within 30 days of the procedure.) Nothing essential changes for outcome variables measured on other scales, such as continuous or survival data. The dichotomous outcome (i.e., presence or absence of a complication) is then aggregated across patients into a complication rate (e.g., 9 complications for 300 patients = 3-percent complication rate).

As a general principle, sample size calculations depend on the study design, the study question, and the scale of measurement of the variables being measured. Indeed, one of the benefits of performing a sample size calculation is the requirement that each of these be specified, thus increasing the likelihood that the proper variables will be measured on the proper patients in the proper manner.

For CE, some registry-based designs and study questions that might be of interest include the following.

Design 1: For patients at high risk of stroke, perhaps using an operational definition of "symptomatic with 70-99 percent stenosis of the carotid artery," the study question is whether the surgeons within a larger entity (e.g., a national chain of hospitals) are, in aggregate, achieving similar complication rates to those who participated in the randomized trials demonstrating the efficacy of CE. (The reason that this is an open question is that the surgeons and institutions in these randomized trials underwent a high degree of selection, thus raising the concern that surgical outcomes were better than could be expected in usual practice.) The patient inclusion criteria for the registry are selected to be as close as possible to those of the randomized trials; thus, while various characteristics might be collected on each patient, no formal adjustment for case mix is required. For the present purposes,

"case-mix adjustment" is the inclusion of various patient characteristics believed to influence complications of CE into a mathematical model used to predict the likelihood of these complications. Here, the most natural such model is a logistic regression. In Design 1, it is assumed that the characteristics of the registry patients are so similar to those of patients in the original randomized trials that no such adjustment is required.

Further, suppose that the 30-day complication rate of CE in the randomized trials was 3 percent. The study question can then be translated into a statistical hypothesis of a one-sample comparison of an observed complication rate vs. a prespecified value. In other words, the null hypothesis is that surgeons within the larger entity are, in aggregate, achieving complication rates that are the same (3 percent) as those of surgeons who participated in the randomized trials. The final input required to perform the sample size calculation is the complication rate under the alternative hypothesis. For example, if it is determined that the goal of the registry is to have high power to flag results as statistically significant if the true complication rate is 6 percent or higher, then the complication rate under the alternative hypothesis is 6 percent.

In general, the value of the complication rate under the alternative hypothesis is derived using a combination of quantitative and qualitative reasoning. (The precise methods used to derive the alternative hypothesis are context dependent and thus not discussed in detail here.) In the present example, a cost-effectiveness analysis might suggest that complication rates of 6 percent and above would call into question the efficacy of CE. Given these inputs, it can be shown that the effect size is 0.21, and the sample size required for 80-percent power is approximately 370.

Design 2: Continuing to follow patients at high risk of stroke, now suppose that the goal of the registry is to compare complication rates across hospitals.

For simplicity, we continue to assume that patients are sufficiently similar to the comparator patients that no explicit adjustment for case mix is required.

Design 2 is a simple form of benchmarking application. For example, the CE complication rates for each hospital might be reported to a regulatory agency and/or the general public, the presumption being that statistically significant differences between complication rates can be used to identify hospitals with differences in quality of care. The particular danger in this design is that the complication rate for any particular hospital might be estimated with relatively little precision, thus generating results that have more noise than signal. (Another danger, discussed later, is that case-mix adjustment is required and not performed, or performed but not adequate.)

We assume that the benchmarking will focus on comparing specific hospitals—i.e., in the underlying statistical model, hospital will represent a "fixed" rather than "random" effect. The null hypothesis is that the complication rates for all the hospitals are identical, and the alternative hypothesis is that the complication rates follow some pattern other than being identical. In this design, specifying the alternative hypothesis of interest is a potentially formidable task. One way to formulate this hypothesis is to focus on outlier hospitals. For example, suppose that there are 10 hospitals in the registry, the overall complication rate among 9 of these is expected to be 3 percent, and the complication rate at the tenth hospital is 10 percent. This information, along with expected number of cases in each hospital, is sufficient to calculate an effect size and thus perform the sample size calculation.

When comparing complication rates among specific hospitals, some adjustment may be made for multiple comparisons—that is, in any group of hospitals, there will always be a hospital with the highest complication rate, and focusing on differences between the outcomes of this particular hospital vs. outcomes of the others will overstate the level of statistical significance. The initial statistical test used to assess the homogeneity of complication rates across all the hospitals in the registry

implicitly takes this multiple-comparison problem into account. Subsequent tests, in particular those tests that compare apparent outlier hospitals with others, should include an explicit adjustment for multiple comparisons, and the sample size calculations should reflect the fact that an adjusted comparison is being made.

In practice, the approach to this design might reasonably depend on whether registry data are being collected electronically or manually. If data are being collected electronically, then the most sensible policy is to collect information on all CE procedures performed within each hospital and to use the sample size formula as an assessment of whether the registry as a whole is likely to produce results that are sufficiently accurate to support decisionmaking. This assessment can be framed in terms of statistical power (as discussed above) or precision.

Considering precision, a 95-percent confidence interval for a nonzero complication rate for any hospital is $p \pm 1.96 \sqrt{(pq/n)}$, where p is the observed complication rate, $q = 1 - p$, and n is the sample size. Supposing that $p = 3$ percent and $n = 300$ per hospital, within any particular hospital, the width of this confidence interval is expected to be approximately ± 1.9 percent. If data are being collected manually, and thus the marginal cost of data collection per patient is high, then a reasonable policy would be to collect data on enough patients per hospital so that the precision of estimates of the complication rate within that hospital is considered adequate.

As with hypothesis testing, in deriving the width of the confidence interval, the analysis usually applies a combination of qualitative and quantitative insights. In particular, the question can be reframed as the following: For what values of the complication rate will my decision (whether taken from the perspective of clinical medicine, public health, etc.) be the same? For example, if the decision is the same regardless of where the complication rate falls within the range of 2-4 percent, then an interval of this width is "sufficiently precise."

Unless sample sizes are large, using registries to compare individual hospitals is potentially quite problematic. Although determining the inputs to the power calculations is not always a straightforward task, performing this analysis is quite useful, even if the result is only to suggest extreme caution in the interpretation of between-hospital differences.

Design 3: Continuing to follow patients undergoing CE, now suppose that the goal of the registry is to compare two different versions of the surgical procedure. For simplicity, continue to assume that patients are sufficiently similar to the comparator patients that no explicit adjustment for case mix is required. The following discussion (after including an adjustment for case mix, if appropriate) also applies to comparing two different versions of a medical device and similar applications. The key distinction between this design and Design 2 is that the primary comparison or comparisons can be stated ahead of time and that the number of comparisons is relatively small, thus implying that the issue of multiple comparisons can be ignored.

The analytic approach to this design is a logistic regression, with the input file having one record per patient. The outcome variable is the presence or absence of a complication, the categorically scaled control variable is the hospital, and the primary predictor is the categorically scaled coding of the type of surgical procedure (i.e., CE using version A vs. CE using version B). The null hypothesis is that, after accounting for any differences in hospitals, the two different versions of the procedure have identical complication rates. The alternative hypothesis is that the rates differ by a specified amount, this amount being the "minimum clinically significant difference" interpreted to be of concern. Power calculations proceed in the same fashion as for logistic regression with multiple predictors.

The main pitfall in this design is that patients who receive version A of the surgical procedure might differ from those who receive version B of the procedure along some dimension that has an impact on outcomes. (This pitfall is discussed in more detail under Design 4.)

In this application, the null and alternative hypotheses are sometimes structured the same way as in an equivalence trial—that is, differences in complication rates are not expected, and the goal of the study is to demonstrate that complication rates for the two versions of the surgical procedure are similar within a certain level of precision. The structure of the analysis is not fundamentally different. Indeed, sample size calculations for equivalence trials sometimes are not performed within a hypothesis-testing framework but instead are performed by identifying a sample size of sufficient magnitude to make the confidence interval for the difference in the complication rates between the two versions of the surgical procedure a certain width. For simplicity of presentation, from now on, assume that any equivalence-trial-type calculations can be reframed into confidence interval format, and thus need not be discussed separately.

Design 4: Continuing to follow patients at high risk of stroke and continuing to assume that the goal of the registry is to compare two different versions of the surgical procedure, now additionally assume that this comparison will adjust for case mix.

Within the logistic regression paradigm, variables used to adjust for case mix are accounted for as covariates (i.e., additional predictors). Alternatively, propensity-scoring methods could be used to adjust for those variables that predict the assignment of patients to particular versions of the procedure. For concreteness, focus on logistic regression. In order to perform a sample size calculation for a logistic regression, the analyst must specify the predictive ability of the covariates and the odds ratio associated with the predictor of interest. (For example, version B of the procedure might increase the odds of complications by a factor of 1.5.) Once these inputs are specified, the sample size calculation is straightforward.

Both the logistic regression and propensity-scoring approaches suffer from the fundamental drawback that they can adjust only for covariates that are observed. In particular, if there are variables that predict outcome that are unmeasured (e.g., physician's assessment of a patient's likelihood to

215

comply with treatment or stroke in evolution not included in the administrative database used as the source of data for the registry), then the comparison between the two versions of the surgical procedure is potentially biased. Accordingly, before proposing to use a registry to compare complication rates (e.g., across different versions of a procedure or a device) or other outcomes, it is critical to determine that the following three conditions do not all hold: (1) a patient, provider, system or other characteristic affects the complication rate; (2) this characteristic is unmeasured within the registry; and (3) there is a reasonable likelihood that this characteristic might be differentially distributed across the different versions of the procedure or the device. If all three conditions (in epidemiologic terms, the conditions for "confounding") hold, use of the registry to compare outcomes is potentially dangerous.

Critical to Designs 1-4 is the assumption that the CE complication rate is stable over time. Thus, for example, it is appropriate to use the registry to estimate a single complication rate associated with version A of the procedure, estimate another single complication rate associated with version B of the procedure, and compare the rates. On the other hand, if the technology of CE (e.g., physical materials, surgical technique) is improving, then the registry should continue to monitor the performance of CE over time. Such an ongoing monitoring function seems particularly relevant for medical devices and similar applications.

Even when the associated technology is assumed to be stable, some registries are intended to provide ongoing assessments of outcomes. For example, in a quality assurance context, CE complication rates might be assessed at individual hospitals on an annual basis (e.g., in order to check for problems that have recently arisen). On the other hand, a registry whose purpose is to assess whether the complication rates that were observed in randomized trials could be achieved in usual practice could be designed with a sunset provision to cease operation once this question is answered. The latter type of registry might, for example, accompany a conditional coverage decision by the Centers for Medicare & Medicaid Services.

Having an ongoing monitoring function induces additional analytical complications, among others a multiple-comparisons problem. Traditional statistical power calculations are performed under the assumption that the sample size is fixed and that (unless otherwise noted) multiple comparisons are not a major issue. Sequential testing methods associated with randomized trials (where, for example, the type I error of .05 is apportioned into an early test with alpha = .001 and a subsequent test with alpha = .499) do not apply to this particular design, since most of these methods assume that the maximum sample size is fixed. (Some methods assume that what is fixed is not the number of patients but the number of events, but these methods are not a good match for registry applications either.)

Design 5: Suppose the goal is to estimate the complication rate associated with CE at multiple time points for the foreseeable future.

Control chart methodology might reasonably be applied to this class of problems. This methodology, often used in the quality assurance and quality improvement context, was originally developed for industrial applications. In this example, the null hypothesis, under which the system in question is "in control," is that the CE complication rate remains at the desired value of 3 percent throughout the entire followup period. Samples are taken at each point in time (e.g., monthly). As an example, if these monthly samples are of size 100, then the standard error is approximately 1.7 percent. The analyst then creates a "control chart" by plotting these monthly complication rates over time and forming "channels" based on the standard error. In this example, the channel extending from the point estimate to 1 standard error above the point estimate is 3 percent to 4.7 percent.

Once the basic control chart (which goes by different names depending on the scale of measurement of the outcome variable) is formed, the plot is checked for various violations of the null hypothesis of constant complication rates. The set of possible violations to be flagged as statistically significant might include (1) any observation more than 3 standard errors from the mean; (2) two of three consecutive observations more than 2 standard errors from the mean; (3) eight observations in a row that increase or decrease; and (4) eight observations in a row on one side of the mean. These rules of thumb implicitly take into account the multiple-comparisons problem by requiring noteworthy departures from the null hypothesis in order to be flagged, and they are based on the observed properties of physical machines as they fall out of adjustment (suddenly breaking down and producing an extreme outlier, gradually heating and thus producing sequentially higher readings, etc.). Complication rates of CE might or might not follow the properties of physical machines, but the decision rules from control chart methodology are at least a good place to start.